Common Problems in Cardiology

Common Problems in Cardiology

Kanu Chatterjee
Clinical Professor of Medicine
The Carver College of Medicine
University of Iowa, USA

Emeritus Professor of Medicine
University of California, San Francisco, USA

Byron F Vandenberg
Associate Professor of Medicine
The Carver College of Medicine
University of Iowa, USA

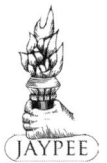

The Health Sciences Publisher

New Delhi | London | Philadelphia | Panama

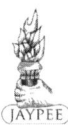 **Jaypee Brothers Medical Publishers (P) Ltd**

Headquarters
Jaypee Brothers Medical Publishers (P) Ltd
4838/24, Ansari Road, Daryaganj
New Delhi 110 002, India
Phone: +91-11-43574357
Fax: +91-11-43574314
Email: jaypee@jaypeebrothers.com

Overseas Offices

J.P. Medical Ltd
83 Victoria Street, London
SW1H 0HW (UK)
Phone: +44 20 3170 8910
Fax: +44 (0)20 3008 6180
Email: info@jpmedpub.com

Jaypee-Highlights Medical Publishers Inc
City of Knowledge, Bld. 237, Clayton
Panama City, Panama
Phone: +1 507-301-0496
Fax: +1 507-301-0499
Email: cservice@jphmedical.com

Jaypee Medical Inc.
The Bourse
111 South Independence Mall East
Suite 835, Philadelphia, PA 19106, USA
Phone: +1 267-519-9789
Email: jpmed.us@gmail.com

Jaypee Brothers Medical Publishers (P) Ltd
17/1-B Babar Road, Block-B, Shaymali
Mohammadpur, Dhaka-1207
Bangladesh
Mobile: +08801912003485
Email: jaypeedhaka@gmail.com

Jaypee Brothers Medical Publishers (P) Ltd
Bhotahity, Kathmandu
Nepal
Phone: +977-9741283608
Email: kathmandu@jaypeebrothers.com

Website: www.jaypeebrothers.com
Website: www.jaypeedigital.com

© 2016, Jaypee Brothers Medical Publishers

The views and opinions expressed in this book are solely those of the original contributor(s)/author(s) and do not necessarily represent those of editor(s) of the book.

All rights reserved. No part of this publication may be reproduced, stored or transmitted in any form or by any means, electronic, mechanical, photocopying, recording or otherwise, without the prior permission in writing of the publishers.

All brand names and product names used in this book are trade names, service marks, trademarks or registered trademarks of their respective owners. The publisher is not associated with any product or vendor mentioned in this book.

Medical knowledge and practice change constantly. This book is designed to provide accurate, authoritative information about the subject matter in question. However, readers are advised to check the most current information available on procedures included and check information from the manufacturer of each product to be administered, to verify the recommended dose, formula, method and duration of administration, adverse effects and contraindications. It is the responsibility of the practitioner to take all appropriate safety precautions. Neither the publisher nor the author(s)/editor(s) assume any liability for any injury and/or damage to persons or property arising from or related to use of material in this book.

This book is sold on the understanding that the publisher is not engaged in providing professional medical services. If such advice or services are required, the services of a competent medical professional should be sought.

Every effort has been made where necessary to contact holders of copyright to obtain permission to reproduce copyright material. If any have been inadvertently overlooked, the publisher will be pleased to make the necessary arrangements at the first opportunity.

Inquiries for bulk sales may be solicited at: jaypee@jaypeebrothers.com

Common Problems in Cardiology

First Edition: **2016**

ISBN 978-93-5152-852-4

Printed at Rajkamal Electric Press, Plot No. 2, Phase-IV, Kundli, Haryana.

Contributors

Alexander Mazur MD
Associate Professor of Medicine
The Carver College of Medicine
University of Iowa, USA

Amandeep Dhaliwal MD
Physician
The Carver College of Medicine
University of Iowa, Iowa, USA

Andres Vargas-Estrada MD
Physician
The Carver College of Medicine
University of Iowa, Iowa City, USA

Ankur Vyas MD
Physician
The Carver College of Medicine
University of Iowa, Iowa, USA

Basil Abu-El-Haija MD
Cardiac Specialist
3901 Rainbow Blvd, Kansas City,
USA

Belal Al Khiami MD
Physician
The Carver College of Medicine
University of Iowa, Iowa City, USA

Byron F Vandenberg MD
Associate Professor of Medicine
The Carver College of Medicine
University of Iowa, USA

Denice Hodgson-Zingman MD
Associate Professor of Internal
Medicine-Cardiovascular Medicine
Associate Professor of Biomedical
Engineering
University of Iowa Hospitals and Clinics
Iowa City, USA

Dwayne N Campbell MD
The Carver College of Medicine
University of Iowa, USA

Hardik Doshi MD
Clinical Professor of Internal Medicine
The Carver College of Medicine
University of Iowa, Iowa City, USA

Hosam M Moustafa MD
Pediatric Radiologist
301 W Bastanchury Rd Ste 130
Fullerton, CA, USA

Jayasheel O Eshcol MD
Physician
The Carver College of Medicine
University of Iowa, Iowa City, USA

Jeffrey S Wilson MD
Clinical Professor of Internal Medicine
The Carver College of Medicine
University of Iowa, Iowa City, USA

Kanu Chatterjee MBBS
Professor of Medicine
The Carver College of Medicine
University of Iowa
Emeritus Professor of Medicine
University of California
San Francisco, USA

Lee Joseph MD
Assistant Attending Physician
NewYork-Presbyterian Hospital/
Columbia University Medical Center,
Department of Medicine
USA

Manish Suneja MD
Clinical Professor of Internal Medicine - Nephrology
University of Iowa Hospitals and Clinics
Iowa City, USA

Michael C Giudici MD
Clinical Professor of Internal Medicine
University of Iowa Hospitals and Clinics
Iowa City, USA

Min Luo DO PhD
Cardiology Fellow
The Carver College of Medicine
University of Iowa, Iowa City, USA

Nathan Funk MD
Consultant Cardilogist
520 Medical Center
Medford, Oregon, USA

Olurotimi Mesubi MBBS
Consultant Cardiologist
Johns Hopkins School of Medicine
Baltimore, Maryland, USA

Omer Iqbal MD
Clinical Professor of Internal Medicine
University of Iowa Hospitals and Clinics
Iowa City, USA

Paul D Lindower MD
Clinical Professor of Internal Medicine
The Carver College of Medicine
University of Iowa, USA

Prashant Bhave MD FHRS
Clinical Professor of Internal Medicine - Cardiovascular Medicine
The Carver College of Medicine
University of Iowa, Iowa City, USA

Ravinder Kumar MD
Consultant Cardiologist
West Patel Nagar
New Delhi, India

Rudhir Tandon MD
Clinical Professor of Internal Medicine
University of Iowa Hospitals and Clinics
Iowa City, USA

Saket Girotra MBBS
Cardiology Division
The Carver College of Medicine
University of Iowa, USA

Seth Maliske MD
Clinical Professor of Internal Medicine
University of Iowa Hospitals and Clinics
Iowa City, USA

Sif Hansdottir MD
Pulmonologist
University of Iowa Hospitals and Clinics
Iowa City, USA

Siva Krothapalli MBBS
Cardiology Fellow
University of Iowa Hospitals and Clinics
Iowa City, USA

Tariq Hamid MD
Specialist of General Family Medicine
Keene, New Hampshire, USA

Uzodinma C Emerenini MD
Cardiologist
University of Iowa Hospitals and Clinics
Iowa City, USA

Preface

Approximately 600,000 people die from cardiac disease in the United States every year, according to the Centers for Disease and Control and Prevention (CDC) estimation. It is a leading cause of death in both men and women. Cardiac disease is often called a "silent killer". Symptoms of cardiac disease vary depending on the specific condition, and physicians often find problems in diagnosing this specific condition. All types of cardiac diseases share some common traits with a few key differences.

Common Problems in Cardiology deals with all the common topics in cardiology with a focus on main problem areas of general practitioners. All the chapters covered in the book present the signs and symptoms, etiological causes, diagnostic methods and management approaches of the various heart diseases. The main topics discussed are on chest pain, ischemic heart disease, coronary and pulmonary artery diseases, dyspnea, heart failure, hypertension and hypotension, shock, diseases of heart valve, infective endocarditis, pericardial diseases, syncope, palpitations, bradyarrhythmias, atrial fibrillation, tachyarrhythmia, claudication, aortic disease, stroke, dyslipidemias, etc.

All the chapters are written by internationally and nationally recognized experts in their respective fields. We are very appreciative and grateful to the contributors for their sine qua non contributions. We sincerely thank Shri Jitendar P Vij (Group Chairman), Mr Ankit Vij (Group President), Mr Tarun Duneja (Director-Publishing), and the expert team of M/s Jaypee Brothers Medical Publishers (P) Ltd, New Delhi, India for their hard work and professional expertise, without which the book could not have been published.

Kanu Chatterjee
Byron F Vandenberg

Contents

1. **Chest Pain** 1
   Hosam Maustafa
   - Acute Coronary Syndrome   2
   - Pulmonary Embolism   4
   - Acute Pericarditis   5
   - Musculoskeletal Chest Pain   6
   - Esophageal Diseases   6

2. **Stable Ischemic Heart Disease** 8
   Amandeep Dhaliwal
   - Testing   8
   - Treatment   11

3. **Acute Coronary Syndromes** 20
   Ankur Vyas, Saket Girotra
   - Pathophysiology   20
   - Clinical Presentation   21
   - Diagnostic Evaluation   23
   - Risk Stratification   23
   - Management   25
   - Treatment Strategy in Nsteacs   29
   - Complications   31
   - Long-term Management   32

4. **Dyspnea: Evaluation and Management** 35
   Ankur Vyas, Jeffrey S Wilson, Paul D Lindower
   - Pathophysiology   35
   - Primary Etiologies of Dyspnea   36
   - History and Physical Examination   37
   - Laboratory Studies   39
   - Management   41

5. **Heart Failure with Reduced Ejection Fraction** 43
   Omer Iqbal
   - Definition   43
   - Classifications and Staging   44

6. **Heart Failure with Preserved Ejection Fraction** 63
   Ravinder Kumar
   - Definition of Heart Failure   63

- Epidemiology 64
- Clinical Features (Demographic Features and Comorbid Conditions) 64
- Stages of Heart Failure 65
- Assessment of Diastolic Dysfunction 65
- Pathophysiology 66
- Management of HFPEF 68

7. Hypotension and Shock 73
Jayasheel O Eshcol
- Physiology 73
- Classification 74
- Cardiogenic Shock – Background, Physical Examination and Diagnostics 75

8. Hypertension 84
Manish Suneja, Seth Maliske
- Hemodynamic Determinants of Blood Pressure and the Variables Affected in Systemic Hypertension 84
- Determinants of Arterial Blood Pressure in the Younger as Well as Aged Circulatory System 85
- Methods of Measuring BP 85
- Measurement Protocol for Accurate Blood Pressure Recording
- Diagnosis and Classification of Hypertension 87
- Physical Examination in a Patient with Hypertension 89
- Clues for Previously Uncontrolled Hypertension 91
- Lifestyle Factors in the Hypertensive Patient Contributing to Elevated Blood Pressure 92
- Lifestyle Interventions to Lower the Risk of Developing Hypertension 92
- Target Goals and Treatment Recommendations for Hypertension Based on Eight Joint National Committee (JNC 8) Guidelines 93
- Mechanisms of Action for the Pharmacologic Treatment of Hypertension 95
- Resistant Hypertension 96
- Evaluation for Secondary Causes of Hypertension 98
- What are Common Causes of Secondary Hypertension 99
- How Does one Diagnose and Treat Primary Hyperaldosteronism? 99

9. Essentials of Pulmonary Hypertension 102
Rudhir Tandon, Sif Hansdottir
- Clinical Classification and Epidemiology 102
- Hemodynamic Classification 104
- Pathology and Pathogenesis 105
- Genetics 105
- Diagnosis 105
- Treatment 110

10. Aortic and Mitral Valve Disease 118
Byron F Vandenberg, Kanu Chatterjee
- Aortic Stenosis 118
- Aortic Regurgitation 122

- Mitral Regurgitation *125*
- Mitral Stenosis *129*

11. Infective Endocarditis **133**
Andres Vargas-Estrada
- Predisposing Conditions *133*
- Etiology and Prognosis *133*
- Clinical Manifestations *134*
- Physical Examination *135*
- Diagnosis *136*
- Treatment *138*
- Recommendations for Surgical Intervention *144*
- Infective Endocarditis Prophylaxis *144*
- Cardiac Implanted Electronic Device Infections *145*

12. Prosthetic Heart Valves **149**
Byron F Vandenberg
- Types of Prosthetic Valves *149*
- Selecting the Optimal Prosthesis *151*
- Prosthesis–Patient Mismatch *152*
- Long-term Management *153*
- Long-term Complications *159*

13. Pericardial Diseases **165**
Tariq Hamid
- Acute Pericarditis and Pericardial Effusion *165*
- Chronic Relapsing/Recurrent Pericarditis *170*
- Pericardial Effusion and Tamponade *171*
- Constrictive Pericarditis *174*
- Transient Constrictive Pericarditis *178*
- Effusive Constrictive Pericarditis *178*

14. Syncope **181**
Olurotimi Mesubi, Alexander Mazur
- Classification and Types of Syncope *181*
- Other Causes of T-LOC *185*
- Evaluation of Patients With T-LOC and Syncope *187*
- Risk Assessment *193*
- Treatment *194*
- Syncope and Driving *198*

15. Palpitations **199**
Uzodinma C Emerenini, Denice Hodgson-Zingman
- Etiology *199*
- Evaluation *200*
- Physical Examination *201*
- Testing *201*
- Palpitations during Pregnancy *203*

16. Bradyarrhythmias **205**
Hardik Doshi, Prashant Bhave
- Sinus Pause/Sinus Arrest and Sinoatrial Exit Block *205*

- Sinus Node Dysfunction *207*
- Sinus Bradycardia *207*
- Atrioventricular Conduction Block *211*

17. Atrial Fibrillation 223
Michael C Giudici, Basil Abu-El-Haija
- Incidence *223*
- Presentation *223*
- Pathophysiology *224*
- Epidemiology *224*
- Management *224*

18. Tachyarrhythmia 238
Min Luo, Dwayne Campbell
- Division *238*
- Narrow Complex Tachycardias *238*
- Wide Complex Tachycardia *243*

19. Claudication and Peripheral Artery Disease 250
Lee Joseph
- Epidemiology and Risk Factors *250*
- Clinical Presentation and Natural History *250*
- Diagnostic Methods *250*
- Management *251*

20. Acute Aortic Syndromes 259
Belal Al Khiami
- Epidemiology *259*
- Aortic Dissection Classification *260*
- Risk Factors and Pathogenesis *261*
- Clinical Manifestations *261*
- Diagnostic Evaluation *264*
- Management *267*
- Prognosis *268*
- Aortic Dissection Variants *269*

21. Cardioembolic Stroke 271
Siva Krothapalli
- Initial Evaluation and Workup *272*

22. Assessment of the Cardiac Patient for Noncardiac Surgery 283
Nathan Funk
- Cardiovascular Risk and Noncardiac Surgery *283*
- Preoperative Cardiac Diagnostic Testing *285*
- Preoperative Assessment of Patients with Valvular Heart Disease *287*
- Revascularization and Noncardiac Surgery *288*
- Perioperative Management of Coronary Stents *288*
- Perioperative Beta-blockade *290*
- Perioperative Statin Use *291*
- Perioperative Anticoagulation Management *291*
- Perioperative Management of Pacemakers *293*
- Preoperative Assessment of Candidates for Kidney or Liver Transplantation *293*

23. Dyslipidemias **297**
Byron F Vandenberg
- Secondary Prevention/Patients with Atherosclerotic CV Disease   *298*
- Primary Prevention   *301*
- Statin Intolerance   *302*
- Familial Hypercholesterolemia   *303*
- Diabetes Mellitus   *303*
- Very High Triglycerides, Severe Hypertriglyceridemia and the Chylomicronemia Syndrome   *304*
- Metabolic Syndrome and/or High Triglycerides   *308*

Index *311*

PLATE 1

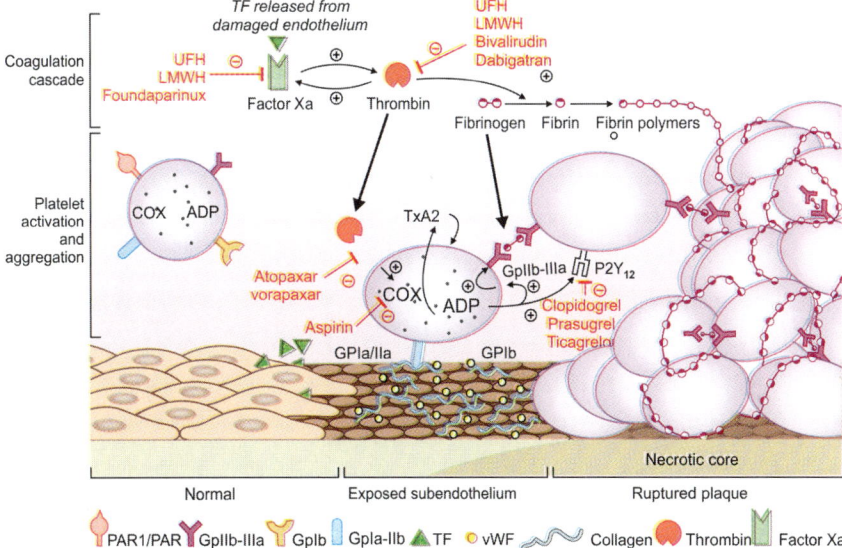

Fig. 3.1: Mechanism of acute coronary syndromes and targets of antiplatelet and antithrombotic agents

UFH, unfractionated heparin; LMWH, low molecular weight heparin; TF, tissue factor.

Source: Reprinted from Lilly SM, Wilensky RL. Emerging therapies for acute coronary syndromes. Front Pharmacol. 2011;2:61. Published online Oct 24, 2011. doi: 10.3389/fphar.2011.00061.

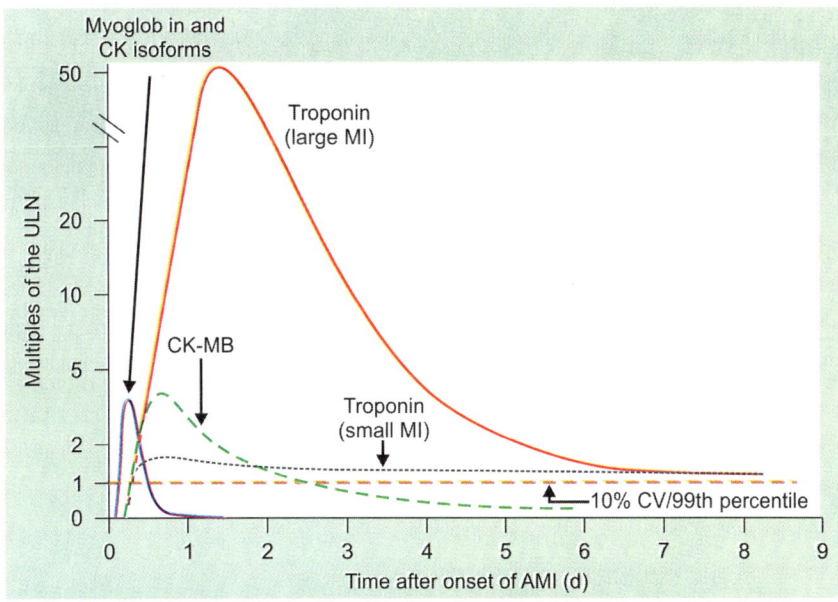

Fig. 3.2: Timing of release of various biomarkers after acute myocardial infarction

ULN, upper limit of normal (defined as the 99th percentile from a normal reference population without myocardial necrosis); CK, creatine kinase; CK-MB, CK muscle and brain fraction.

Source: Reprinted with permission from Kumar, Cannon CP. Acute coronary syndromes: diagnosis and management, part I. Mayo Clin Proc. 2009;84(10):917-38, Elsevier.

PLATE 2

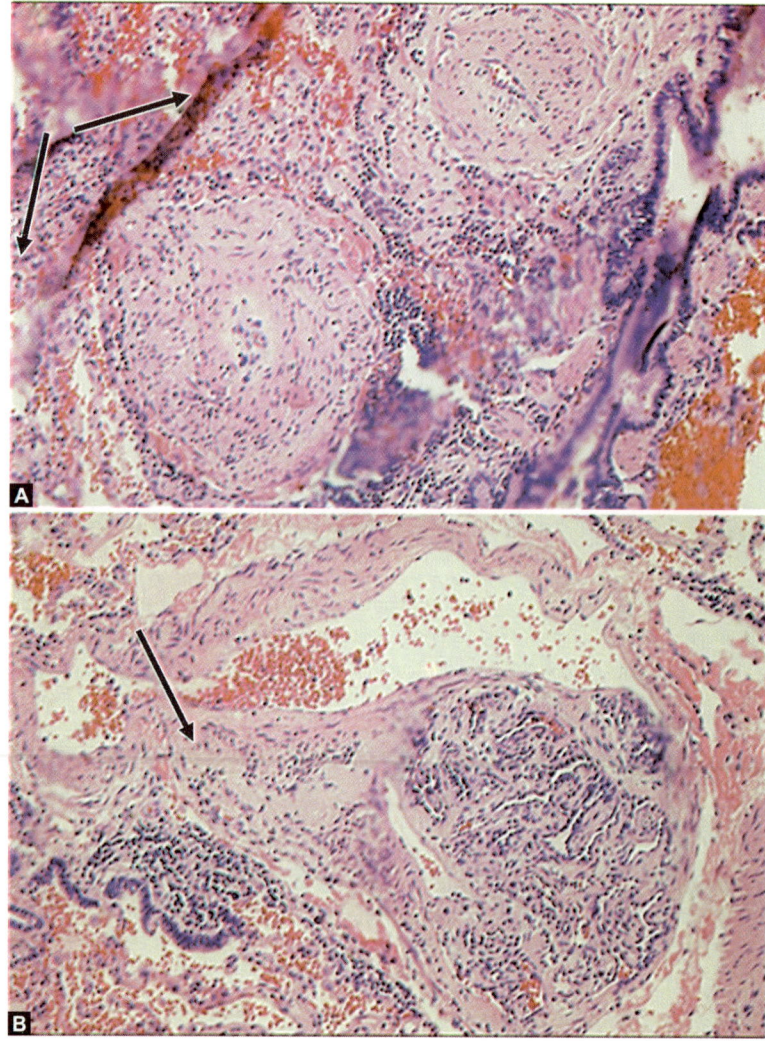

Fig. 9.1: H&E stained section (200 X) of pulmonary artery in a patient with idiopathic PAH. (A) Concentric laminar intimal fibrosis (arrows) characterized by markedly thickened intima with dramatically narrowed lumen; (B) Complex glomeruloid vascular structures (arrow) originating from pulmonary arteries (plexiform lesion), characteristic of idiopathic PAH and hereditary PAH

PLATE 3

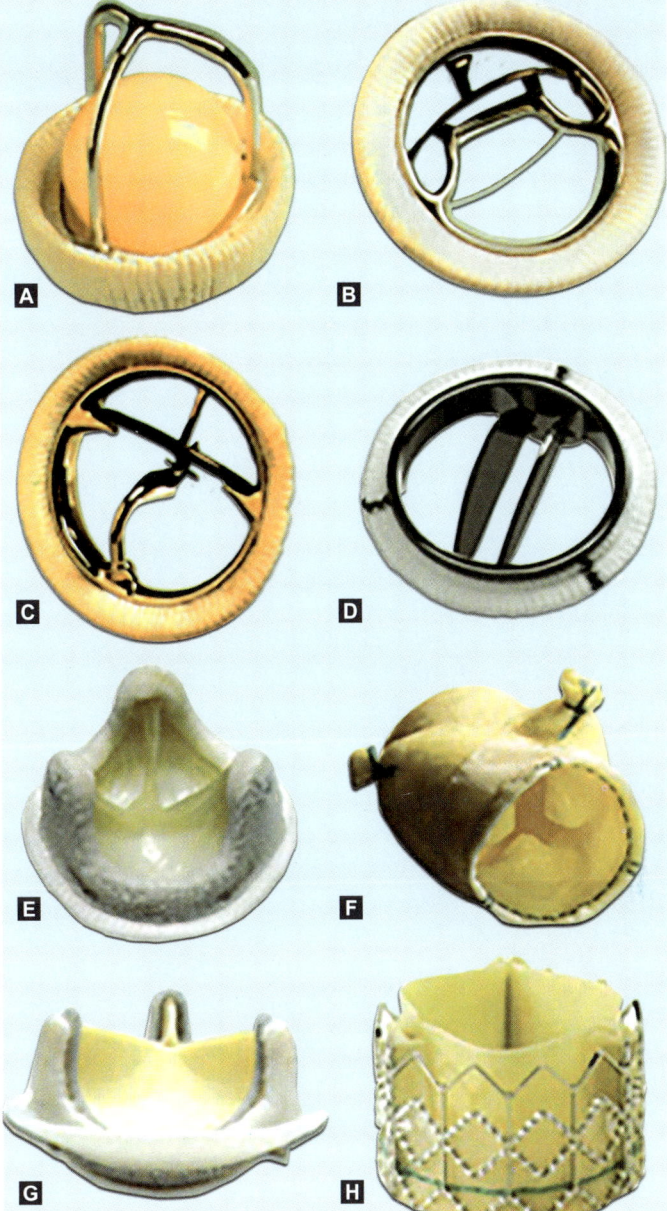

Fig. 12.1: Different models of prosthetic heart valves. (A) Starr–Edwards caged-ball valve; (B) Bjork–Shiley tilting disk valve; (C) Medtronic–Hall tilting disk valve; (D) St. Jude Medical bileaflet valve; (E) Medtronic Hancock II porcine valve; (F) Medtronic Freestyle porcine valve; (G) Carpentier-Edwards Perimount bovine pericardial valve; (H) Edwards SAPIEN transcatheter pericardial aortic valve.

Source: Reprinted with permission from Sun JCJ, Davidson MJ, Lamy A, Eikelboom JW. Antithrombotic management of patients with prosthetic heart valves: current evidence and future trends. Lancet. 2009;374:565-76, Davidson MJ, Lamy A, Eikelboom JW, Elsevier.

Chest Pain

Chapter 1

Hossam Mustafa

INTRODUCTION

Chest pain is one of the major symptoms of cardiovascular disease. It may be caused by a myriad of conditions. Since it may be the initial symptom of a potentially lethal medical condition, it is generally considered a symptom that needs prompt evaluation.

Chest pain has a wide differential diagnosis. It is well recognized as a common presentation of acute coronary syndrome (ACS). A patient with known coronary artery disease (CAD) remains at high risk for recurrent coronary events. Nonetheless, similar to any other patient presenting with a clinical problem, a systematic diagnostic approach is needed.

Chest pain is a common symptom leading to hospital visit. Less than one-third of patients evaluated in the emergency room for chest pain have known CAD. Among patients hospitalized for the evaluation of chest pain, 49% have a history of known CAD. Among patients undergoing percutaneous coronary interventions, 6.7% are readmitted within 30 days with chest pain. In patients undergoing coronary arterial bypass surgery, 30% reported frequent episodes of chest pain 2 years post-bypass.

Overall, there were 5.8 million annual visits to the emergency department for the evaluation of chest pain. Current statistics show that an estimated >16 million American adults have CAD. Therefore, chest pain in a patient with known CAD is a commonly encountered medical problem. Patients with a history of myocardial infarction (MI) are a high-risk group with approximately one in three presenting with a recurrent MI within 5 years. Owing to the high-risk nature of this patient population, ACS is foremost in the differential (Table 1.1).

Table 1.1: Causes of chest pain	
Acute coronary syndrome	Esophageal spasm
Aortic dissection	Costochondritis
Acute pulmonary embolism	Osteoarthritis of the spine
Pericarditis	Psychogenic
Hypertrophic cardiomyopathy	Peptic ulcer disease
Mitral valve prolapse	Pancreatitis
Pulmonary arterial hypertension	Acute cholecystitis
Gastroesophageal reflux	

This chapter discusses the differential diagnosis of chest pain symptomatology with emphasis on the life-threatening causes of chest pain, keeping in mind the severity of chest pain and seriousness of the cause are not necessarily correlated. For any particular patient complaining of chest pain, the time that should be spent in obtaining history and performing physical examination should be directly proportionate to the clinical condition of the patient. In a clinically unstable patient, therapeutic measures will need to be started even before a thorough history and physical examination has been completed. Physical examination should start with assessment of vital signs. If the patient is hemodynamically unstable, attention should be turned to resuscitative measures.

ACUTE CORONARY SYNDROME

Acute coronary syndrome comprises a wide spectrum of conditions that includes unstable angina at one end, non-ST-elevation MI and ST-elevation MI (STEMI) at the other end. The most common pathophysiologic mechanism in ACS is rupture or erosion of a vulnerable atherosclerotic plaque.

Former reports have demonstrated that descriptors of chest pain predict ACS weakly or not at all. Variability in taking the history leads to poor interobserver reliability. Despite these limitations, chest pain described as pressure, similar to that of prior MI, accompanied by other symptoms, such as nausea, vomiting, or diaphoresis or chest pain that radiates to one or both shoulders or arms and increases with exertion has a higher probability of being coronary ischemia. The usual location of anginal chest pain is central/retrosternal and may spread all over the precordium to the neck, jaw or arm. Short duration of chest pain that lasts only for seconds is rarely indicative of ischemic chest pain. The association between coronary ischemia and relief of chest pain with nitroglycerin is unreliable as this can also happen with esophageal causes of chest pain, such as spasms. Unfortunately, there is no sign on physical examination that establishes a diagnosis of ACS. In the stable patient, evaluation of vital signs will provide important information that aids diagnosis and decision making. Jugular venous distension in a patient with history suggestive of an ACS may suggest a right ventricular infarct particularly in the presence of hypotension and clear lung fields.

In every patient presenting with ongoing chest pain, an electrocardiogram (ECG) should be obtained immediately. Certain ECG features, such as ≥ 1 mm ST segment elevation in two contiguous leads (except ≥ 2 mm in V1-V3) or new left bundle branch block suggest an occluded coronary artery. However, it must be remembered that ST segment elevation on an ECG has a wide range of differential diagnoses (Table 1.2). However, 50% of patients with ongoing coronary ischemia may not have significant ischemic ST segment changes on an ECG. The abnormal ECG should always be compared to previous available reference ECGs. An ECG is of value even in the absence of ongoing symptoms, as signs of recent MI, such as new Q waves can be identified.

Patients with known CAD and reduced left ventricular systolic function may have implanted intracardiac defibrillators or pacemakers. In an underlying ventricular-paced rhythm, interpreting ischemic ST segment

Table 1.2: Causes of ST elevation

ST segment elevation myocardial infarction	Left ventricular hypertrophy
Pericarditis	Early repolarization
Ventricular aneurysm	

changes reliably is not possible. Underlying coronary ischemia may present as recurrent defibrillator discharges for ventricular tachycardia. Baseline comprehensive lab work is of value as anemia, electrolyte, endocrine, hepatic and renal abnormalities might be related to the genesis of chest pain symptom.

Cardiac troponin (cTn) has been by far the preferred diagnostic marker for diagnosis of MI. The risk of missing an MI when using a single cTn test upon arrival at the hospital's emergency department is 10-15%. American and European guidelines recommend repeat tests for cTn elevation up to 12 hours after the onset of symptoms. Myocardial damage results in elevation of cTn within 6-10 hours after symptom onset and cTn values return to normal in 10-14 days. Other biomarkers, such as creatinine kinase MB (CKMB) fraction and serum myoglobin have different pharmacokinetic profiles. Serum myoglobin is the first biomarker to rise after myocardial damage (within 30-60 minutes). However, its diagnostic utility is limited owing to low specificity and false-positive values seen with rhabdomyolysis, alcohol intake and skeletal muscle trauma. Creatinine kinaseMB is also less specific than cTn for diagnosis of myocardial damage. This biomarker rises within 6-8 hours of symptom onset and returns to normal in 12-24 hours. Thus, CKMB was traditionally used to diagnose recurrent MI in a patient with recent ACS or periprocedural MI.

Recent guidelines state that recurrent infarction can also be diagnosed by cTn, provided there is a >20% increase in the value of the second cTn sample. Elevations of cardiac biomarkers reflect myocardial damage but do not suggest mechanisms. Elevated cTn is seen with myocardial damage due to ruptured plaque as well as supply demand mismatch and a wide variety of other medical problems, including anemia, sepsis, hypertensive crisis, heart failure exacerbation, acute pulmonary embolism (PE), and acute myocarditis. Therefore, biomarker elevation needs to be interpreted within the clinical context and should be remembered as being one of the tools for assessment and management of patients with chest pain.

When history, physical examination, and basic laboratory investigations do not establish or rule out ACS, stress testing has a diagnostic role. It should be performed when the patient is symptom-free and an evolving MI has been ruled out. The type of test ordered depends on an individual patient's profile. Exercise ECG is preferred whenever feasible as it also provides an estimation of the patient's functional capacity. If the ECG has baseline ST-T segment changes or is otherwise uninterpretable, then an echocardiogram to visualize wall motion changes with peak stress or nuclear imaging scan to visualize perfusion deficits with stress is recommended. In patients unable to exercise, pharmacological agents, such as adenosine, regadenoson or dobutamine can be used as stressors. Nuclear imaging stress test is preferred to stress echocardiogram in those with underlying left bundle branch block, paced rhythm and multiple wall motion abnormalities at rest. Emerging newer modalities of stress testing are cardiac magnetic resonance and positron emission tomography.

Additional information is provided in Chapter 3: Acute Coronary Syndromes.

Aortic Dissection

Aortic dissection almost invariably includes chest pain. It is most commonly seen in patients with hypertension or congenital weakness of the aortic media. In patients with known atherosclerosis or history of a recent intra-aortic catheterization or cardiac surgery, the risk of ascending aortic dissection increases. In patients presenting with acute aortic dissection, physicians correctly suspected the diagnosis in as few as 15–43% of patients. The chest pain characteristic (especially intensity and onset) of aortic dissection sets it apart from other etiologies. It is often described as very intense tearing/ripping chest pain of sudden onset, with lack of gradual crescendo onset. The pain location is usually described in the anterior chest, interscapular region, epigastrium and lumbar area. Involvement of multiple sites is an important characteristic of aortic dissection. Unlike effort angina, the pain of aortic dissection is not predictably triggered by any specific activity or event, except rarely when it occurs during intense isometric exercise. Syncope can occur with aortic dissection and there may be rupture of the ascending aorta into the pericardial space.

Two physical findings can support the diagnosis of aortic dissection: (i) absence of peripheral pulses in half of the patients with ascending aortic dissection and (ii) murmur of aortic regurgitation, due to distortion of the aortic root by dissection. Blood pressure should be measured in all four extremities. A blood pressure difference of ≥ 20 mm Hg is considered an independent predictor of dissection.

Chest X-ray findings, such as abnormal aortic contour, wide mediastinum and new pleural effusion can suggest the presence of aortic dissection. A completely normal chest X-ray lowers the probability of aortic dissection, although it does not rule it out. Electrocardiogram is of limited utility for the diagnosis of aortic dissection. Computed tomography, transesophageal echocardiography or magnetic resonance imaging has high sensitivity and specificity for aortic dissection. The choice of imaging modality should be dictated by the availability, patient characteristics and local expertise in addition to hemodynamic stability of the patient.

Additional information is provided in Chapter 3: Acute Aortic Syndromes.

PULMONARY EMBOLISM

Pulmonary embolism is an often underdiagnosed cause of chest pain. It occurs in patients with one or more of the risk factors defined as Virchow's triad: venous stasis, endothelial damage, or a hypercoagulable state.

Chest pain is encountered in only 49% of patients with PE. Interestingly, chest pain was inversely associated with 3 months mortality in some studies, possibly reflecting smaller and more distal embolization. Pleuritic chest pain is the second most common clinical symptom of PE (66%), and angina-like chest pain occurred in only 4%.

Large PE usually causes sudden shortness of breath; retrosternal pressure may also take place due to associated myocardial ischemia. Dyspnea as the presenting symptoms of acute myocardial ischemia in elderly is also relatively common. The separation of PE from ACS is not always easy based on pain characteristics.

The pleuritic chest pain by definition is aggravated by inspiration; it is knife-like quality discomfort that continues for hours or days. Dyspnea otherwise dominates the clinical picture. The clinical setting surrounding the chest pain onset may give a clue to PE as the etiology. Risk factors, such as immobilization, a long period of travel or postpartum period may raise suspicion of the diagnosis. Compared to angina, pain due to PE is not precipitated by effort, and exercise might aggravate pleuritic pain due to increase in frequency of respiratory rate.

Other associated symptoms in PE apart from dyspnea include hypotension and syncope, which indicate severe hemodynamic compromise.

The physical examination findings in acute massive PE are dominated by findings of acute right ventricular failure as a result of acute severe pulmonary hypertension. These include tachypnea, tachycardia, hypotension and jugular venous distension. Pulmonary infarction less commonly results in a pleural rub.

ACUTE PERICARDITIS

Chest pain due to acute pericarditis accounts for only 5% of emergency room visits. Chest pain in acute pericarditis is usually the initial presentation except in rare entities, such as rheumatoid pericarditis. The pain is characteristically "sharp" in quality, sudden in onset and increased in a recumbent position, by body movements and with inspiration. Sitting up and leaning forward typically relieve the discomfort. Rarely, the pain is described as "dull" in patients with large pericardial effusion due to stretch of the pericardium. The pain can radiate in all over the typical locations of angina creating a diagnostic dilemma in differentiating it from angina. Low-grade fever is common and may precede the onset of chest pain. Physical examination, classically pericardial rub may be transient or intermittent. Blood pressure should be evaluated for the presence of pulsus paradoxus (i.e. a 10 mm Hg drop in systolic blood pressure with inspiration), which indicates pericardial effusion with tamponade physiology. The typical ECG abnormalities in acute pericarditis include diffuse ST segment elevation in all leads except in V1 and aVR with PR segment depression in all leads except V1 and aVR. These ECG changes are found in the majority of patients with acute pericarditis although atypical patterns or absent changes are noted in up to 40–50% of patients. Troponin can rise due to subepicardial myocarditis. Leukocytosis and acute phase reactant, such as the erythrocyte sedimentation rate and C-reactive protein are typically elevated.

Additional information is provided in Chapter 13: Pericardial Diseases.

MUSCULOSKELETAL CHEST PAIN

Many disorders of the chest wall, such as costochondritis and thoracic outlet syndromes can result in chest pain. Costochondritis is an inflammatory process of the cartilage of the costochondral joints and its prevalence is not known. Pain is usually described as "sharp" rather than "pressure. It is frequently well localized and may radiate extensively due to multiple joint involvement. The most common locations are the second through the fifth costochondral junctions. Movements of the chest wall, such as lifting, deep inspiration and torso turning aggravate the pain. Tenderness of the costochondral joints is essentially diagnostic of this disorder.

ESOPHAGEAL DISEASES

Many esophageal disorders can give rise to chest pain that closely mimics the pain of angina and ACS. These include gastroesophageal reflux diseas, motility disorders, namely, diffuse esophageal spasm and achalasia. Gastroesophageal reflux disease pain is typically burning sensation (possibly described as "heartburn") or indigestion. The pain is in the retrosternal area, radiates straight through to the back, usually aggravated by supine position after a large meal, not related to effort. This can be a helpful differentiating point from angina if the patient is active but not in individuals with sedentary lives. Relief of pain by antacids might not differentiate it from angina if the latter is intermittent. It should be remembered that angina can also be triggered by a heavy meal. Tenderness to palpation of the epigastric area may help guide diagnosis.

Esophageal motility disorders are quite rare. Chest pain due to these disorders may not be indistinguishable from angina pectoris or ACS. The pain is centrally locate and may radiate throughout the chest. The pain duration is variable, with no obvious precipitating cause, and not necessarily related to food ingestion. Nitroglycerin relieves pain of esophageal spasm similar to angina. Patients with esophageal spasm commonly describe dysphagia in addition to typical reflux symptoms. Due to the similarities of symptoms in angina and esophageal motility disorders, appropriate studies to rule CAD are often indicated before performing tests for esophageal motility disorders.

SUGGESTED READING

1. Anderson JL, Adams CD, Antman EM, Bridges CR, Califf RM, Casey DE, et al. ACCF/AHA focused update incorporated into the ACCF/AHA 2007 guidelines for the management of patients with unstable angina/non-ST-elevation myocardial infarction: a report of the American College of Cardiology Foundation/American Heart Association Task Force on Practice Guidelines. Circulation. 2013;127(23):e66--e828.

2. Brandrup-Wognsen G, Berggren H, Caidahl K, Karlsson T, Sjöland H, Herlitz J. Predictors for recurrent chest pain and relationship to myocardial ischaemia during long-term follow-up after coronary artery bypass grafting. Eur J Cardiothorac Surg. 1997 Aug;12(2):304-11.
3. Constant J. The diagnosis of nonanginal chest pain. Keio J Med. 1990;39(3):187192.
4. Curtis JP, Schreiner G, Wang Y, Chen J, Spertus JA, Rumsfeld JS, et al. All-cause readmission and repeat revascularization after percutaneous coronary intervention in a cohort of medicare patients. J Am Coll Cardiol. 2009;54(10):903-7.
5. De Winter RJ, Koster RW, Sturk A,lSanders GT. Value of myoglobin, troponin T, and CK-MB mass in ruling out an acute myocardial infarction in the emergency room. Circulation. 1995 15;92(12):340107.
6. Diercks DB, Boghos E, Guzman H, Amsterdam EA, Kirk JD. Changes in the numeric descriptive scale for pain after sublingual nitroglycerin do not predict cardiac etiology of chest pain. Ann Emerg Med. 2005;45(6):581-5.
7. Hamm CW. Cardiac biomarkers for rapid evaluation of chest pain. Circulation. 2001;104(13):1454-56.
8. Henrikson CA, Howell EE, Bush DE, Miles JS, Meininger GR, Friedlander T, et al. Chest pain relief by nitroglycerin does not predict active coronary artery disease. Ann Intern Med. 2003;139(12):979-86.
9. Hickam DH, Sox H, J., Sox CH. Systematic bias in recording the history in patients with chest pain. J Chronic Dis. 1985;38(1):91-100.
10. Hofgren C, Karlson BW, Herlitz J. Prodromal symptoms in subsets of patients hospitalized for suspected acute myocardial infarction. Heart Lung. 1995;24(1):3-10.
11. Jneid H, Anderson JL, Wright RS, Adams CD, Bridges CR, Casey DE, et al. 2012 ACCF/AHA focused update of the guideline for the management of patients with unstable angina/non-ST-elevation myocardial infarction (updating the 2007 guideline and replacing the 2011 focused update): a report of the American College of Cardiology Foundation/American Heart Association Task Force on Practice Guidelines. J Am Coll Cardiol. 2012;60(7):645-81.
12. Lee TH, Rouan GW, Weisberg MC, Brand DA, Acampora D, Stasiulewicz C, et al. Clinical characteristics and natural history of patients with acute myocardial infarction sent home from the emergency room. Am J Cardiol. 1987;60(4):219-24.
13. Nawar EW, Niska RW, Xu J. National Hospital Ambulatory Medical Care Survey: 2005 emergency department summary. Adv Data. 2007;(386):1-32.
14. Panju AA, Hemmelgarn BR, Guyatt GH, Simel DL. The rational clinical examination. Is this patient having a myocardial infarction? JAMA. 1998;280(14):1256-63.
15. Pope JH, Aufderheide TP, Ruthazer R, Woolard RH, Feldman JA, Beshansky JR, et al. Missed diagnoses of acute cardiac ischemia in the emergency department. N Engl J Med. 2000;342(16):1163-70.
16. Sonel A, Sasseen BM, Fineberg N, Bang N, Wilensky RL. Prospective study correlating fibrinopeptide A, troponin I, myoglobin, and myosin light chain levels with early and late ischemic events in consecutive patients presenting to the emergency department with chest pain. Circulation. 2000;102(10):1107-13.
17. Swap CJ, Nagurney JT. Value and limitations of chest pain history in the evaluation of patients with suspected acute coronary syndromes. JAMA. 2005;294(20):2623-9.
18. Thygesen K, Alpert JS, Jaffe AS, Simoons ML, Chaitman BR, White HD, et al. Third universal definition of myocardial infarction. J Am Coll Cardiol. 2012;60(16):1581-98.

Stable Ischemic Heart Disease

Chapter 2

Amandeep Dhaliwal

INTRODUCTION

Angina pectoris, the prototypical symptom of stable ischemic heart disease (SIHD), occurs when myocardial oxygen demand exceeds supply. Stable angina is *stable* because the onset of symptoms occurs predictably and is reproducible at a certain level of exertion or provoked by emotional stress. Further, symptoms are relieved with rest or use of nitroglycerin. Stable ischemic heart disease typically results from a fixed *stable* stenosis within the coronary artery, resulting in limitation of coronary blood flow and should be distinguished from unstable angina that results from an *unstable* plaque associated with acute thrombosis. In practice, in *unstable* angina, the pain is typically prolonged (>20 minutes), occurring at rest and recurring or displaying an accelerating tempo (generally within 48 hours). New onset angina that is *severe* (at least Canadian Cardiovascular Society Class III) within 2 months of presentation or previously diagnosed angina that is distinctly more frequent, longer in duration or lower in threshold also suggests *unstable* angina.

Not uncommonly, certain intercurrent illnesses may unmask coronary artery disease (CAD), such as the development of severe anemia or an arrhythmia—in this instance it may be difficult to determine whether CAD is stable or otherwise (Table 2.1). Many patients can be diagnosed based on a history of angina (or an anginal equivalent, such as dyspnea on exertion), in the presence of risk factors for CAD or CAD equivalents, such as a history of cerebrovascular vascular accidents or peripheral artery disease.

TESTING

All patients should have an electrocardiogram (ECG). An assessment of left ventricular (LV) systolic function is not necessary, unless the patient has prior myocardial infarction, symptoms of heart failure or a murmur on physical examination. Cardiac enzymes do not need to be checked unless the history suggests that the presentation is *unstable*. Patients with suspected and known SIHD should have stress testing for diagnosis and prognostication (Figs 2.1 and 2.2).

If the baseline ECG is interpretable (i.e. no baseline ST or T wave abnormalities and no left bundle branch block (LBBB)) and the patient can exercise, a graded exercise treadmill test (GXT) should be performed.

Table 2.1: Conditions provoking or exacerbating ischemia oxygen demand

Increased oxygen demand	Decreased oxygen supply
Cardiac	Cardiac
Hypertrophic cardiomyopathy	Hypertrophic cardiomyopathy
Aortic stenosis	Aortic stenosis
Dilated cardiomyopathy	Significant coronary obstruction
Tachycardia	Microvascular disease
Noncardiac	Noncardiac
Hyperthermia	Anemia
Hyperthyroidism	Hypoxemia
Sympathomimetic toxicity	Hyperviscosity
Hypertension	
Anxiety	
Arteriovenous fistulae	

Source: Adapted from Fihn SD, Gardin JM, Abrams J, Berra K, Blankenship JC, Dallas AP, et al. 2012 ACCF/AHA/ACP/AATS/PCNA/SCAI/STS guideline for the diagnosis and management of patients with stable ischemic heart disease: a report of the American College of Cardiology Foundation/American Heart Association Task Force on Practice Guidelines, and the American College of Physicians, American Association for Thoracic Surgery, Preventive Cardiovascular Nurses Association, Society for Cardiovascular Angiography and Interventions, and Society of Thoracic Surgeons. J Am Coll Cardiol. 2012;60(24):e44-e164

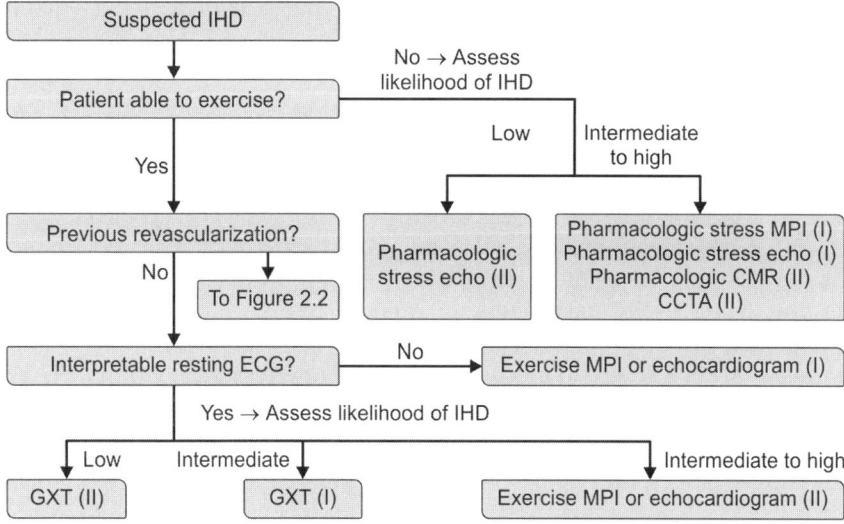

Fig. 2.1: Diagnostic algorithm for patients with suspected ischemic heart disease

I, recommended; II, reasonable; IHD, ischemic heart disease; ECG, electrocardiogram; GXT, graded exercise treadmill; MPI, myocardial perfusion imaging; CMR, cardiac magnetic resonance; CCTA, cardiac computed tomographic angiography.

Source: Adapted from Fihn SD, Gardin JM, Abrams J, Berra K, Blankenship JC, Dallas AP, et al. 2012 ACCF/AHA/ACP/AATS/PCNA/SCAI/STS guideline for the diagnosis and management of patients with stable ischemic heart disease: a report of the American College of Cardiology Foundation/American Heart Association Task Force on Practice Guidelines, and the American College of Physicians, American Association for Thoracic Surgery, Preventive Cardiovascular Nurses Association, Society for Cardiovascular Angiography and Interventions, and Society of Thoracic Surgeons. J Am Coll Cardiol. 2012;60(24):e44-e164.

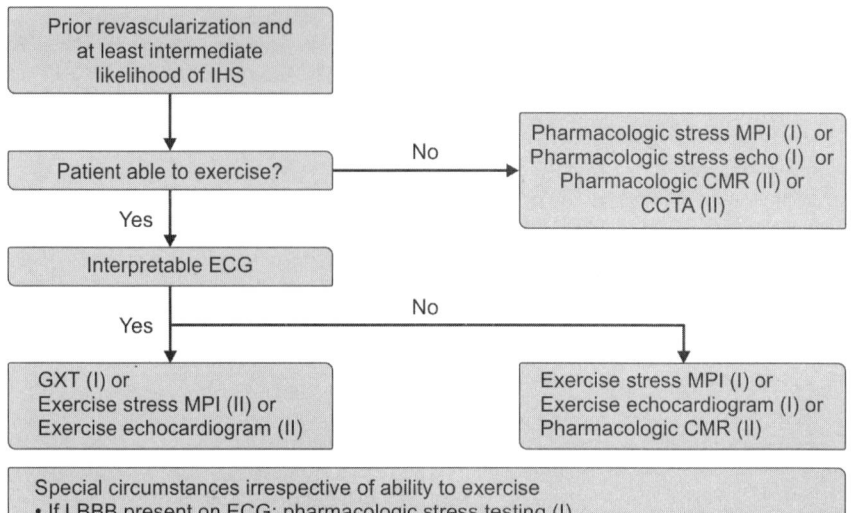

Fig. 2.2: Diagnostic algorithm for patients with known ischemic heart disease

I, recommended; II, reasonable; IHD, ischemic heart disease; ECG, electrocardiogram; GXT, graded exercise treadmill; MPI, myocardial perfusion imaging; CMR, cardiac magnetic resonance; CCTA, cardiac computed tomographic angiography; LBBB, left bundle branch block.

Source: Adapted from Fihn SD, Gardin JM, Abrams J, Berra K, Blankenship JC, Dallas AP, et al. 2012 ACCF/AHA/ACP/AATS/PCNA/SCAI/STS guideline for the diagnosis and management of patients with stable ischemic heart disease: a report of the American College of Cardiology Foundation/American Heart Association Task Force on Practice Guidelines, and the American College of Physicians, American Association for Thoracic Surgery, Preventive Cardiovascular Nurses Association, Society for Cardiovascular Angiography and Interventions, and Society of Thoracic Surgeons. J Am Coll Cardiol. 2012;60(24):e44-e164

A GXT is considered positive for ischemia if there is significant horizontal or downsloping ST segment depression (≥1 mm) in contiguous leads with testing. Other useful parameters on exercise testing that suggest adverse prognosis or multivessel CAD include effort tolerance <5 metabolic equivalent or tasks (METs); failure to increase systolic blood pressure ≥ 120 mm Hg or a sustained ≥10 mm Hg decrease below rest levels; ST segment depression ≥2 mm starting at <5 METs, involving ≥5 leads and persisting ≥5 minutes into recovery; any ST elevation and reproducible sustained or symptomatic ventricular tachycardia. The Duke treadmill score can be used to integrate some of these findings and is calculated as score = exercise time – (5 × ST segment deviation) – (4 × angina index). The angina index is 0 if there is no chest pain, 1 if there is nonlimiting chest pain and 2 if there is limiting chest pain. A low-risk score corresponds to a value of 5 or greater whereas a high-risk score corresponds to value of –11 or lower; the 5-year survival in the former is 97% compared to 72% in the latter.

Exercise with imaging may be used if the patient can exercise, but the baseline ECG has changes that will interfere with interpretation. Pharmacologic stress testing should be used if the patient cannot exercise

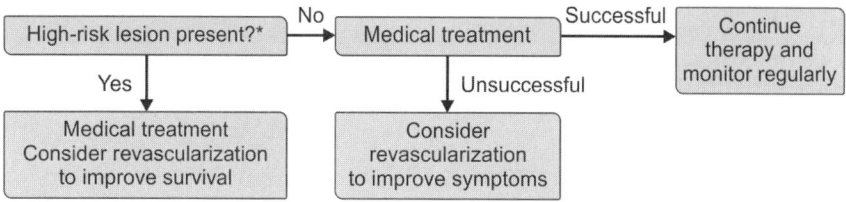

Fig. 2.3: Management algorithm for patients based on diagnostic testing

Source: Adapted from Fihn SD, Gardin JM, Abrams J, Berra K, Blankenship JC, Dallas AP, et al. 2012 ACCF/AHA/ACP/AATS/PCNA/SCAI/STS guideline for the diagnosis and management of patients with stable ischemic heart disease: a report of the American College of Cardiology Foundation/American Heart Association Task Force on Practice Guidelines, and the American College of Physicians, American Association for Thoracic Surgery, Preventive Cardiovascular Nurses Association, Society for Cardiovascular Angiography and Interventions, and Society of Thoracic Surgeons. J Am Coll Cardiol. 2012;60(24):e44-e164.

or has a LBBB, as the latter results in an artifactual defect in the ventricular septum. Coronary angiography should be performed if a high-risk feature (or certain intermediate-risk features) on stress testing is present, whereas low-risk features can be treated medically, at least initially (Fig. 2.3) (Table 2.2 and next section on Treatment).

In some instances, the choice of stress testing should be guided by the pretest probability of disease, which is determined from a description of symptoms and largely by the age and gender of the patient (Tables 2.3 and 2.4). Current American College of Cardiology Foundation (ACCF)/American Heart Association (AHA) guidelines generally discourage use of cardiac computed tomographic angiography (CCTA) as the initial investigation for patients with SIHD.

TREATMENT

Clinical trial data support medical therapy as the first line strategy for patients with SIHD. Coronary angiography should be done in patients with angina that limits lifestyle despite maximal medical therapy, patients with high-risk features and selected patients with intermediate-risk criteria on noninvasive stress testing (see section on Testing). Coronary angiography, where performed, provides prognostic information where patients with more extensive CAD (indicating a larger area of myocardium at risk) have poorer 5 year survival rates (Table 2.5).

Percutaneous and surgical revascularization results in better angina relief upfront; however, there is no difference in other clinical endpoints over moderate to long-term follow-up. Revascularization is reserved when medical therapy fails. There is, however, a strong preference for surgical revascularization—coronary artery bypass grafting (CABG) —if the following coronary anatomy is seen:
- Significant (≥50%) left main coronary artery stenosis
- Significant (≥70%) three vessel CAD, with or without involvement of the proximal left anterior descending artery to improve survival

Table 2.2: Noninvasive stress testing risk stratification

High risk features (>3% annual risk of death or myocardial infarction (MI)	Intermediate-risk features (1-3% annual risk of death or MI)	Low-risk features (<1% annual risk of death or MI)
Severe resting LV systolic dysfunction [ejection fraction (EF) < 35%]	Mild-to-moderate resting LV systolic dysfunction (EF 35–49%)	Low-risk Duke score or no new ST segment changes or exercise induced chest pain when achieving maximal exertion
Resting perfusion abnormalities involving at least 10% of the myocardium	Resting perfusion abnormality involving 5–9.9% of the myocardium	Normal or small perfusion defect involving <5% of the myocardium
Stress ECG findings including ≥2 mm ST segment depression at <5 METs or persisting >5 minutes into recovery, exercise-induced ST segment elevation or VT/VF	≥1 mm ST depression with exertional symptoms	Normal stress or no change in limited wall motion abnormality during stress
Severe stress-induced LV dysfunction (peak exercise LVEF <45% or drop in LVEF with stress ≥ 10%),	Stress-induced perfusion abnormalities involving 5–9.9% of the myocardium in 1 vascular territory without LV dilatation	CAC score <100 Agatston units
Stress-induced perfusion abnormalities involving at least 10% of the myocardium in multiple vascular territories	Small wall motion abnormality involving 1–2 segments limited to 1 coronary bed	CCTA: No coronary stenosis > 50%
Stress-induced LV dilatation	CAC Score 100–399 Agatston units	
Inducible wall motion abnormalities involving >2 segments or 2 coronary beds or a wall motion abnormality	CCTA: one vessel CAD (≥70% stenosis) or moderate CAD (50–69%) in ≥2 arteries	
Wall motion abnormality developing at low dose dobutamine or a low heart rate		
CAC score > 400 Agatston units		
CCTA: Multivessel obstructive CAD (≥70% stenosis) or left main stenosis (≥50%).		

LV, left ventricle; ECG, electrocardiogram; LVEF, left ventricular ejection fraction; CAC, coronary artery calcium; CCTA, cardiac computed tomographic angiography; CAD, coronary artery disease.

Source: Adapted from Fihn SD, Gardin JM, Abrams J, Berra K, Blankenship JC, Dallas AP, et al. 2012 ACCF/AHA/ACP/AATS/PCNA/SCAI/STS guideline for the diagnosis and management of patients with stable ischemic heart disease: a report of the American College of Cardiology Foundation/American Heart Association Task Force on Practice Guidelines, and the American College of Physicians, American Association for Thoracic Surgery, Preventive Cardiovascular Nurses Association, Society for Cardiovascular Angiography and Interventions, and Society of Thoracic Surgeons. J Am Coll Cardiol. 2012;60(24):e44-e164

Table 2.3: Pretest likelihood of coronary artery disease (CAD) in symptomatic patients according to age and gender

Age (years)	Nonanginal chest pain* (%)		Atypical chest pain* (%)		Typical angina* (%)	
	Men	Women	Men	Women	Men	Women
30–39	4	2	34	12	76	26
40–49	13	3	51	22	87	55
50–59	20	7	65	31	93	73
60–69	27	14	72	51	94	86

*Typical angina involves (i) substernal chest discomfort with characteristic quality and duration that is (ii) provoked by exertion or emotional stress and (iii) relieved by rest or nitroglycerin. Atypical chest pain meets two of these characteristics. Nonanginal chest pain meets none or one characteristic. Each value in the table represents the percent of patients with significant CAD on coronary angiography.

Source: Adapted from Fihn SD, Gardin JM, Abrams J, Berra K, Blankenship JC, Dallas AP, et al. 2012 ACCF/AHA/ACP/AATS/PCNA/SCAI/STS guideline for the diagnosis and management of patients with stable ischemic heart disease: a report of the American College of Cardiology Foundation/American Heart Association Task Force on Practice Guidelines, and the American College of Physicians, American Association for Thoracic Surgery, Preventive Cardiovascular Nurses Association, Society for Cardiovascular Angiography and Interventions, and Society of Thoracic Surgeons. J Am Coll Cardiol. 2012;60(24):e44-e164.

Table 2.4: Pretest probability of coronary artery disease (CAD) in low-risk versus high-risk patients*

Age (years)	Nonanginal chest pain (%)		Atypical chest pain (%)		Typical angina (%)	
	Men	Women	Men	Women	Men	Women
35	3–35	1–19	8–59	2–39	30–88	10–78
45	9–47	2–22	21–70	5–43	51–92	20–79
55	23–59	4–21	45–79	10–47	80–95	38–82
65	49–69	9–29	71–86	20–51	93–97	56–84

*Values represent the percent of patients with significant CAD. The first value in the range is for a low-risk patient without diabetes, smoking or hyperlipidemia. The second value is for the same patient but with diabetes, smoking and hyperlipidemia.

Source: Adapted from Fihn SD, Gardin JM, Abrams J, Berra K, Blankenship JC, Dallas AP, et al. 2012 ACCF/AHA/ACP/AATS/PCNA/SCAI/STS guideline for the diagnosis and management of patients with stable ischemic heart disease: a report of the American College of Cardiology Foundation/American Heart Association Task Force on Practice Guidelines, and the American College of Physicians, American Association for Thoracic Surgery, Preventive Cardiovascular Nurses Association, Society for Cardiovascular Angiography and Interventions, and Society of Thoracic Surgeons. J Am Coll Cardiol. 2012;60(24):e44-e164

- Significant (≥70%) two vessel CAD with involvement of the proximal left anterior descending artery to improve survival
- Patient with significant CAD (≥70%) amenable to revascularization with medically refractory angina.

Weaker preferences for surgical revascularization include:
- Significant (≥70%) two vessel CAD with *extensive ischemia* but without involvement of the proximal left anterior descending artery

Table 2.5: Coronary artery disease prognosis based on extent of disease, assuming medical treatment only

Extent of CAD	5-year survival rate (%)
One vessel disease, 75%	93
One vessel disease, 50–74%	93
One vessel disease, ≥95%	91
Two vessel disease	88
Two vessel disease, both ≥95%	86
One vessel disease, ≥95% proximal LAD artery	83
Two vessel disease, ≥95% LAD artery	83
Two vessel disease, ≥95% proximal LAD artery	79
Three vessel disease	79
Three vessel disease, ≥95% in ≥ 1 vessel	73
Three vessel disease, 75% proximal LAD artery	67
Three vessel disease, ≥ 95% proximal LAD artery	59

CAD, coronary artery disease; LAD, left anterior descending.

Source: Adapted from Fihn SD, Gardin JM, Abrams J, Berra K, Blankenship JC, Dallas AP, et al. 2012 ACCF/AHA/ACP/AATS/PCNA/SCAI/STS guideline for the diagnosis and management of patients with stable ischemic heart disease: a report of the American College of Cardiology Foundation/American Heart Association Task Force on Practice Guidelines, and the American College of Physicians, American Association for Thoracic Surgery, Preventive Cardiovascular Nurses Association, Society for Cardiovascular Angiography and Interventions, and Society of Thoracic Surgeons. J Am Coll Cardiol. 2012;60(24):e44-e164.

- Significant (≥70%) proximal left anterior descending artery disease if a left internal mammary artery graft can be placed, with evidence of extensive ischemia
- Mild-to-moderate LV systolic dysfunction [ejection fraction (EF) 35–50%] with multivessel or proximal left anterior descending CAD with viable myocardium in the territory to be revascularized

A caveat to the above recommendations is that data supporting these recommendations are largely based on older studies that compared revascularization to suboptimal (certainly not contemporary) medical therapy. It should be noted that revascularization is *not* indicated for significant one vessel CAD involving the circumflex or right coronary artery and SIHD.

Coronary artery bypass grafting or percutaneous coronary intervention (PCI) may be considered for subjects who continue to have unacceptable angina despite medical therapy who have significant CAD amenable to revascularization with the following exceptions:

- Coronary artery bypass grafting is preferred over PCI for complex three-vessel CAD
- Percutaneous coronary intervention is preferred over CABG for patients who have had prior CABG
- *Beta blockers* are first line therapy (Fig. 2.4 and Table 2.6) to decrease angina frequency and improve exercise tolerance; mechanisms of action

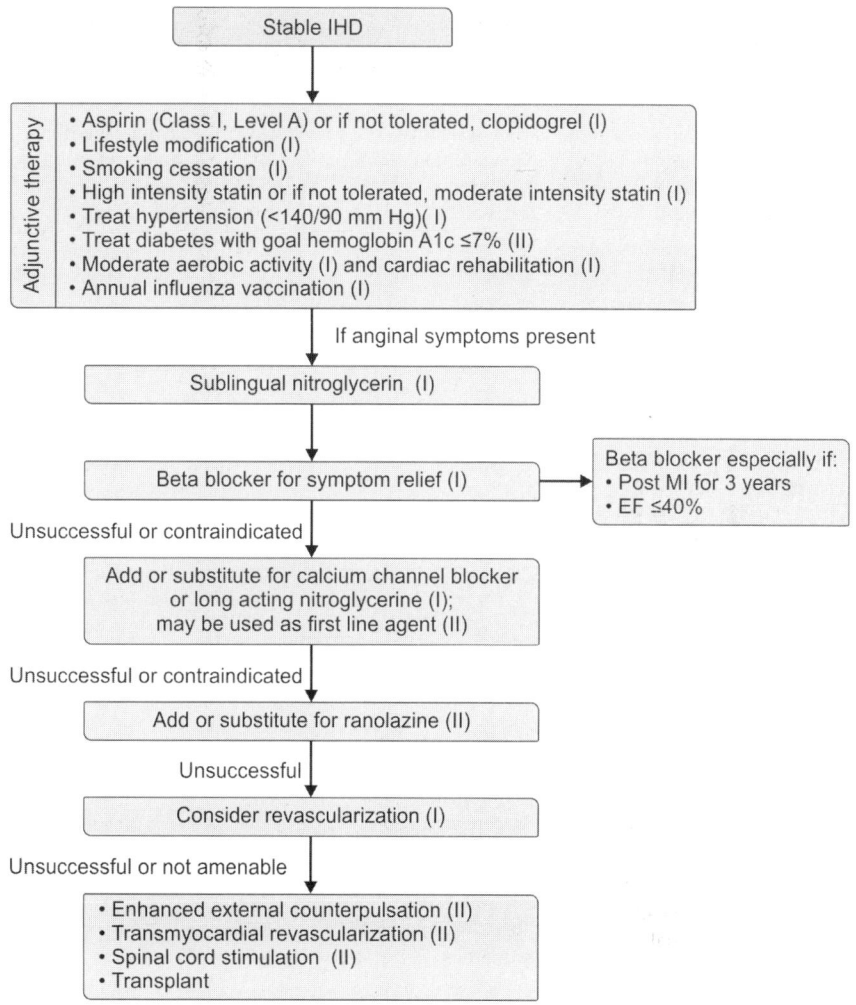

Fig. 2.4: Treatment algorithm for stable ischemic heart disease
MI; myocardial infraction; EF, ejection fraction; I, recommended; II; reasonable

Source: Adapted from Fihn SD, Gardin JM, Abrams J, Berra K, Blankenship JC, Dallas AP, et al. 2012 ACCF/AHA/ACP/AATS/PCNA/SCAI/STS guideline for the diagnosis and management of patients with stable ischemic heart disease: a report of the American College of Cardiology Foundation/American Heart Association Task Force on Practice Guidelines, and the American College of Physicians, American Association for Thoracic Surgery, Preventive Cardiovascular Nurses Association, Society for Cardiovascular Angiography and Interventions, and Society of Thoracic Surgeons. J Am Coll Cardiol. 2012;60(24):e44-e164

include decreasing the heart rate-blood pressure product. Beta blockers are preferred over calcium channel blockers due to the survival benefit observed in patients with prior myocardial infarction or impaired LV systolic function—benefits that have not been observed with other agents
- *Calcium channel blockers*—such as long acting diltiazem or verapamil or a second generation dihydropyridine—may be used when β-blockers are

Table 2.6: Specific anti-anginal agents

Pharma-ceutical class	Dose range	Contra-indications	Major adverse effects	Comments
Isosorbide dinitrate	Initial: 5–20 mg bid-tid Usual: 10–40 mg bid-tid	Hypersensitivity Concomitant PDE5 inhibitor Increased intracranial pressure	Headache	Nitrate-free interval (see text)
Isosorbide mononitrate (extended release)	Initial: 30–60 mg daily Usual: 60–120 mg daily Max: 240 mg daily			
Nitroglycerin				
Transdermal patch	Initial: 0.2–0.4 mg/h Usual: 0.4–0.8 mg/h			
Sublingual	0.3–0.6 mg every 5 min for max three doses			Prophylactic use 5–10 min prior to angina provoking activity
Metoprolol	Initial: 12.5–25 mg bid Usual: 50–200 mg bid Max: 400 mg/day	Sinus bradycardia 2nd or 3rd degree heart block Cardiogenic shock Decompensated heart failure Severe peripheral arterial disease Reactive airway disease Sick sinus syndrome (except with pacemaker)	Hypotension Bradycardia	
Atenolol	Initial: 12.5–25 mg daily Usual: 25–50 mg daily Max: 200 mg/day			Caution in renal failure
Diltiazem SR	Initial: 120 mg daily Usual: 120–360 mg daily Max: 480 mg daily	2nd or 3rd degree heart block Sick sinus syndrome (except with pacemaker) Severe hypotension Left ventricular systolic dysfunction	Headache Pedal edema Bradycardia Hypotension Constipation	Immediate release formulation available (start 30 mg qid)
Verapamil SR	Initial: 180 mg qhs Usual: 180–360 mg daily Max: 480 mg daily		Constipation Headache Gingival hyperplasia Peripheral edema Hypotension Bradycardia	

Contd...

Contd...

Pharma-ceutical class	Dose range	Contra-indications	Major adverse effects	Comments
Nifedipine SR	Initial: 30–60 mg daily Usual: 60–120 mg daily Max: 180 mg daily	Concomitant strong CYP3A4 inducers Cardiogenic shock	Flushing Pedal edema Nausea Heartburn Hypotension Palpitations	
Amlodipine	Initial: 5 mg daily Usual: 5–10 mg daily Max: 10 mg daily	Hypersensitivity to formulation		
Ranolazine	Initial: 500 mg bid Usual: 1,000 mg bid Max: 2,000 mg/day (1,000 mg/day with moderate CYP3A inhibitors)	Liver cirrhosis Concomitant strong CYP3A inhibitors Concomitant CYP3A inducers	Dizziness Headache Constipation Nausea QT prolongation	Caution in renal failure May prolong QT interval
Ivabradine	Initial: 5 mg bid Max: 7.5 mg bid	Hypersensitivity Bradycardia/AV block Hypotension or shock Myocardial ischemia Sick sinus syndrome CYP3A inhibitors	Luminous phenomena ("phosphenes") Bradycardia Headache	Use in patients with intolerance of beta blockers Avoid concomitant QT prolonging pharmaceuticals
Nicorandil	Initial: 10 mg bid Max: 30 mg bid	Hypersensitivity Cardiogenic shock Concomitant PDE5 inhibitor	Headache Dizziness Nausea Flushing	
Trimetazidine	30 mg tid	Hypersensitivity Parkinson's Severe renal impairment	Headache Dyspepsia Rash	Not primary agent

PDE5, phosphodiesterase 5; SR, sustained release; CYP, cytochrome; AV, atrioventricular; bid, twice daily; tid, thrice daily; qid, four times daily; qhs, at bed time

not tolerated or in combination with β-blockers. Mechanisms of action include decreasing the heart rate-blood pressure product and causing coronary vasodilatation and decreasing contractility
- *Nitrates* are recommended for treatment of acute symptoms (i.e. sublingual), and are added to β blockers for treatment of chronic symptoms. Synergistic effects are noted when added to β blockers or calcium channel blockers, with greater anti-ischemic effect. Chronic exposure to nitrates

results in tolerance that cannot be overcome by dose escalation. Hence, a period—typically when activity is the least (i.e. at night)—of no exposure to nitrates is incorporated into the dosing regimen of most long acting nitrate formulations to minimize the risk of tolerance
- *Ranolazine* may be considered in refractory angina alone (in subjects intolerant to the previous agents) or in combination with other agents. Outside the United States, ivabradine may be used to decrease heart rate and thus angina threshold
- *Nonpharmacologic therapies* for refractory angina include enhanced external counterpulsation, spinal cord stimulation and transmyocardial revascularization. Currently stem cell therapy for treatment of refractory angina is investigational with cardiac transplantation occasionally performed as a last resort
- All patients should receive an *aspirin, or clopidogrel if allergic* to or intolerant of aspirin. As these patients have established CAD, all should receive high intensity statin therapy or if intolerant, moderate intensity therapy (see Chapter 23: Dyslipidemias—for details on statin dosing). All patients should be counseled to cease smoking and avoid second-hand smoke exposure. Lifestyle modification, primarily adopting a healthful diet and losing weight, should be encouraged
- *Angiotensin converting enzyme (ACE) inhibitors* should be considered for blood pressure management in patients with hypertension. Patients with SIHD with diabetes, EF ≤40% or having chronic kidney disease should be on ACE inhibitors. Additionally, the use of ACE inhibitors is reasonable in patients with SIHD and other vascular disease.
  Diabetes mellitus should be treated with a goal hemoglobin A1c of ≤7%
- An *annual influenza vaccine* is recommended for patients with SIHD
- All patients should be counseled to participate in *regular aerobic exercise*, specifically 30-60 minutes of moderate intensity activity for at least 5 days and preferably 7 days per week. Exercise can improve exercise tolerance and reduce symptoms. Patients should be referred to a cardiac rehabilitation program where appropriate.
- *Dietary therapy* includes reduced intake of saturated fats (to <7% of total calories), transfatty acids (to <1% of total calories) and cholesterol (to <200 mg/day).

Finally, patients with SIHD should generally be followed up every 6–12 months.

SUMMARY

Stable ischemic heart disease is characterized by angina, which occurs when myocardial oxygen demand exceeds supply, in a manner that is generally predictable and reproducible. Patients with suspected or known SIHD should have stress testing for diagnosis and prognostication. The choice of test depends on the underlying ECG, the patient's ability to exercise and the need for concomitant imaging. Clinical trial data support medical therapy as the first line strategy for patients with SIHD. However, there is a strong preference for surgical revascularization in the presence of more extensive coronary disease. Contemporary medical therapy should include anti-anginal pharmaceuticals as well as appropriate treatment of underlying risk factors such as hypertension, hyperlipidemia, diabetes and cigarette smoking.

SUGGESTED READING

1. Fihn SD, Gardin JM, Abrams J, Berra K, Blankenship JC, Dallas AP, et al. 2012 ACCF/AHA/ACP/AATS/PCNA/SCAI/STS guideline for the diagnosis and management of patients with stable ischemic heart disease: a report of the American College of Cardiology Foundation/American Heart Association Task Force on Practice Guidelines, and the American College of Physicians, American Association for Thoracic Surgery, Preventive Cardiovascular Nurses Association, Society for Cardiovascular Angiography and Interventions, and Society of Thoracic Surgeons. J Am Coll Cardiol. 2012;60(24):e44-e164.
2. Stone NJ, Robinson J, Lichtenstein AH, Merz CN, Blum CB, Eckel RH, et al. 2013 ACC/AHA guideline on the treatment of blood cholesterol to reduce atherosclerotic cardiovascular risk in adults: a report of the American College of Cardiology/American Heart Association Task Force on Practice Guidelines. Circulation. 2014;129:S1-S45.

Acute Coronary Syndromes

3

Chapter

Ankur Vyas, Saket Girotra

INTRODUCTION

Acute coronary syndrome (ACS) which represents a spectrum of clinical diagnoses, occurs due to myocardial ischemia resulting from acute coronary artery obstruction, and is a leading cause of morbidity and mortality across the world. It includes unstable angina, non-ST elevation myocardial infarction (NSTEMI) and ST elevation myocardial infarction (STEMI). Unstable angina and NSTEMI are often grouped together as non-ST elevation ACS (NSTEACS), and differ from STEMI with respect to the degree of coronary ischemia, electrocardiographic features and, importantly, prognosis and management.

PATHOPHYSIOLOGY

Rupture of an atherosclerotic plaque is the most common mechanism responsible for ACS. Plaque disruption initiates a cascade of platelet activation, coagulation and thrombosis that results in coronary artery obstruction, reduction in myocardial blood flow and consequently, myocardial ischemia and infarction (Fig. 3.1). Other, less frequent etiologies of ACS include plaque erosion, intraplaque hemorrhage, coronary artery vasospasm, spontaneous coronary artery dissection and, rarely, embolization from a distinct upstream source in absence of atherosclerotic plaque. Finally, in conditions of increased myocardial demand, fixed chronic coronary obstructions may also result in ischemia and infarction.

The degree of coronary artery occlusion determines the clinical presentation. Complete obstruction of a major epicardial coronary artery results in STEMI, and if not promptly relieved, results in significant myocardial necrosis. Partial obstruction may lead to myocardial ischemia that may be accompanied with necrosis (NSTEMI) or without necrosis (unstable angina). While myocardial necrosis is present in both STEMI and NSTEMI, treatment intensity is different. For example, immediate reperfusion is necessary in patients with STEMI in order to restore blood flow in a completely occluded coronary artery, without which significant myocardial damage would result. In contrast, most patients with unstable angina or NSTEMI can undergo a period of medical stabilization (12-24 hours) prior to coronary revascularization because the coronary obstruction is usually not complete, allowing adequate myocardial perfusion at rest.

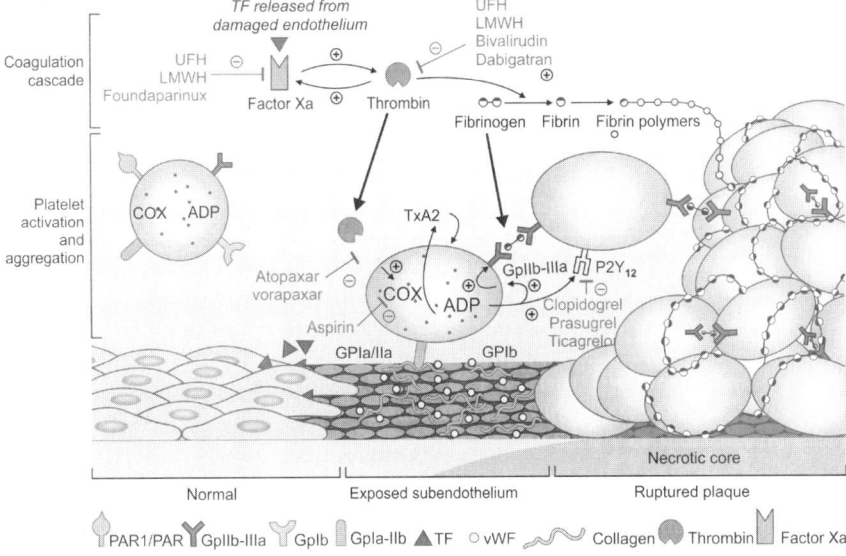

Fig. 3.1: Mechanism of acute coronary syndromes and targets of antiplatelet and antithrombotic agents *(For color version, see Plate 1)*

UFH, unfractionated heparin; LMWH, low molecular weight heparin; TF, tissue factor.

Source: Reprinted from Lilly SM, Wilensky RL. Emerging therapies for acute coronary syndromes. Front Pharmacol. 2011;2:61. Published online Oct 24, 2011. doi: 10.3389/fphar.2011.00061.

The clinical setting, e.g. sudden cardiac death or postcoronary revascularization state, also impacts the diagnosis and management of MI. These factors were thus synthesized recently to create a universal definition of MI, with an aim to improve consistency in reporting as well as in clinical practice. Under this classification, MI ranges from that due to a primary coronary event, such as plaque rupture (Type I), to those associated with myocardial oxygen supply-demand mismatch (Type II), sudden cardiac death (Type III), percutaneous coronary interventions (PCI) (Type IV) and coronary artery bypass grafting (CABG) (Type V) (Table 3.1).

CLINICAL PRESENTATION

The typical presentation in patients with ACS is anginal chest discomfort. This is classically described as precordial chest pressure or squeezing sensation, radiating to the jaw, neck or left arm. In comparison to stable angina, chest discomfort in ACS has a sudden onset, may arise at rest or with minimal exertion, and may last ≥30 minutes. In addition to chest discomfort, patients may also experience shortness of breath, nausea, vomiting and diaphoresis. These symptoms may sometimes be the sole presenting features of acute cardiac ischemia, and thus a high degree of clinical suspicion is warranted in the appropriate settings. Certain populations, such as women and the elderly, are more likely to present in such an atypical fashion. When the burden of ischemia is significant, patients may present with syncope or cardiac arrest.

Table 3.1: Universal classification of myocardial infarction

Type 1: Spontaneous myocardial infarction

Spontaneous myocardial infarction related to atherosclerotic plaque rupture, ulceration, assuring, erosion or dissection with resulting intraluminal thrombus in one or more of the coronary arteries leading to decreased myocardial blood flow or distal platelet emboli with ensuing myocyte necrosis. The patient may have underlying severe CAD but on occasion nonobstructive or no CAD.

Type 2: Myocardial infarction secondary to an ischemic imbalance

In instances of myocardial injury with necrosis where a condition other than CAD contributes to an imbalance between myocardial oxygen supply and/or demand, e.g. coronary endothelial dysfunction, coronary artery spasm, coronary embolism, tachy-/brady-arrhythmias, anemia, respiratory failure, hypotension and hypertension with or without LVH.

Type 3: Myocardial infarction resulting in death when biomarker values are unavailable

Cardiac death with symptoms suggestive of myocardial ischemia and presumed new ischemic ECG changes or new LBBB, but death occurring before blood samples could be obtained, before cardiac biomarker could rise or in rare cases cardiac biomarkers were not collected.

Type 4a: Myocardial infarction related to PCI

Myocardial infarction associated with PCI is arbitrarily defined by elevation of cTn values >5 x 99th percentile URL in patients with normal baseline values (<99th percentile URL) or a rise of cTn values >20% if the baseline values are elevated and are stable or falling. In addition, either (i) symptoms suggestive of myocardial ischemia, or (ii) new ischemic ECG changes or new LBBB or (iii) angiographic loss of patency of a major coronary artery or a side branch or persistent slow-or no-flow or embolization or (iv) imaging demonstration of new loss of viable myocardium or new regional wall motion abnormality are required.

Type 4b: Myocardial infarction related to stent thrombosis

Myocardial infarction associated with stent thrombosis is detected by coronary angiography or autopsy in the setting of myocardial ischemia and with a rise and/or fall of cardiac biomarkers values with at least one value above the 99th percentile URL.

Type 5: Myocardial infarction related to coronary artery bypass grafting (CABG)

Myocardial infarction associated with CABG is arbitrarily defined by elevation of cardiac biomarker values >10 × 99th percentile URL in patients with normal baseline cTn values (<99th percentile URL). In addition, either (i) new pathological Q waves or new LBBB, or (ii) angiographic documented new graft or new native coronary artery occlusion or (iii) imaging evidence of new loss of viable myocardium or new regional wall motion abnormality.

CAD, coronary artery disease; LVH, left ventricular hypertrophy; ECG, electrocardiogram; LBBB, left bundle branch block; URL, upper reference limit; cTn, cardiac troponin; PCI, percutaneous coronary intervention.

Source: Reprinted with permission from Thygesen K, Alpert JS, Jaffe AS, Simoons ML, Chaitman BR, White HD, et al. Third universal definition of myocardial infarction. J Am Coll Cardiol. 2012;60(16):1581-98, Elsevier

Physical examination findings often vary with the degree of ischemia, and may serve as a guide to determine possible etiologies or precipitating conditions and, more importantly, hemodynamic consequences that would affect further management. Signs of significant hemodynamic compromise include sinus tachycardia, hypotension and shock, jugular venous distension, cool extremities and third and fourth heart sounds. Mechanical complications of acute MI may also be detected using a careful physical examination, and these include murmur of acute mitral regurgitation or ventricular septal defect. Finally, physical examination may also help distinguish between ACS and other etiologies of chest discomfort, such as pericarditis (e.g. presence of a pericardial rub) or aortic dissection (e.g. unequal pulses and blood pressure in the upper extremities).

DIAGNOSTIC EVALUATION

- A *12-lead electrocardiogram* (ECG) is perhaps the single most important test in patients with suspected ACS and should be performed within 10 minutes of patient arrival to the hospital. Presence of new ST segment elevation of ≥0.1 mV in two or more contiguous leads, or a new left bundle branch block identifies patients with STEMI who would benefit from immediate reperfusion therapy. Findings in patients with NSTEACS are more varied, and range from transient ST-elevation, ST depression, T wave inversion or other nonspecific changes. Because ECG findings can evolve over time in the setting of acute ischemia, obtaining serial ECGs is important and should be considered in patients even if the initial ECG is unremarkable
- *Cardiac troponins* (T and I) are preferred biomarkers for detection of myocardial necrosis. Troponin levels usually rise by about 6 hours of onset of symptoms, and elevated levels persist for 5–14 days. Therefore, a negative troponin in a patient with suspected ACS should be confirmed with a repeat test. Levels of creatine kinase muscle and brain (CK-MB fraction) are less sensitive and specific than troponins, and therefore have largely been replaced by troponin in the initial diagnosis of ACS. However, compared to troponin, CK-MB has a shorter half-life (i.e. 2–3 days), and therefore is more useful for detection of recurrent infarction. Myoglobin, which rises in 1–4 hours and peaks at 6–7 hours, is the earliest marker to be detected in the bloodstream and therefore may have value in the emergency department for early diagnosis of myocardial infarction (Fig. 3.2)
- *Echocardiography* is a very useful diagnostic test in patients with ACS. It provides an assessment of left ventricular systolic function, which has significant prognostic value. Moreover, it can help identify other comorbid cardiac conditions (e.g. aortic stenosis) that can influence therapeutic decisions (e.g. PCI vs. CABG surgery). Even in the acute setting, echocardiography can be used, especially when there is diagnostic uncertainty. For example, detection of a regional wall motion abnormality could help confirm myocardial ischemia when the ECG is nondiagnostic (e.g. high lateral myocardial infarction due to an occluded left circumflex artery). Finally, echocardiography is also very helpful in diagnosing mechanical complications of acute MI such as acute mitral regurgitation or ventricular septal defect.

RISK STRATIFICATION

The risk of short-term mortality in patients with ACS varies widely and therefore appropriate risk stratification of patients helps to tailor treatment

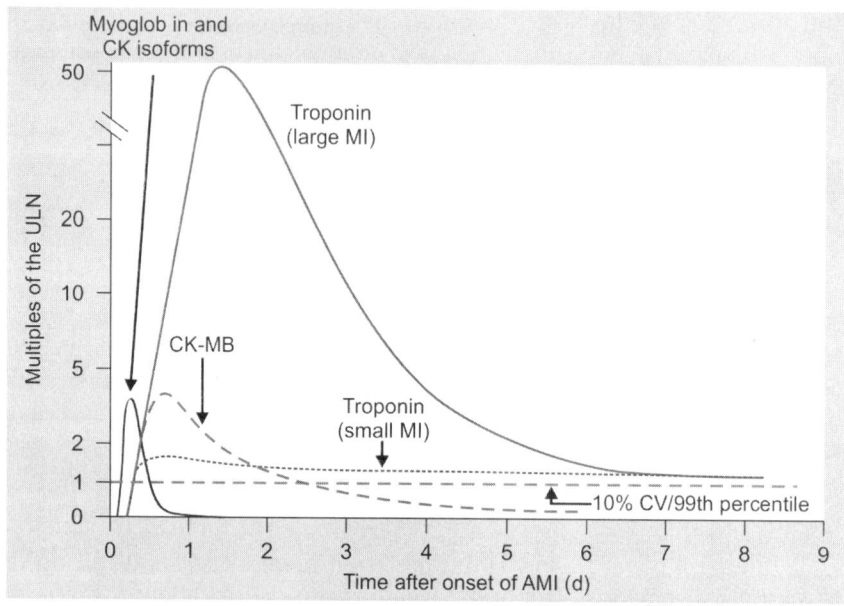

Fig. 3.2: Timing of release of various biomarkers after acute myocardial infarction
(For color version, see Plate 1)

ULN, upper limit of normal (defined as the 99th percentile from a normal reference population without myocardial necrosis); CK, creatine kinase; CK-MB, CK muscle and brain fraction.

Source: Reprinted with permission from Kumar, Cannon CP. Acute coronary syndromes: diagnosis and management, part I. Mayo Clin Proc. 2009;84(10):917-38, Elsevier.

intensity according to patient's risk. As a first step, it is important to determine whether the clinical presentation is consistent with an ischemic coronary event. A good history and physical examination are an integral part of this process. Presence of ischemia on ECG (e.g. ST-segment deviation and T wave inversion) and elevation in cardiac biomarkers not only helps in diagnosis, but also has important prognostic implications. Patients with a clinical presentation that suggests a low likelihood of ACS (e.g. atypical chest pain, normal exam, no ischemic changes on ECG, and negative biomarkers) can be treated conservatively. After two negative troponins 6-8 hours apart, such patients can either get stress testing in the emergency department, or be safely discharged with outpatient evaluation if necessary.

Among patients with likely or definite ACS, further risk stratification into low, intermediate or high risk should be performed based on the risk of short-term mortality. In general, all patients with STEMI inherently fall in the high-risk category and in the absence of contraindications should receive immediate reperfusion therapy with either primary PCI, or thrombolytics. Although a number of risk assessment scores for the NSTEACS population are available (e.g. global registry of acute coronary events (GRACE), thrombolysis in myocardial infarction (TIMI) risk score) (Table 3.2), the presence of significant ECG changes (e.g. ST-segment depression or diffuse T-wave inversions) and/or elevation of cardiac biomarkers elevation are perhaps the most important variables that identify patients at high-risk of short-term mortality and recurrent MI. Studies have shown that an early invasive strategy

Table 3.2: Thrombolysis in myocardial infarction (TIMI) risk score for UA/NSTEMI

Characteristics included in TIMI risk score for UA/NSTEMI*	TIMI risk score	Rates of all-cause mortality, myocardial infarction and severe recurrent ischemia prompting urgent revascularization through 14 days (in TIMI 11B test cohort)
Age ≥65 years		
≥3 risk factors for coronary artery disease†	0/1	4.3%
Prior coronary artery stenosis ≥50%	2	8.3%
Use of aspirin in previous 7 days	3	13.2%
≥2 anginal events in previous 24 hours	4	19.9%
ST segment deviation on electrocardiogram	5	26.2%
Elevated serum cardiac markers	6/7	40.9%

*1 point awarded for each characteristic present.
†Risk factors: Family history of coronary artery disease, patient history of hypertension, hypercholesterolemia, diabetes or being a current smoker.
TIMI, thrombolysis in myocardial infarction.

Source: Adapted from Antman EM, Cohen M, Bernink PJ, McCabe CH, Horacek T, Papuchis G, et al. The TIMI risk score for unstable angina/non-ST elevation MI: a method for prognostication and therapeutic decision making. JAMA. 2000;284(7):835-42

(i.e. coronary angiography within 24–48 hours followed by revascularization as indicated) in patients with high-risk NSTEACS is associated with higher survival and lower rates of recurrent MI. In contrast, patients with low-risk NSTEMI can be treated with an initial conservative strategy (i.e. period of medical stabilization followed by risk stratification with a noninvasive stress test).

MANAGEMENT

Since ACS occurs most commonly due to plaque disruption, which leads to platelet activation, coagulation and subsequently ischemia due to reduction in myocardial blood flow, initial pharmacotherapy includes antiplatelets, anticoagulants, and anti-ischemic drugs. The need and urgency of myocardial reperfusion depends on the underlying syndrome. Patient with STEMI generally have complete coronary artery occlusion, and therefore require prompt reperfusion to limit further myocardial damage. In contrast, most patients with NSTEACS can be treated with a strategy of initial medical stabilization, and further treatment strategy (i.e. early invasive vs. conservative) is based on their underlying risk.

Initial Medical Therapy

- Antithrombotic therapy (antiplatelet and anticoagulant agents) (Table 3.3)
  - *Aspirin*, 162–325 mg, in a nonenteric formulation, is recommended in all patients with suspected ACS. Aspirin irreversibly blocks the platelet

Table 3.3: Antithrombotic agents

Agent	Mechanism	Dose	Comments
Unfractionated heparin	Binds antithrombin, which inactivates thrombin (IIa), and activated factor Xa	Bolus: 60–70 units/kg Maintenance: 12–15 units/kg/hour	• Widely used, inexpensive • Anticoagulant activity can be easily monitored using activated clotting time (ACT) or partial thromboplastin time (PTT), which makes it attractive for use in cath lab. • Risk of heparin-induced thrombocytopenia (HIT)
Enoxaparin	Similar to unfractionated heparin except greater specificity for Xa, and reduced anti-IIa activity	1 mg/kg twice a day Prior to percutaneous coronary interventions (PCI): administer 0.3 mg/kg bolus if last dose of enoxaparin was >8 hours ago	• More predictable anticoagulant activity (does not require routine monitoring). Anti-Xa levels can be used to monitor, however not widely available. • Dose response unpredictable in obese patients • Contraindicated in patients with advanced renal failure or dialysis • Lower risk of HIT • ST-elevation myocardial infarction: not commonly used especially in patients undergoing PCI due to difficulty in monitoring anticoagulant activity • Non-ST-elevation myocardial infarction: may be used as an alternative to heparin especially in patients treated with an initial conservative strategy
Bivalirudin	Direct thrombin inhibitor	Initial: bolus 0.1 mg/kg followed by 0.25 mg/kg/hour Prior to PCI: additional bolus of 0.5 mg/kg followed by 1.75 mg/kg/hour	• Superior to heparin or enoxaparin due to lower risk of bleeding • Anticoagulant activity can be monitored using ACT • Can be used in patients with HIT • No antidote available • Expensive • Should not be used in patients treated with a conservative strategy (not studied)
Fondaparinux	Factor Xa inhibitor	2.5 mg once daily	• Low risk of bleeding • Can be used in patients with HIT • Not recommended in patients undergoing invasive treatment

Source: Adapted from Makki N, Brennan TM, Girotra S. Acute coronary syndrome. J Intensive Care Med. 2013 (published online before print) doi: 10.1177/0885066613503294.

enzyme cyclooxygenase 1 and prevents collagen-induced platelet activation as well as the synthesis and release of thromboxane A2—a potent activator of platelets. In the Second International Study of Infarct Survival (ISIS-2) randomized trial, early treatment with aspirin in patients with suspected acute MI was associated with a 23% reduction in risk of vascular mortality compared to placebo. The benefit was even greater in the Veteran's Administration Cooperative Study, where patients with unstable angina who were administered aspirin had a 51% reduction in risk of death or MI. Although aspirin irreversibly blocks thromboxane induced platelet aggregation, it has no effect on platelet aggregation that is mediated by adenosine dinucleotide phosphate (ADP) on the P2Y12 receptors. Therefore, therapy with a 2nd antiplatelet agent is warranted.

- Currently, three *P2Y12 inhibitors* are available (*clopidogrel, prasugrel* and *ticagrelor*). Clopidogrel and prasugrel belong to the same class (i.e. thienopyridines) and cause irreversible inhibition of the P2Y12 receptor, and therefore inhibit ADP-induced platelet aggregation. Since binding of these agents on the P2Y12 receptor is irreversible, the antiplatelet effect of these drugs lasts for the life of the platelet. Both clopidogrel and prasugrel are prodrugs and undergo metabolic activation by the cytochrome P450s in the intestine and liver to their active metabolites. A number of well-conducted randomized trials have showed that clopidogrel (with a loading dose of 300 mg followed by 75 mg daily) significantly reduces the risk of mortality, recurrent MI and stroke in patients with STEMI, NSTEMI and unstable angina. This benefit is present regardless of treatment strategy in both STEMI (i.e. thrombolytics and primary PCI) and NSTEACS patients (i.e. early invasive and conservative treatment). The reduction in ischemic endpoints is achieved at an increased risk of bleeding especially in patients who need to undergo CABG. Therefore, it is recommended that clopidogrel be discontinued for a period of 5 days prior to elective CABG.

Due to its dependence on the cytochrome P450s for metabolic activation, there is significant interindividual heterogeneity in responsiveness to clopidogrel (i.e. "clopidogrel resistance"). A number of factors [i.e. age, smoking, diabetes mellitus, high body mass index and genetic polymorphism in enzymes that metabolize clopidogrel to its active metabolite (e.g. CYP2C19 gene)] have been associated with clopidogrel resistance. As a result, some patients continue to have high platelet reactivity to ADP despite adequate therapy with clopidogrel. In recent years, platelet function assays that can determine platelet reactivity in clopidogrel treated patients (e.g. VerifyNow) as well as genetic testing for polymorphisms of the important cytochrome P450s (e.g. CYP2C19*2 allele) have become available that can help identify patients who may not achieve adequate platelet inhibition despite therapeutic doses of clopidogrel. However, clinical trials so far have not conclusively proven whether modifying antiplatelet strategy (e.g. higher dose of clopidogrel or using alternative antiplatelet agents) based on results of platelet function or genetic testing is associated with a reduction in ischemic endpoints.

Prasugrel is also a thienopyridine drug and is more potent compared to clopidogrel. Prasugrel is also less dependent on cytochrome P450s for enzymatic activation, which leads to a more rapid onset of its antiplatelet action. Due to both these reasons, prasugrel is an alternative option in patients suspected to have resistance to clopidogrel (e.g. patients with stent thrombosis while taking clopidogrel). In a clinical trial of 13,608 patients with ACS, prasugrel in a loading dose of 60 mg followed by 10 mg daily was superior to clopidogrel in reducing the risk of a composite endpoint of cardiovascular death, MI and stroke (hazard ratio 0.81; 95% CI [0.73–0.90]). However, the risk of bleeding in prasugrel treated patients was significantly higher. In subgroup analyses, it was found that patients with a prior history of stroke or transient ischemic attack had net harm on prasugrel therapy and therefore prasugrel is contraindicated in such patients. Moreover, prasugrel should also be avoided in elderly patients (age >75 years) and patients with body weight <60 kg, as in both these groups the reduction in ischemic endpoints was counterbalanced with an increased risk of bleeding leading. Also, given the high risk of bleeding, it is recommended that prasugrel be withheld for at least 7 days prior to elective CABG.

Ticagrelor on the other hand, is a nonthienopyridine drug and reversibly inhibits the P2Y12 receptor. The agent is orally active, and does not require metabolic activation and therefore is also an alternative in patients with resistance to clopidogrel or allergy to thienopyridines. It is administered in a loading dose of 180 mg followed by 90 mg twice a day. In a large clinical trial of patients with ACS, ticagrelor significantly reduced major adverse cardiovascular events compared to clopidogrel (hazard ratio 0.84; 95% CI [0.77–0.92]). Although rates of fatal intracranial and non-CABG related major bleeding were higher with ticagrelor, overall rates of major bleeding were similar in both groups. As a result, the trial also showed that ticagrelor was also associated with a net reduction in mortality compared to clopidogrel (4.5% vs. 5.9%, $p < 0.0001$). Current guidelines recommend discontinuing ticagrelor for 5 days prior to elective CABG; however, given its reversible inhibition of the P2Y12 receptor and its short half-life (of 7–8 hours), earlier performance of CABG may be a consideration in selected patients. Finally, both ticagrelor and prasugrel have only been studied in patients with ACS and it remains unclear whether similar benefit is also present in patients undergoing PCI for other indications.

- *Anti-ischemic therapy*
    - *Nitroglycerin*, given sublingually (0.4 mg, and repeated every 5 minutes up to 3 times), spray or as an intravenous infusion (at a starting dose of 5–10 mg/min), can relieve chest discomfort secondary to cardiac ischemia. It improves myocardial blood flow by causing coronary vasodilation, and reduces myocardial oxygen demand by reducing preload and afterload. However, it should be avoided in the presence of systemic hypotension, or when right ventricular infarction is suspected, where reduction in preload may lead to significant worsening of cardiac output. Adjuvant therapy with morphine may be useful if nitroglycerin is unable to relieve pain. Supplemental oxygen to maintain systemic arterial oxygen saturation is also indicated in all patients with ACS.

- Beta-blockers reduce heart rate, blood pressure and myocardial contractility and thereby can significantly reduce myocardial oxygen demand. They are recommended in patients with ACS, however should not be used in patients with bradycardia, hypotension, heart failure as they can precipitate cardiogenic shock. Oral agents (e.g. metoprolol 25–50 mg) are acceptable and can be switched to intravenous agents if needed. If β-blockers are contraindicated, nondihydropyridine calcium channel blockers (e.g. verapamil or diltiazem) may be used instead, in the absence of contraindications.

- *Immediate reperfusion therapy in STEMI*

Emergent reperfusion is the cornerstone of treatment in patients with acute STEMI and it reduces infarct size and mortality. Reperfusion therapy can be performed using mechanical (i.e. primary PCI), or pharmacological (i.e. thrombolytics) means. The importance of timely reperfusion in patients with STEMI is recognized as an important goal for the healthcare system. It is recommended that, for patients treated with primary PCI, balloon inflation in the infarct-related artery be accomplished within 90 minutes of patient arrival to the hospital (door-to-balloon time), whereas for patients treated with thrombolytics, treatment should be started within 30 minutes of patient arrival (door-to-needle time). The choice of treatment strategy depends on duration of symptoms, availability of cardiac catheterization and degree of hemodynamic compromise.

In general, primary PCI is more effective at restoring coronary flow and therefore superior to thrombolytics in reducing the risk of mortality, recurrent MI, stroke and is also associated with a lower risk of bleeding complications. Moreover, there are few absolute contraindications for primary PCI compared to thrombolytics. Therefore, whenever available, primary PCI is the treatment of choice.

However, a major limitation of primary PCI is that it is not available at all hospitals and at all times. For STEMI patients presenting to hospitals without PCI capability, treatment options include on-site thrombolytics or transfer to a primary PCI-capable hospital. Broadly speaking, interhospital transfer for primary PCI is preferable if transfer to a PCI-capable hospital can be achieved rapidly such that the overall door-to-balloon time (i.e. from presentation at initial hospital to balloon inflation in the infarct-related artery) is ≤20 minutes. If rapid transfer is not feasible, then initial treatment with thrombolytics followed by transfer to a PCI-capable center should be instituted. Table 3.4 provides a list of commonly used thrombolytic drugs in the United States, and Table 3.5 includes the absolute and relative contraindications. All patients treated with thrombolytics should be transferred to a PCI-capable center, since there is a 30% chance that patients may not achieve reperfusion and may require rescue PCI.

TREATMENT STRATEGY IN NSTEACS

Patients with NSTEACS can generally undergo a period of medical stabilization prior to revascularization, unless recurrent or refractory symptoms are

Table 3.4: List of available thrombolytic agents

Agent	Dose	Fibrin-specific	Comments
Streptokinase	1.5 million units for 30–60 minutes	No	• Lower cost • Neutralizing antibodies may limit subsequent use • Risk of hypersensitivity • Less effective compared to fibrin-specific agents
Tissue plasminogen activator (t-PA, alteplase)	15 mg bolus → 0.75 mg/kg over 30 min → 0.5 mg/kg over 60 min	Yes	• More effective than streptokinase • Costly • Short half-life, requires continuous infusion
Reteplase	Two boluses 10 units each 30 min apart	Yes	• Outcomes similar to alteplase • Short half-life, allows bolus dosing
Tenecteplase	Single bolus <60 kg: 30 mg 60–9 kg: 35 mg 70–9 kg: 40 mg 80–9 kg: 45 mg >90 kg: 50 mg	Yes	• As effective as alteplase • Can be administered as a bolus due to longer half-life

Source: Adapted from Makki N, Brennan TM, Girotra S. Acute coronary syndrome. J Intensive Care Med. 2013 (published online before print) doi: 10.1177/0885066613503294.

Table 3.5: Contraindications of thrombolytic agents

Absolute contraindications	Relative contraindications
• Any previous history of hemorrhagic stroke • History of stroke, dementia or central nervous system damage within 1 year • Head trauma or brain surgery within 6 months • Known intracranial neoplasm • Suspected aortic dissection • Internal bleeding within 6 weeks • Active bleeding or known bleeding disorder • Major surgery, trauma or bleeding within 6 weeks • Traumatic cardiopulmonary resuscitation within 3 weeks	• Oral anticoagulant therapy • Acute pancreatitis • Pregnancy or within 1 week postpartum • Active peptic ulceration • Transient ischemic attack within 6 months • Dementia • Infective endocarditis • Active cavitating pulmonary tuberculosis • Advanced liver disease • Intracardiac thrombi • Uncontrolled hypertension (systolic blood pressure >180 mmHg, diastolic blood pressure >110 mm Hg) • Puncture of noncompressible blood vessel within 2 weeks • Previous streptokinase therapy

Source: Adapted from Makki N, Brennan TM, Girotra S. Acute coronary syndrome. J Intensive Care Med. 2013 (published online before print) doi: 10.1177/0885066613503294.

present. Thrombolytics are contraindicated in patients with NSTEACS. Initial treatment with antiplatelets, anticoagulants and anti-ischemic agents should be started as outlined above which generally leads to resolution of angina. Further management depends on the underlying risk of short-term mortality, which can be estimated using validated tools (e.g. TIMI or GRACE risk score, as discussed above). In patients with intermediate to high risk of short-term mortality, an early invasive strategy comprised of coronary angiography with intent of PCI within 24-48 hours is recommended. In contrast, patients who are at low risk, a conservative strategy comprised of medical therapy and noninvasive risk stratification before discharge is recommended. In conservatively treated patients, angiography should be considered if the patient has recurrent symptoms or high-risk findings on noninvasive stress testing (e.g. large ischemic burden).

COMPLICATIONS

- *Cardiogenic shock* after acute MI may occur secondary to extensive myocardial damage leading to pump failure, or due to mechanical complications and carries a very high mortality (~50%). Immediate revascularization, preferably by primary PCI, is recommended in patients who present with cardiogenic shock as part of their initial STEMI presentation. Mechanical circulatory support devices, such as intraaortic balloon pump or percutaneous ventricular assist devices (e.g. Impella), may also be useful in temporarily stabilizing patients and providing adequate systemic perfusion. (Refer to Chapter 7: Hypotension and Shock—for additional information on this subject)
- *Right ventricular infarction* occurs in about one-third of patients with inferior STEMI, and presents with hypotension and elevated jugular venous distension in the absence of pulmonary congestion. Diagnosis can be confirmed using echocardiography. Right ventricular output in these patients is dependent on preload, so nitroglycerin and other agents that decrease preload should be avoided as they may worsen hypotension Treatment includes hemodynamic support with appropriate volume loading to maintain right ventricular filling well as inotropes if necessary.
- *Mechanical complications* may occur either within the first 24 hours after STEMI, or after the initial presentation but within the first week. These include papillary muscle rupture leading to acute mitral regurgitation, ventricular septal rupture and left ventricular free wall rupture. All are potentially catastrophic events, and therefore a high degree of clinical suspicion must be maintained in the event of acute clinical decompensation of a patient post-MI. Echocardiography is the cornerstone for diagnosis, and emergent surgery is required in most cases, although clinical outcomes are uniformly poor. While awaiting surgery, patients can be temporarily stabilized with an intra-aortic balloon pump (or other mechanical circulatory support device)
- *Ventricular arrhythmias* may be provoked by myocardial ischemia. Premature ventricular complexes and short runs of ventricular tachycardia are quite common in patients with ACS and generally subside within the first 48 hours. Treatment with β-blockers is usually sufficient, and specific antiarrhythmic therapy is generally not required. If patients develop sustained ventricular tachycardia and/or develop hemodynamic compromise, treatment with intravenous lidocaine or amiodarone can be helpful. Defibrillation is necessary in patients with ventricular fibrillation or when accompanied by hemodynamic compromise.

LONG-TERM MANAGEMENT

All patients with ACS should undergo assessment of left ventricular function prior to discharge. Left ventricular ejection fraction is a very strong prognostic indicator following ACS. The importance of smoking cessation, exercise-based cardiac rehabilitation, healthy diet and aggressive management of comorbidities needs to be emphasized.

As discussed in the antithrombotic therapy section, all patients with ACS should receive aspirin lifelong and a second antiplatelet agent (clopidogrel, prasugrel or ticagrelor) for at least 1 year. Beta-blockers are also recommended especially in patients with heart failure. All patients with decreased ejection fraction (<40%) should also receive treatment with angiotensin converting enzyme-inhibitors unless contraindicated, and may also be beneficial in patients with diabetes or peripheral vascular disease. In the Eplerenone Post-Acute Myocardial Infarction Heart Failure Efficacy and Survival trial, therapy with eplerenone (an aldosterone blocker) led to a reduction in mortality by 15% in patients with left ventricular systolic dysfunction (ejection fraction <40%) or decompensated heart failure in the setting of an acute MI and is therefore recommend in that setting. There are compelling data for the clinical benefits of high intensity statin therapy (e.g. atorvastatin in a dose of 40-80 mg or rosuvastatin 20-40 mg) following ACS. The PROVE-IT TIMI 22 (Pravastatin or atorvastatin evaluation and infection therapy—thrombolysis in myocardial infarction 22) trial randomized patients hospitalized with ACS to atorvastatin 80 mg or pravastatin 40 mg, and demonstrated a 16% reduction in risk of cardiovascular events and mortality in the high potency group. Therefore, the most recent clinical practice guidelines from the American Heart Association and the American College of Cardiology on lipid management recommend that following an ACS, all patients should be treated with high intensity statin therapy regardless of their baseline low-density lipoprotein-cholesterol. Finally, patients with decreased left ventricular function immediately after an acute MI require close follow-up to assess improvement in cardiac function. If left ventricular systolic dysfunction persists (with ejection fraction <35%) even after 6 weeks following revascularization and medical therapy, an implantable cardioverter-defibrillator for primary prevention of sudden cardiac death is recommended.

SUMMARY

Acute coronary syndrome is a spectrum that includes STEMI, NSTEMI and unstable angina and results due to acute obstruction in a major epicardial coronary artery obstruction leading to myocardial ischemia. Patients usually present with chest discomfort of varying severity, and require immediate evaluation with a history and physical examination, ECG and cardiac biomarkers. Appropriate medical therapy for initial management of ACS includes antianginal agents, antiplatelet agents, and systemic anticoagulation. Patients with STEMI require emergent revascularization, either via primary PCI or fibrinolytics. Treatment strategy in patients with NSTEACS depends on the patient's risk of short-term mortality. Early invasive management, with coronary angiography performed within 24-48 hours is recommended in high-risk patients whereas low-risk patients may undergo risk stratification with noninvasive stress testing. Patient with ACS are at an increased risk of future recurrent ischemic coronary events. Aggressive risk factor modification (e.g. smoking cessation) and secondary prevention therapy (e.g. aspirin and statin) are effective in reducing the risk and should be instituted in all patients.

SUGGESTED READING

1. Antman EM, Cohen M, Bernink PJ, McCabe CH, Horacek T, Papuchis G, et al. The TIMI risk score for unstable angina/non-ST elevation MI: a method for prognostication and therapeutic decision making. JAMA. 2000;284(7):835-42.
2. Anderson JL, Adams CD, Antman EM, Bridges CR, Califf RM, Casey DE, et al. 2012 ACCF/AHA focused update incorporated into the ACCF/AHA 2007 guidelines for the management of patients with unstable angina/non-ST-elevation myocardial infarction: a report of the American College of Cardiology Foundation/American Heart Association Task Force on Practice Guidelines. Circulation. 2013;127(23):e663-e828.
3. Cannon CP, Braunwald E, McCabe CH, Rader DJ, Rouleau JL, Belder R, et al. Intensive versus moderate lipid lowering with statins after acute coronary syndromes. N Engl J Med. 2004;350(15):1495-504.
4. ISIS-2 (Second International Study of Infarct Survival) Collaborative Group. Randomised trial of intravenous streptokinase, oral aspirin, both, or neither among 17,187 cases of suspected acute myocardial infarction: ISIS-2. Lancet. 1988;2(8607):349-60.
5. James S, Akerblom A, Cannon CP, Emanuelsson H, Husted S, Katus H, et al. Comparison of ticagrelor, the first reversible oral P2Y(12) receptor antagonist, with clopidogrel in patients with acute coronary syndromes: rationale, design, and baseline characteristics of the PLATelet inhibition and patient Outcomes (PLATO) trial. Am Heart J. 2009;157(4):599-605.
6. Jneid H, Anderson JL, Wright RS, Adams CD, Bridges CR, Casey DE, et al. 2012 ACCF/AHA focused update of the guideline for the management of patients with unstable angina/non-ST-elevation myocardial infarction (updating the 2007 guideline and replacing the 2011 focused update): a report of the American College of Cardiology Foundation/American Heart Association Task Force on Practice Guidelines. J Am Coll Cardiol. 2012;60(7):645-81.
7. Kumar A, Cannon CP. Acute coronary syndromes: diagnosis and management, part I. Mayo Clin Proc. 2009;84(10):917-38.
8. Kumar A, Cannon CP. Acute coronary syndromes: diagnosis and management, part II. Mayo Clin Proc. 2009;84(11):1021-36.
9. Lewis HD Jr,<AQ5> Davis JW, Archibald DG, Steinke WE, Smitherman TC, Doherty JE 3rd, et al. Protective effects of aspirin against acute myocardial infarction and death in men with unstable angina. Results of a veterans administration cooperative study. N Engl J Med. 1983;309(7):396-403.
10. Lilly SM, Wilensky RL. Emerging therapies for acute coronary syndromes. Front Pharmacol. 2011;2:61. Published online Oct 24, 2011. doi: 10.3389/fphar.2011.00061
11. Libby P, Theroux P. Pathophysiology of coronary artery disease. Circulation. 2005;111(25):3481-8.

12. Makki N, Brennan TM, Girotra S. Acute coronary syndrome. J Intensive Care Med. 2013 (published online before print) doi: 10.1177/0885066613503294.
13. O'Gara PT, Kushner FG, Ascheim DD, Casey DE, Chung MK, de Lemos JA, et al. 2013 ACCF/AHA guideline for the management of ST-elevation myocardial infarction: a report of the American College of Cardiology Foundation/American Heart Association Task Force on Practice Guidelines. Circulation. 2013;127(4):e362-e425.
14. Pitt B, Remme W, Zannad F, Neaton J, Martinez F, Roniker B, et al. Eplerenone, a selective aldosterone blocker, in patients with left ventricular dysfunction after myocardial infarction. N Engl J Med. 2003;348(14):1309-21.
15. Rajappa M, Sharma A. Biomarkers of cardiac injury: an update. Angiology. 2005;56(6):677-91.
16. Siller-Matula JM, Trenk D, Schrör K, Gawaz M, Kristensen SD, Storey RF, et al. Response variability to P2Y12 receptor inhibitors: expectations and reality. JACC Cardiovasc Interv. 2013;6(11):1111-28.
17. Stone NJ, Robinson JG, Lichtenstein AH, Merz CNB, Blum CB, Eckel RH, et al. 2013 ACC/AHA guideline on the treatment of blood cholesterol to reduce atherosclerotic cardiovascular risk in adults: a report of the American College of Cardiology/American Heart Association Task Force on Practice Guidelines. Circulation. 2014;129(25 Suppl 2):S1-S45.
18. Thygesen K, Alpert JS, Jaffe AS, Simoons ML, Chaitman BR, White HD, et al. Third universal definition of myocardial infarction. J Am Coll Cardiol. 2012;60(16):1581-98.
19. Wallentin L, Becker RC, Budaj A, Cannon CP, Emanuelsson H, Held C, et al. Ticagrelor versus clopidogrel in patients with acute coronary syndromes. N Engl J Med. 2009;361(11):1045-57.
20. Wiviott SD, Braunwald E, McCabe CH, Montalescot G, Ruzyllo W, Gottlieb S, et al. Prasugrel versus clopidogrel in patients with acute coronary syndromes. N Engl J Med. 2007;357(20):2001-15.

Dyspnea: Evaluation and Management

Chapter 4

Ankur Vyas, Jeffrey Wilson, Paul Lindower

INTRODUCTION

Dyspnea may be defined as an uncomfortable sensation of breathing and is a fairly common symptom in patients who have either cardiovascular or pulmonary disease. An American Thoracic Society consensus statement describes dyspnea as a "subjective experience of breathing discomfort that consists of qualitatively distinct sensations that vary in intensity." Further, the experience of dyspnea derives from interactions among multiple physiological, psychological, social and environmental factors, and may induce secondary physiologic and behavioral responses.

The perception of dyspnea is subjective and can be modulated by a variety of factors including emotion, memory, activity level as well as individual variability. Normal breathing is automatic and unconscious. When shortness of breath is greater than expected for a given level of activity, it is considered to be abnormal. Therefore, it would not be abnormal to experience dyspnea in the face of vigorous exercise. However, dyspnea that occurs in the context of only modest activity would more likely be considered abnormal.

PATHOPHYSIOLOGY

The sensation of dyspnea is the result of a complex integrative process in the central nervous system where afferent sensory information from multiple receptors is processed in the brainstem with resultant efferent output to both the ventilatory muscles and cerebral cortex. Accordingly, dyspnea may result from one or often more mechanisms in a variety of different circumstances.

Chemoreceptors located both centrally in the medulla oblongata of the brainstem and peripherally in the aortic arch and carotid body are sensitive to oxygen and carbon dioxide tension, as well as acid-base status. Hypercapnia, hypoxemia and acidemia all promote increased respiratory drive and the sensation of dyspnea.

Further afferent sensory input is provided to the central nervous system by airway irritant and stretch receptors, juxtapulmonary capillary or J-receptors and respiratory muscle and chest wall mechanoreceptors. These monitor changes in pressure, flow, volume and metabolism throughout the respiratory system. Upper airway receptors, when stimulated, reduce the sensation of dyspnea. Cool air blowing on the face stimulates the trigeminal nerve and has been shown to reduce the sensation of breathlessness.

PRIMARY ETIOLOGIES OF DYSPNEA

In a series of patients seen in a pulmonary subspecialty clinic, approximately two-thirds of the cases of dyspnea were due to either pulmonary or cardiovascular disorders. However, it is important to recognize that there are multiple potential causes of dyspnea that do not involve the heart or lungs (Table 4.1).

Cardiovascular

The cardiovascular system pumps oxygenated blood from the left ventricle to the vital organs of the body. It also circulates deoxygenated blood back to the right heart, where it is then pumped by the right ventricle to the lungs. Gas exchange occurs in the alveoli of the lungs with diffusion of oxygen to the blood and carbon dioxide to the environment. Optimally, this system

Table 4.1: Some disorders that cause dyspnea

Pulmonary	Vascular
Airway	Pulmonary hypertension
Airway mass	Thromboembolic disease
Asthma	Vasculitis
Bronchiolitis obliterans	Veno-occlusive disease
Chronic bronchitis	**Neuromuscular**
Laryngeal disease	Central nervous system disorders
Tracheal stenosis	Myopathy and neuropathy
Tracheomalacia	Phrenic nerve and diaphragmatic disorders
Parenchymal	Spinal cord disorders
Acute alveolitis	Systemic neuromuscular disorders
Drug-induced conditions	**Cardiac**
Emphysema	Arrhythmia
Lymphangitic carcinomatosis	Coronary artery disease
Metastatic disease	Intracardiac shunt
Pneumonitis	Left ventricular failure
Pulmonary edema	Myxoma
Pulmonary fibrosis	Pericardial disease
Pleural or chest wall	Valvular disease
Abdominal distention	**Other**
Chest wall injury	Anemia
Effusion	Deconditioning
Fibrothorax	Gastroesophageal reflux
Kyphoscoliosis	Hyperthyroidism or hypothyroidism
Pleural mass	Metabolic acidosis
Pneumothorax	Psychogenic

Source: Adapted from Gillespie DJ, Staats BA. Unexplained dyspnea. Mayo Clin Proc. 1994;69(7):657-63

functions to provide adequate cardiac output without needing to generate high pulmonary capillary pressures.

Heart failure is a clinical syndrome that can result from a variety of abnormalities that impair the heart's ability to fill or empty normally. This may promote varying symptoms of reduced cardiac output, increased pulmonary congestion and increased peripheral congestion. Cardiovascular diseases that result in a reduced pumping ability of the heart, or that require its operation at increased filling pressures leading to lung edema, cause dyspnea by stimulating pulmonary capillary receptors from stretch and congestion and chemoreceptors from hypoxemia. Common cardiovascular causes of dyspnea include valvular disease, cardiomyopathy, ventricular dysfunction and pericardial disease. These subjects are discussed in more detail in other chapters in this book.

Pulmonary

The ventilatory pump system moves air in and out of the lungs providing oxygen from the environment to the blood and removing carbon dioxide produced by cellular metabolism from the blood. This exchange of gases occurs by diffusion across the alveolar-capillary membrane.

Pulmonary disorders leading to dyspnea are often associated with both increased ventilatory demand and altered ventilatory or gas exchange mechanics. Common pulmonary diagnoses associated with dyspnea include obstructive airway disease [such as asthma and chronic obstructive pulmonary disease (COPD)], restrictive lung diseases and pulmonary vascular disease.

Other

There are multiple additional etiologies for dyspnea including neuromuscular disorders, anemia, deconditioning, obesity, gastroesophageal reflux, thyroid disorders, metabolic acidosis and psychogenic factors.

HISTORY AND PHYSICAL EXAMINATION

A complete history and physical examination should be performed in all patients with dyspnea. Pratter et al. reported that findings on history and physical examination in conjunction with a chest X-ray (CXR), revealed the diagnosis in two-thirds of patients with dyspnea in a university-based pulmonary practice, highlighting the importance of a thorough clinical assessment.

History

The characteristics of dyspnea that should be elicited include its onset, duration, quality, frequency, severity, exercise capacity, associated symptoms and provocative or relieving activities. The abrupt onset of dyspnea usually represents a sudden clinical event that leads to severe pathophysiologic disturbances at rest (e.g. pulmonary embolism, pneumothorax, acute asthma or pulmonary edema). Temporally related events, such as weight gain, fever or medication change may explain the cause of dyspnea. The activity level of the patient should be determined as this is often reduced to minimize symptoms. A smoking history and any environmental exposures or triggers should also be assessed. Associated symptoms of cough, sputum production, wheezing or paroxysmal nocturnal dyspnea may provide insight to the differential diagnosis.

Physical Examination

The physical examination should be directed toward the heart and lungs as well as any other organ systems uncovered in the history (Table 4.2). The patient's general appearance and vital signs including oxygen saturation are used to determine the severity of illness. Cyanosis may be present with severe hypoxia. An increase in accessory respiratory muscle use is seen most often in severe airflow obstruction and in neuromuscular diseases causing diaphragmatic weakness. A pulsus paradoxus may be seen in patients with a pericardial effusion and tamponade physiology. Jugular venous distension and peripheral edema suggest (but are not specific for) congestive heart failure. Inspection of the chest may reveal hyperinflation of the lungs or a chest wall deformity (e.g. scoliosis). Stridor suggests obstruction of the upper airway. Decreased breath sounds in both lungs may be seen in COPD and absent breath sounds with dullness to percussion may indicate a pleural effusion. Wheezing is heard most commonly in asthma and COPD and can also be heard in patients with heart failure with pulmonary edema. Inspiratory crackles may suggest either interstitial lung disease or pulmonary edema.

The cardiac point of maximal impulse is downwardly and laterally displaced in heart failure. An increased pulmonic closure sound (P2) may be heard with pulmonary hypertension. A rapid or irregular heart rate may indicate significant dysrhythmia. Auscultation of a heart murmur may indicate significant valvular disease. Detection of a third heart sound (S3)

Table 4.2: Physical examination of dyspnea	
Diagnosis	Findings
CHF	Edema, jugular venous distension, S3 or S4, hepatojugular reflux, murmurs, rales, wheezing, hypertension
ACS	Tachycardia, heart failure findings
PE	Wheezing, lower extremity swelling, friction rub
COPD/asthma	Wheezing, barrel chest, clubbing, decreased breath sounds, pulsus, paradoxical, accessory muscle use
Pneumonia	Fever, crackles, increased fremitus
Pneumothorax	Absent breath sounds, hyper-resonance, jugular venous distension, tracheal deviation

CHF, congestive heart failure; ACS, acute coronary syndrome; PE, pulmonary embolism; COPD, chronic obstructive pulmonary disease.

Source: Adapted from Shiber JR, Santana J. Dyspnea. Med Clin North Am. 2006;90:453-79

gallop suggests ventricular dysfunction in an older patient, but may be normal in a young person.

Digital clubbing can be seen in several disorders including chronic respiratory conditions, pulmonary malignancy, congenital heart disease and others.

LABORATORY STUDIES

Laboratory testing for dyspnea should be driven by the history and physical examination findings. For patients with a suspected cardiac condition, a CXR and electrocardiogram are common initial tests. For many patients, an echocardiogram gives important information about cardiac structure, function and hemodynamics with data regarding chamber dimensions, ventricular function, wall motion abnormalities, valvular abnormalities, pericardial effusion, intracardiac shunting, masses, filling parameters, pulmonary hypertension and volume state.

Brain-type natriuretic peptide (BNP) levels are especially useful in evaluating the diagnosis of congestive heart failure in patients with acute dyspnea. Brain-type natriuretic peptide levels <100 pg/mL or N-terminal pro BNP (NT-proBNP) levels <300 ng/mL have a very high negative predictive value for heart failure, and can be used to essentially exclude this diagnosis. Brain-type natriuretic peptide levels >400 pg/mL or age-adjusted NT-proBNP values of >450 pg/mL (in patients aged <50 years), >900 pg/mL (in patients aged 50–75 years), or >1800 pg/mL (in patients aged >75 years) are highly suggestive of congestive heart failure as the etiology of dyspnea. Intermediate values of BNP and NT-proBNP levels require clinical judgment and further evaluation with other appropriate modalities.

For patients with suspected pulmonary disease, a CXR and pulmonary function studies are common initial tests. Spirometry is essential in the diagnosis of obstructive lung disorders (e.g. asthma and COPD), and can suggest restrictive physiology (e.g. parenchymal, pleural or chest wall disorders) that can then be confirmed by measuring lung volumes. The flow volume loop obtained during spirometry can demonstrate evidence of an upper airway obstruction (i.e. a narrowing of the trachea or glottis) caused most commonly by tumors, inflammation and vocal cord dysfunction. The diffusing capacity of the lung for carbon monoxide (DL_{CO}) reflects both the integrity of the alveolar-capillary membrane and the pulmonary-capillary blood volume. It is reduced in many conditions including interstitial lung disease, emphysema, pulmonary vascular disease and heart failure.

A simplified algorithm (from the American Thoracic Society and European Respiratory Society Task Force) may be used to assess lung function in clinical practice (Fig. 4.1). It presents classic patterns for various pulmonary disorders. The forced expiratory volume in 1 second/vital capacity (FEV_1/VC) ratio and VC should be considered first. Total lung capacity is necessary to confirm or exclude the presence of a restrictive defect when VC is below the lower limit of normal. The algorithm also includes DL_{CO} measurement with the predicted value adjusted for hemoglobin. However, the flowchart (Fig. 4.1) does not assess the severity of upper airway obstruction, and more details on interpretation of pulmonary function tests can be obtained from the reference to Table 4.1.

A high-resolution chest computed tomography scan is a standard test for aiding in the diagnosis of specific forms of interstitial lung disease and is the most commonly performed test to evaluate for pulmonary embolism.

Both anemia and thyroid disease may cause dyspnea and should be excluded when the initial diagnosis is not obvious.

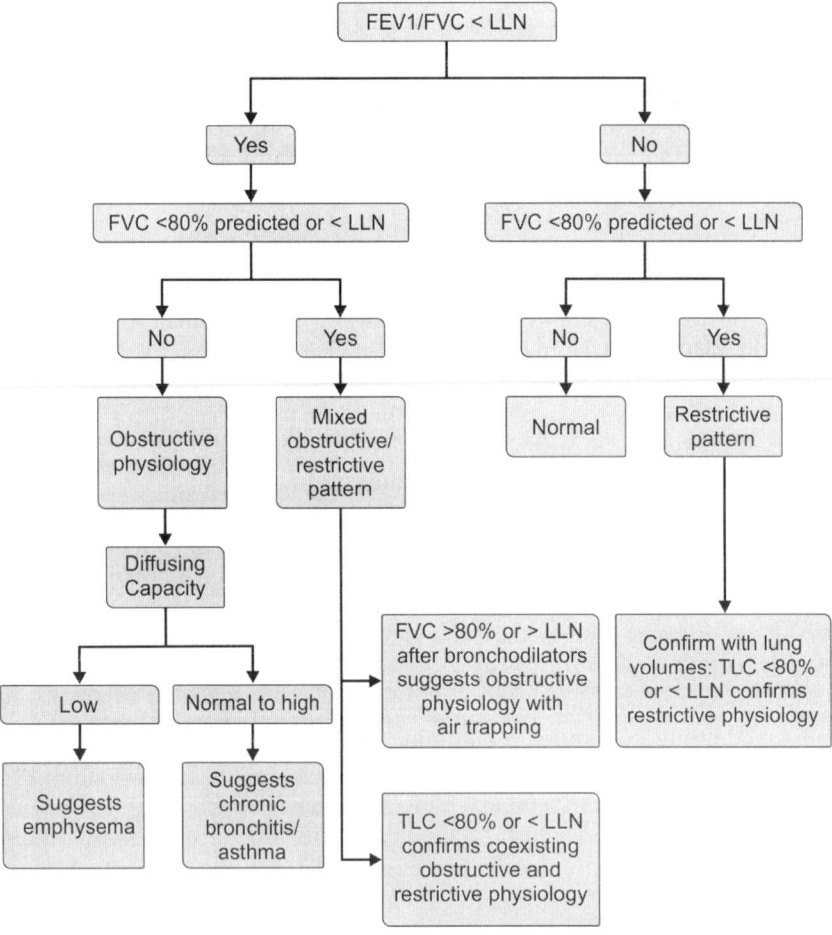

Fig. 4.1: A simplified algorithm that may be used to assess lung function in clinical practice

FEV1, forced expiratory volume in one second; VC, vital capacity; LLN, lower limit of normal; DL_{CO}, diffusing capacity for carbon monoxide measurement (with the predicted value adjusted for hemoglobin); PV, pulmonary vascular; CW, chest wall; NM, neuromuscular; ILD, interstitial lung diseases.

Source: Adapted from the recommendations of the American Thoracic Society and European Respiratory Society Task Force on Standardization of Lung Function Testing, Pellegrino R, Viegi G, Brusasco V, Crapo RO, Burgos F, Casaburi R, et al. Interpretative strategies for lung function tests. Eur Resp J. 2005;26(5):948-68

When dyspnea remains unexplained despite extensive testing, a cardiopulmonary exercise test can be helpful by quantifying exercise capacity and providing both respiratory and cardiac physiologic responses to exercise.

MANAGEMENT

The management of dyspnea is primarily directed at the identification and treatment of the underlying cause. For the specific treatment of dyspnea due to a cardiovascular etiology, refer to the relevant chapter in this book. The treatment of pulmonary disease causing dyspnea is outside the scope of this book and other resources should be consulted.

Many patients with dyspnea become deconditioned that further contributes to their dyspnea. A rehabilitation program can be very beneficial in reversing deconditioning. Oxygen therapy is useful in hypoxemic patients and has been shown to reduce mortality in chronically hypoxemic patients with COPD. Opioids are potent suppressors of dyspnea and can be used carefully in end-of-life settings to palliate severe dyspnea.

SUMMARY

Dyspnea is a common clinical problem and is the result of a complex interaction of sensory input to the central nervous system. It is a subjective perception that can result from a wide variety of disorders. The majority of patients with dyspnea will have abnormalities of the cardiovascular or pulmonary systems. A systematic diagnostic approach including a thorough history and physical examination, and basic laboratory studies will usually establish the diagnosis in the majority of patients. More extensive investigation, including cardiopulmonary exercise testing may be performed when the etiology remains unexplained. Therapy should be directed at the underlying cause.

SUGGESTED READING

1. DePaso WJ, Winterbauer RH, Lusk JA, et al. Chronic dyspnea unexplained by history, physical examination, chest roentgenogram, and spirometry. Analysis of a seven year experience. Chest. 1991;100:1293-9.
2. Gillespie DJ, Staats BA. Unexplained dyspnea. Mayo Clin Proc. 1994;69(7): 657-63.
3. Mahler DA, Horowitz MB. Clinical evaluation of exertional dyspnea. Clin Chest Med. 1994;15:259-69.
4. Maisel AS, Krishnaswamy P, Nowak RM, et al. Rapid measurement of B-type natriuretic peptide in the emergency diagnosis of heart failure. N Engl J Med. 2002;347:161-7.
5. Maisel A, Mueller C, Adams K Jr, et al. State of the art: using natriuretic peptide levels in clinical practice. Eur J Heart Fail. 2008;10(9):824-39.
6. Manning HL, Schwartzstein RM. Pathophysiology of dyspnea. N Engl J Med. 1995;333:1547-53.
7. Parshall MB, Schwartzstein RM, Adams L, et al. An official American Thoracic Society Statement: Update on the mechanisms, assessment, and management of dyspnea. Am J Respir Crit Care Med. 2012;185:435-52.

8. Pellegrino R, Viegi G, Brusasco V, Crapo RO, Burgos F, Casaburi R, et al. Interpretative strategies for lung function tests. Eur Resp J. 2005;26(5):948-68.
9. Pratter MR, Curley FJ, et al. Cause and evaluation of chronic dyspnea in a pulmonary disease clinic. Arch Intern Med. 1989;149:2277-82.
10. Pratter MR, Bartter T, Akers SM, et al. A clinical approach to chronic dyspnea. Clin Pulm Med. 2006;13(3):149-63.
11. Schwartzstein R, Lahive K, Pope A, et al. Cold facial stimulation reduces breathlessness induced in normal subjects. Am Rev Respir Dis. 1987;136:58-61.
12. Shiber JR, Santana J. Dyspnea. Med Clin North Am. 2006;90:453-79.

Heart Failure with Reduced Ejection Fraction

Chapter 5

Omer Iqbal

INTRODUCTION

In the past half century, there have been major improvements in the treatment of most cardiac disorders. The prognosis and mortality rates have fallen dramatically for patients with acute coronary syndrome (ACS), congenital and valvular heart disease, uncontrolled hypertension and many arrhythmias. In addition, age-adjusted cardiovascular disease-related deaths have declined by about two-thirds in industrialized nations. However, heart failure (HF) is an exception. Its prevalence is rising and there has been only a small prolongation in survival. Annual hospital discharges in patients with a primary diagnosis of HF have risen steadily since 1975, and now exceed 1 million discharges per year in the United States.

Several pathogenic mechanisms appear to be operative in HF including increased hemodynamic overload, ischemia-related dysfunction, ventricular remodeling, excessive neurohumoral stimulation, abnormal myocyte calcium cycling, and inadequate proliferation of the extracellular matrix, accelerated apoptosis and genetic mutations. There are many therapies for systolic HF, both medical and mechanical, which directly or indirectly affect these mechanisms and thus, slow or occasionally reverse the process of HF.

Promising new therapies that are now undergoing intensive investigation include an angiotensin receptor neprilysin inhibitor, a naturally occurring vasodilator peptide, a myofilament sensitizer and several drugs that enhance Ca^{++} uptake by the sarcoplasmic reticulum. Cell therapy, using autologous bone marrow and cardiac progenitor cells, appears to be promising, as does gene therapy. Chronic left ventricular (LV) assistance with continuous flow pumps is being applied more frequently and successfully as destination therapy, as a bridge to transplantation, and even as a bridge to recovery. While many of these therapies will improve the care of patients with HF, significant reductions in prevalence will require vigorous, multifarious and preventive approaches.

DEFINITION

Systolic HF, also called as HF with reduced ejection fraction (HFrEF) is a syndrome caused by cardiac dysfunction, generally resulting from myocardial muscle dysfunction or loss and usually characterized by reduced left ventricular ejection fraction (LVEF) and LV dilation with or without LV hypertrophy. It leads to neurohormonal and circulatory abnormalities, usually resulting in characteristic symptoms, such as fluid retention, shortness of breath and fatigue, especially on exertion. In the absence of appropriate therapeutic intervention, this syndrome is usually progressive at the level of both cardiac function and clinical symptoms. The severity of clinical symptoms may vary substantially during the course of the disease process and may not correlate with changes in underlying cardiac function. Although it is progressive and often fatal, patients can be stabilized and myocardial dysfunction and remodeling may improve, either spontaneously or as a consequence of therapy.

CLASSIFICATIONS AND STAGING

There are various ways that HFrEF has been staged and classified in the literature. The most common and universally recognized ones include subjective classification [e.g. New York Heart Association (NYHA) functional classification] and objective staging [e.g. American College of Cardiology/American Heart Association (ACC/AHA) HF staging].

- *NYHA functional classification* assigns patients to one of four functional classes, depending on the degree of effort needed to elicit symptoms. Patients with very low LVEF may be asymptomatic, whereas patients with preserved LV systolic function may have following symptoms:
  - Class I (asymptomatic LV dysfunction)
    - Symptoms of HF only at levels that would limit normal individuals
    - Achieve >7 metabolic equivalent (METs)
  - Class II (mild HF)
    - Symptoms of HF on ordinary exertion
    - Achieve 5 METs
  - Class IIIa (moderate HF)
    - Symptoms of HF on less than ordinary exertion
    - Achieve 3 METs
  - Class IIIb
    - Significant symptoms of HF on mild exertion
    - Achieve 2 METs
  - Class IV (severe HF)
    - Symptoms of HF at rest
    - Achieve <1.6 METs
- *ACC/AHA HF staging* emphasizes the evolution and progression of the disease. Only stages C and D qualify for the traditional clinical diagnosis of HF. This classification is intended to complement but not to replace the NYHA functional classification.
  - Stage A: Patients who are at high risk for developing HF but have no structural disorder of the heart
  - Stage B: Patients with structural disorders of the heart who have never had symptoms of HF
  - Stage C: Patients with past or current symptoms of HF associated with underlying structural heart disease.

Heart Failure with Reduced Ejection Fraction **45**

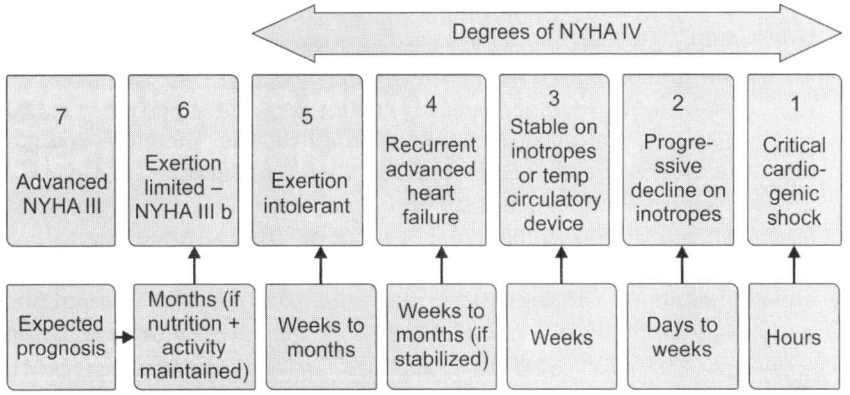

Fig. 5.1: The classification of stage D heart failure; the upright pointing arrows define the expected prognosis if the patient in respective profile or status.

INTERMACS, Patient profile/status (Interagency Registry for mechanically assisted circulatory support)

- Stage D: Patients with end-stage disease who require specialized treatment strategies such as mechanical circulatory support, continuous intravenous (IV) inotrope infusions, cardiac transplantation, or hospice care.

The Interagency Registry for Mechanically Assisted Circulatory Support (INTERMACS) has further classified stage D or end stage HF. Interagency Registry for Mechanically Assisted Circulatory Support is a national registry for patients with the Food and Drug Administration (FDA)-approved mechanical circulatory support devices that treat advanced HF (Fig. 5.1). This registry was devised as a joint effort of the National Heart, Lung and Blood Institute, the Centers for Medicare and Medicaid Services and the FDA, in conjunction with the University of Alabama at Birmingham and the United Network for Organ Sharing.

Biomarkers

Biomarkers aid in the diagnosis of HF, provide an estimate of prognosis and help in the identification of apparently healthy people who are at excessive risk for this condition. The available biomarkers reflect pathobiological processes operative in systolic HF, help to identify the specific ones involved in individual patients and aid in guiding management plans.
- *Biomarkers of myocardial stretch:* Atrial natriuretic peptide (ANP) was the first NP elaborated by stretched cardiac tissue to be identified and studied in patients with HF; however, it was soon replaced due to its instability and other analytic problems. B-type Natriuretic Peptide (BNP) and its pro hormone fragment, N-terminal pro BNP (NT-proBNP), are widely used markers in the care of patients with known or suspected HFrEF. These are peptides derived largely from the ventricles.

  Low plasma BNP or NT-proBNP concentration has a high negative predictive value for cardiac dysfunction in patients presenting to the emergency room with dyspnea, and it may therefore be used to exclude

HF as a cause of dyspnea with a relatively high degree of certainty. However, the positive predictive value for these tests in a low-prevalence and asymptomatic population for the purpose of detecting cardiac dysfunction varies among studies, and the possibility of false-positive results has significant cost-effectiveness implications. Therefore, routine determination of plasma BNP or NT-proBNP concentration as part of a screening evaluation for structural heart disease in asymptomatic patients is not yet recommended. Fortunately, a robust, adequately sized multicenter trial of a single-target NP level and the use of guideline-approved therapies in both treatment arms of prespecified subgroups is now underway [GUIDE-IT (Guiding Evidence Based Therapy Using Biomarker Intensified Treatment)] to address these concerns

- *Biomarkers of myocyte injury:* The two cardiac-specific troponins (cTnI and cTnT) have become the most accurate and widely used markers of myocardial necrosis in patients with ACS. However, it has been reported that cTnI is also present in the serum of patients with severe HF without ischemia, and it was then observed that levels of cTnI and cTnT were predictive of adverse clinical outcomes in these patients. This observation has been confirmed, particularly as progressively more sensitive assays for cTn have become available. The release of troponin from the heart in HF has been considered to be due to myocyte injury, apparently irrespective of the mechanism involved, that is, ischemia, necrosis, apoptosis or autophagy

- *Biomarkers of matrix remodeling:* Serum peptides derived from collagen metabolism reflect both the synthesis and degradation of collagen and thus constitute a "window" on the extracellular matrix. The ratio of procollagen type I amino-terminal propeptide (a marker of collagen synthesis) to collagen type I cross-linked carboxy-terminal telopeptide (a marker of collagen breakdown) is a useful serum marker of collagen accumulation.
  Aldosterone is a stimulant of collagen synthesis and enhances cardiac fibrosis in HFrEF. The administration of the aldosterone receptor antagonist in patients with chronic HFrEF reduces elevated levels of markers of collagen synthesis and is associated with clinical benefit

- *Biomarkers of inflammation:* Elevation of an inflammatory biomarker as C-reactive protein (CRP) and proinflammatory cytokines, such as tumor necrosis factor alpha and interleukin-6 have also been reported to have been elevated in HF. In elderly subjects without HF, abnormal elevations in three inflammatory markers (i.e. CRP, tumor necrosis factor alpha and interleukin-6) were reported to have been associated with a fourfold increase in the development of HF

- *Biomarkers of renal dysfunction:* In addition to serum creatinine, neutrophil gelatinase-associated lipocalin is a polypeptide marker of renal injury and is elevated in patients with acutely decompensated (AD) HF and renal failure, that is, with the cardiorenal syndrome.
  Kidney injury molecule-1 is a glycoprotein in proximal renal tubule and its presence in patients with HF as well as its correlation with NT-proBNP suggests that renal involvement occurs in many patients with severe HF.

- *Multimarker strategies:* In a study on ambulatory patients with chronic HF, a group of seven biomarkers, each reflecting a different pathophysiologic pathway of HFrEF could be combined into a multimarker score that would predict the risk for an adverse outcome, defined as death, cardiac transplantation, or placement of a ventricular-assisted device. These biomarkers were BNP (a marker of neurohormonal activation), soluble fat-mobilizing substance-like tyrosine kinase receptor (a marker of vascular remodeling), hs-CRP (a marker of inflammation), ST2 (a marker of myocyte stretch/injury), cTnI (a marker of myocyte injury), uric acid (a marker of oxidative stress) and creatinine (a marker of renal function). The combined multimarker integers score provided an excellent assessment of event-free survival.

Evaluation of Ventricular Dysfunction

Patients undergoing evaluation for ventricular dysfunction and HF fall into three general groups: (i) patients at risk of developing HF, (ii) patients suspected of having HF based. on signs and symptoms or incidental evidence of abnormal cardiac structure or function, and (iii) patients with established symptomatic HF.

- *Patients at risk for HFrEF:* Patients identified to be at risk for HF require aggressive management of modifiable risk factors as outlined in Prevention section. Patients with risk factors may have undetected abnormalities of cardiac structure or function. In addition to risk factor reduction, these patients require careful assessment for the presence of symptoms of HF and, depending on their underlying risk, may warrant noninvasive evaluation of cardiac structure and function. The noninvasive evaluation of cardiac structure and function by echocardiography is recommended for the following conditions:
    - Coronary artery disease (CAD) [e.g. after myocardial infarction (MI) or revascularization]
    - Valvular heart disease
    - Family history of cardiomyopathy in a first degree relative
    - Atrial fibrillation or flutter
    - Electrocardiographic (ECG) evidence of LV hypertrophy, left bundle branch block (LBBB) or pathological Q waves
    - Complex ventricular arrhythmias
    - Cardiomegaly

    The routine determination of plasma BNP or NT-proBNP concentration as part of a screening evaluation for structural heart disease in asymptomatic patients is not yet recommended. However, its assessment is recommended in patients suspected of having HF, especially when the diagnosis is not certain.

- *Patients suspected of having HFrEF:* The evaluation of patients suspected of having HF focuses on interpretation of signs and symptoms that have led to the consideration of this diagnosis. A careful history and physical examination, combined with an evaluation of cardiac structure and function, should be undertaken to determine the cause of symptoms and to evaluate the degree of underlying cardiac pathology.

- *Causes*: There are many causes of myocardial injury involving the above-mentioned mechanisms, which can lead to systolic dysfunction. Approximately two-thirds of these patients will have ischemic cardiomyopathy as a result of CAD. The etiology in the remaining one-third of nonischemic cardiomyopathy patients can be due to multiple etiologies (Table 5.1).
- *Clinical presentation*: The signs and symptoms in a patient being evaluated for suspected HFrEF result from venous congestion and/or low forward output (Table 5.2). The physical examination should focus on the detection and etiology of structural heart disease, current volume status and the severity of HF, as a guide to initiating therapy and a baseline to gauge the effect of that therapy.

- *Patients with established symptomatic HF*: Once the suspected diagnosis is established on clinical grounds and clinical severity of HF is assessed by history and physical examination, initial evaluation should include assessment of cardiac structure and function, determination of the etiology of HF with particular attention to reversible causes, an evaluation of CAD and myocardial ischemia, an evaluation of the risk of life threatening arrhythmias, the identifications of any exacerbating or triggering factors and of any comorbidities that can influence therapy (e.g. sleep disorders, syncope related to cerebral hypoperfusion or embolic events) (Fig. 5.2). Finally, barriers to adherence to treatment should be identified.

Table 5.1: Causes of systolic dysfunction

- Coronary artery disease
- Hypertension
- Myocarditis
  - Infection
  - Autoimmune
- Toxin induced
  - Alcohol
  - Cocaine
  - Amphetamines
  - Chemotherapy (e.g. anthracyclines)
- Postpartum (can occur 1 month before to 5 months after delivery)
- Tachycardia-induced
  - Ectopic atrial tachycardia
  - Permanent junctional reciprocating tachycardia using an accessory pathway
  - Atrial fibrillation with a rapid ventricular response
  - Incessant idiopathic ventricular tachycardias
  - Premature ventricular beats (20–30% of all beats or >10,000/24 hours)
- Noncompaction
  Takotsubo (i.e. stress induced) cardiomyopathy
- Genetic
  - Cardiac specific: (Arrhythmogenic right ventricular dysplasia)
  - Generalized myopathies: (Duchenne or Becker muscular dystrophy).
- Diabetes mellitus
- Idiopathic

Table 5.2: Symptoms and signs to evaluate in patients suspected of systolic dysfunction

Symptoms	• Dyspnea at rest or on exertion • Reduction in exercise capacity • Paroxysmal nocturnal dyspnea or nocturnal cough • Edema • Ascites or scrotal edema
Less specific presentations	• Early satiety, nausea and vomiting, abdominal discomfort • Wheezing or cough • Unexplained fatigue • Confusion/delirium • Depression/weakness (especially in the elderly)
Elevated cardiac-filling pressures and fluid overload	• Elevated jugular venous pressure • S3 gallop • Rales • Hepatojugular reflux • Ascites • Edema
Cardiac enlargement	• Laterally displaced or prominent apical impulse • Murmurs suggesting valvular dysfunction
Reduced cardiac output	• Narrow pulse pressure • Cool extremities • Tachycardia with pulsus alternans
Arrhythmia	• Irregular pulse suggestive of atrial fibrillation or frequent ectopy
Murmurs	• Those of aortic stenosis or mitral regurgitation may provide clues to the etiology of left ventricular dysfunction • Murmurs of tricuspid regurgitation and mitral regurgitation vary depending on the degree of pulmonary or systemic pressure, respectively, volume overload and ventricular dilatation.
Functional assessment	• New York Heart Association functional classification • 6-minute walk test distance.

Source: Reprinted with permission from Lindenfeld J, Albert NM, Boehmer JP, Collins SP, Ezekowitz JA, Givertz MM, et al. Executive Summary: HFSA 2010 comprehensive heart failure practice guideline. J Card Fail. 2010;16:475-539, Elsevier.

The evaluation of patients with an established diagnosis of HF is undertaken to identify the etiology, assess nature of symptom and its severity and establish a prognosis. Follow-up of patients with HF or cardiac dysfunction involves continuing reassessment of symptoms, functional capacity, prognosis and therapeutic effectiveness. In patients with established HFrEF, the current functional status and the rate of decline in their activity level should be assessed periodically. The classification of HF helps in directing therapy and assessing prognosis (Fig. 5.3).

Four Phenotypes of HFrEF

- *Asymptomatic left ventricular dysfunction (ALVD)*

Left ventricular remodeling and reduced EF should be distinguished from the syndrome of clinical HF. When LVEF is reduced to <40%, but there are no

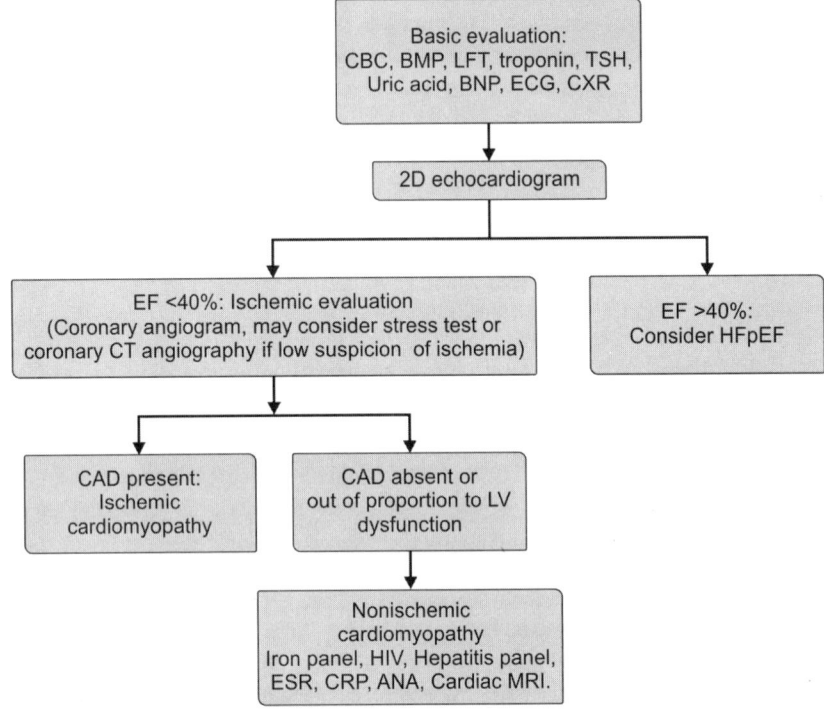

Fig. 5.2: Initial diagnostic evaluation of new onset heart failure.

CBC, complete blood count; BMP, basic metabolic profile; LFT, liver function tests; TSH, thyroid stimulating hormone; BNP, brain naturetic peptide; ECG, electrocardiogram; CXR, chest X-ray; EF, ejection fraction; CT, computed tomography; HFpEF, heart failure with preserved ejection fraction; CAD, coronary artery disease; LV, left ventricle; HIV, human immunodeficiency virus; ESR, erythrocyte sedimentation rate; CRP, C-reactive peptide; ANA, antinuclear antibody; MRI, magnetic resonance imaging

signs and symptoms of HF, the condition frequently is referred to as ALVD. It is important to distinguish between ALVD and patients categorized as NYHA Class I HF. Although patients with NYHA Class I HF do not currently have HF symptoms, they may have ALVD currently, or they may have clinical systolic HF with symptoms in the past. In contrast, patients with ALVD have no past history of HF symptoms. It is now well recognized that there may be a latency period when the LVEF is reduced before the development of symptomatic HF. The recent realization that therapies aimed at symptomatic HF may improve outcomes in patients with ALVD has increased the importance of recognizing and treating patients with this condition.

Patients with ALVD have approximately half the mortality rate (5% annual) of those with overt symptoms of HF, but their risk of death is 5–8 times higher than a normal age-matched population. In the Study of Left Ventricular Dysfunction (SOLVD) prevention study, patients with untreated ALVD developed overt HF at a 10% annual rate; with a further 8% annual risk of

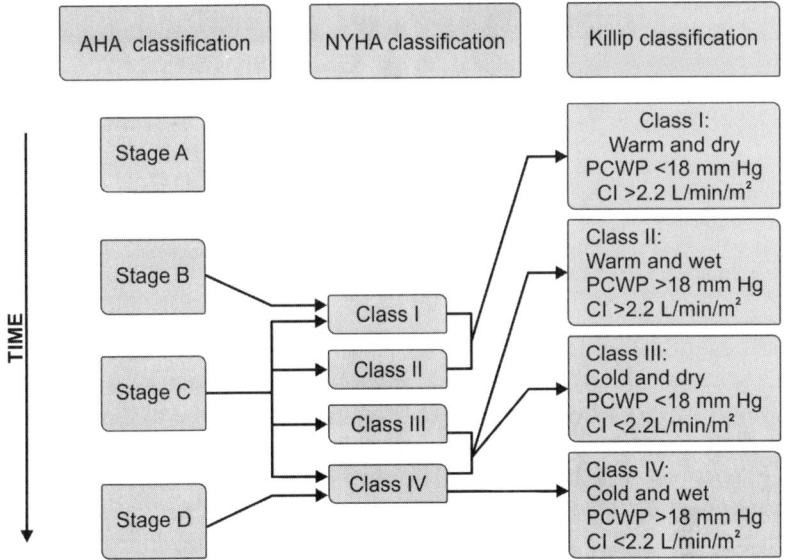

Fig. 5.3: Relationship of functional clinical status (based on AHA, NYHA and Killip classifications) at different stages of systolic heart failure and time.

AHA, American Heart Association; NYHA, New York Heart Association; PCWP, pulmonary capillary wedge pressure; CI, cardiac index.

death or hospitalization for HF. These data indicate that patients with ALVD are at high risk for developing symptomatic HF.

Studies suggest that relatives of those with idiopathic dilated cardiomyopathy often have asymptomatic LV dilatation and may be at increased risk for developing HF. In addition, those exposed to toxins through alcohol overuse, ionizing radiation or chemotherapy with anthracyclines may develop ALVD, which may progress to HF in the absence of intervention.

- *ADHF*

In patients with known cardiomyopathy presenting with ADHF, it is important to identify the potential triggers of acute exacerbation (Table 5.3).

Evaluation begins with major signs and symptoms. When the diagnosis is uncertain, determination of plasma BNP or NT-proBNP concentration is recommended in patients being evaluated for dyspnea who have signs and symptoms compatible with HF. Further evaluation is almost similar to what is mention of new onset or suspected HF; however, management in this group needs to be initiated as soon as possible with hospitalization to improve patient symptoms, correct hemodynamic and volume status, minimize cardiac and multi-organ injury and initiate lifesaving medical therapies.

- *Low cardiac output state*

This condition can be present with or without ADHF. In addition to the basic evaluation, direct hemodynamic monitoring by right heart catheterization has been advocated in the management of hospitalized patients with this advanced HF to (i) guide therapy by permitting direct tracking of filling

> **Table 5.3: Most common triggers of acute decompensated heart failure.**
> - Valvular disease
> - Arrhythmia (atrial fibrillation)
> - Noncompliance (medications; dietary)
> - Ischemia
> - Infection
> - Hypertension
> - Substance abuse
> - Drugs: Nonsteroidal anti-inflammatory agents, calcium channel blockers, antiarrhythmics, thiazolidinediones, pregabalin, tumor necrosis factor antagonists

pressures and systemic vascular resistance until certain specific hemodynamic goals are reached and (ii) assist in understanding volume status and tissue perfusion by direct determination of the extent and type of hemodynamic abnormalities present. The evaluation study of congestive heart failure and pulmonary artery catheterization effectiveness (ESCAPE) trial demonstrated neutral results of this strategy to guide therapy; however, patients with a clear clinical need for right heart catheterization (e.g. cardiogenic shock) were excluded from ESCAPE.

Invasive monitoring may benefit patients who are hypotensive, fail to respond to diuretic therapy or have worsening renal function but unknown filling pressures and cardiac output. The need for invasive hemodynamics often becomes apparent as treatment progresses.

- *Slowly progressive fluid accumulation or chronic HF*

Slowly progressive or chronic HF is the most common phenotype of established HF. These are the patients with systolic dysfunction who get frequently hospitalized with increased fluid accumulation. The goals of treatment in this group include (i) reduction in mortality, (ii) improvement of symptoms, and (iii) reduction in HF hospitalizations. These patients require periodic assessment of their NYHA functional status and 6 minute walk test. Once they reach end-stage HF, they need evaluation for advanced HF therapy. The evaluation can be initiated by performing a 6-minute walk test, cardiopulmonary exercise testing, and calculating prognosis with the Seattle HF model (which is an online comprehensive risk prediction tool for assessing the survival probability in a given individual and is available on the web at http://dept.washington.edu/shfm/index.php).

Serial Assessment of LV Function

The repeat determination of LVEF is usually unnecessary in patients with previously documented LV dilatation and low LVEF who manifest worsening signs or symptoms of HF, unless the information is needed to justify a change in patient management (such as device implantation or advanced HF therapy).

In the absence of deteriorating clinical presentation, repeat measurements of ventricular volume and LVEF should be considered in the following limited circumstances:

- When a prophylactic implantable cardioverter defibrillator (ICD) or cardiac resynchronization therapy device and defibrillator (CRT-D) placement is being considered in order to determine that LVEF criteria for device placement are still met after guideline-directed medical therapy
- When a patient shows substantial clinical improvement (e.g. in response to β-blocker treatment or following pregnancy in a patient with peripartum cardiomyopathy). Such change may denote improved prognosis, although it does not in itself mandate alteration or discontinuation of specific treatments
- In an alcohol or other cardiotoxic substance abuser after having discontinued the abused substance
- In a patient receiving cardiotoxic chemotherapy for surveillance.

Management

The management of HFrEF according to different HF stages has been well documented.

- *Management of stage A:* Epidemiologic, clinical and basic research have identified a number of antecedent conditions that predispose individuals to HFrEF and its predecessors, LV remodeling and dysfunction. Many of these traditional risk factors can be modified resulting in treating HFrEF with less difficulty and cost; this has focused attention on preventive strategies for HF.
- *Management of stage B or ALVD:* The management of patients with stage B HF or ALVD focuses on cardiovascular risk factors (hypertension, CAD, diabetes, obesity and metabolic syndrome) and on preventing, controlling or reducing progressive ventricular remodeling.

    Administration of angiotensin converting enzyme (ACE) inhibitors or angiotensin receptor blocker (ARBs) (if ACE-inhibitor intolerant) reduced the tendency to progressive LV enlargement in patients with ALVD, regardless of symptoms in the SOLVD, Candesartan in Heart Failure Assessment of Reduction in Mortality and Morbidity (CHARM-Alternative) and the Valsartan Heart Failure Trial (Val-HeFT). This beneficial effect on LV remodeling, in combination with prevention of MI, most likely explains the mechanism of reduction of both cardiovascular mortality and progression to HF.

    A strong rationale exists for the use of β-blocker therapy in the management of patients with ALVD and stage B HF from ischemic heart disease, based on the benefits seen in patients with cardiac dysfunction and no overt HF after acute MI. These benefits came from Carvedilol Post-Infarct Survival Control in Left Ventricular Dysfunction (CAPRICORN) study showing all cause mortality and HF hospitalization benefit and Reversal of Ventricular Remodeling with Toprol-XL (REVERT) trial showing attenuation of LV remodeling in patients with ALVD. Also, in patients with asymptomatic LV dysfunction without ischemia, β-blocker therapy is reasonable to use based on guidelines available.

No data is available to support benefit of aldosterone antagonists in ALVD patients
- *Management of stage C:* Once the patient starts having symptoms with LV dysfunction, in addition to pharmacotherapy, significant nonpharmacological management and health care maintenance is needed.
  - *Nonpharmacological management:* It is recommended that patients with HF should receive specific education to facilitate HF self-care. Patients need to understand how to monitor their symptoms and weight fluctuations, restrict their sodium intake, take their medications as prescribed and stay physically active. Education regarding these recommendations is necessary, albeit not always sufficient, to significantly improve outcomes. Also, social support is thought to buffer stress and promote treatment adherence and a healthy lifestyle. Most studies examining the relationship between social support and hospitalization in adults with HF have found that a lack of social support is associated with higher hospitalization rates and mortality risk. Continuous positive airway pressure can be beneficial to increase LVEF and improve functional status in patients with HF and sleep apnea.
  - *Pharmacological management:* Angiotensin converting enzyme inhibitors (or ARBs) and β-blockers are the mainstay of pharmacological therapy for stage C HF (Fig. 5.4). Multiple trials on the HFrEF population

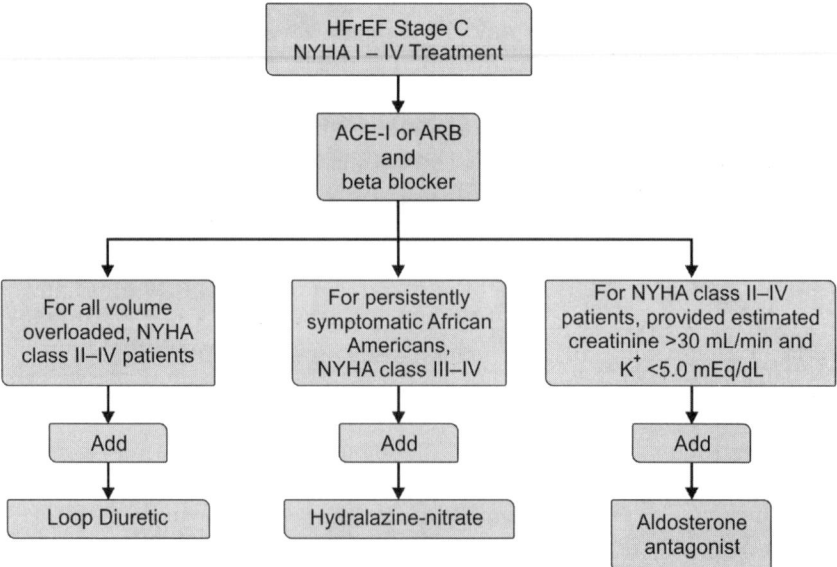

Fig. 5.4: Medical therapy for stage C heart failure.

ACEI, angiotensin-converting enzyme inhibitor; ARB, angiotensin-receptor blocker; HFrEF, heart failure with reduced ejection fraction; NYHA, New York Heart Association.

Source: Reprinted with permission from Yancy CW, Jessup M, Bozkurt B, Butler J, Donald E, Casey DE, et al. 2013 ACCF/AHA Guideline for the management of heart failure: Executive summary: a report of the American College of Cardiology Foundation/American Heart Association Task Force on practice guidelines. J Am Coll Cardiol. 2013;62(16):1495-539, Elsevier.

have been conducted over the years and found the maximum target doses of these medications that can affect remodeling of the heart. The initial and target doses based on clinical trials and current guidelines are shown in Table 5.4.

- *Angiotensin-converting enzyme inhibitors and ARBs*: There is compelling evidence that ACE inhibitors should be used to inhibit the renin–angiotensin–aldosterone system (RAAS) in all HF patients with reduced LVEF, whether or not they are symptomatic. In various trials (e.g. SOLVD, CONSENSUS, SAVE, TRACE, AIRE), ACE inhibitors were consistently associated with a mortality reduction of about 20–25% at 1–5 years. With initiation of ACE inhibitors or ARBs, an increase up to 30% in creatinine is acceptable and should not lead to discontinuation of therapy. Angiotensin receptor blockers are recommended for routine administration to symptomatic and asymptomatic patients with an LVEF ≤40% who are intolerant to ACE inhibitors for reasons other than hyperkalemia or renal insufficiency including angioedema.
- *Betablockers*: In addition to inhibitors of RAAS, β-blocker therapy is recommended in all patients (asymptomatic or symptomatic) with LVEF <40%. It is also recommended for patients with a recent decompensation of HF after optimization of volume status and successful discontinuation of IV diuretics and vasoactive agents, including inotropic support. Beta-blocker therapy should be continued in most patients experiencing a symptomatic exacerbation of HF during chronic maintenance treatment, unless they develop cardiogenic shock, refractory volume overload, or symptomatic bradycardia when a temporary dose reduction should be considered. Use of one of the three β-blockers (i.e. bisoprolol, carvedilol and sustained-release metoprolol succinate) is proven to reduce mortality. In studies, all cause and cardiovascular mortality was consistently reduced by 25–48%.
- *Diuretics*: Despite the lack of randomized studies to guide optimal approach to diuretic therapy, diuretics are the mainstay of medical therapy for volume management in ADHF and chronic HF. Diuretic therapy is recommended to restore and maintain normal volume status in patients with clinical evidence of fluid overload, generally manifested by congestive symptoms (orthopnea, edema and shortness of breath), or signs of elevated filling pressures. Loop diuretics like furosemide rather than thiazide-type diuretics are typically necessary to restore normal volume status in patients with HF. Torsemide or bumetanide should be considered in patients with significant right-sided HF and abdominal venous congestion, where the absorption of furosemide is frequently unpredictable. The conversion from furosemide to torsemide to bumetanide is 40:20:1
- *Aldosterone antagonists*: Aldosterone receptor antagonists (or mineralocorticoid receptor antagonists) are recommended in

Table 5.4: Pharmacological treatment of heart failure with reduced ejection fraction.

Drug	Initial daily dose	Max daily dose	Mean dose achieved in clinical trials
• Angiotensin converting enzyme inhibitors			
Captopril	6.25 mg tid	50 mg tid	122.7 mg/day
Enalapril	2.5 mg bid	10-20 mg bid	16.6 mg/day
Fosinopril	5-10 mg qd	40 mg qd	
Lisinopril	2.5-5 mg qd	20-40 mg qd	35 mg/day
Perindopril	2 mg qd	8-16 mg qd	
Quinapril	5 mg bid	20 mg bid	
Ramipril	1.25-2.5 mg qd	10 mg qd	
Trandolapril	1 mg qd	4 mg qd	
• Angiotensin receptor blocker			
Candesartan	4-8 mg qd	32 mg qd	24 mg/day
Losartan	25-50 mg qd	50-150 mg qd	129 mg/day
Valsartan	20-40 mg bid	160 mg bid	254 mg/day
• Aldosterone antagonists			
Spironolactone	12.5-25.0 mg qd	25 mg qd or bid	26 mg/day
Eplerenone	25 mg qd	50 mg qd	42.6 mg/day
• Beta-blockers			
Bisoprolol	1.25 mg qd	10 mg qd	8.6 mg/day
Carvedilol	3.125 mg bid	50 mg twice	37 mg/day
Carvedilol controlled release	10 mg qd	80 mg qd	
Metoprolol succinate extended release	12.5-25 mg qd	200 mg once	159 mg/day
• Hydralazine/isosorbide dinitrate Fixed dose combination	Hydralazine 25-50 mg + isosorbide dinitrate 20-30 mg tid or qid 37.5 mg hydralazine/20 mg isosorbide dinitrate tid	Hydralazine 300 mg + isorbide dinitrate 120 mg daily in divided doses Hydralazine: 300 mg in divided doses and isosorbide dinitrate: 120 mg in divided doses	175 mg hydralazine + 90 mg isosorbide dinitrate daily
• Digoxin	0.125 mg qd	Dose for digoxin level of 0.5-1.2.	

ACE, angiotensin-converting enzyme; ARB, angiotensin receptor blocker: CR, controlled release.
Source: Reprinted with permission from Yancy CW, Jessup M, Bozkurt B, Butler J, Donald E, Casey DE, et al. 2013 ACCF/AHA Guideline for the management of heart failure: Executive summary: a report of the American College of Cardiology Foundation/American Heart Association Task Force on practice guidelines. J Am Coll Cardiol. 2013;62(16):1495-539, Elsevier.

patients with NYHA class II–IV HF and with a LVEF of 35% or less, unless contraindicated, to reduce morbidity and mortality. Patients with NYHA class II HF should have a history of prior cardiovascular hospitalization or elevated plasma natriuretic peptide levels to be considered for aldosterone receptor antagonists. Creatinine should be $\leq$2.5 mg/dL in men or $\leq$2.0 mg/dL in women (or estimated GFR >30 mL/min/1.73 m^2), and potassium should be less than 5.0 mEq/L. Careful monitoring of potassium, renal function and diuretic dosing should be performed at initiation and closely followed thereafter to minimize risk of hyperkalemia and renal insufficiency. The landmark Randomized Aldactone Evaluation Study (RALES) trial showed a 30% reduction in all-cause mortality as well as a reduced risk of sudden cardiac death and HF hospitalizations with the use of spironolactone in patients with chronic HFrEF and LVEF <35%

- *Hydralazine/Nitrates*: The combination of hydralazine and isosorbide dinitrate is recommended to reduce morbidity and mortality for patients self-described as African Americans with NYHA class III–IV HFrEF receiving optimal therapy with ACE inhibitors and β-blockers, unless contraindicated. A-HEFT trial demonstrated a 43% decrease in mortality and 33% decrease in HF hospitalization in this group of patients. The combination of hydralazine and oral nitrates may also be considered in patients who do not tolerate ACE inhibitor or ARB therapy
- *Digoxin*: Digoxin is a cardiac glycoside, which can be beneficial in patients with HFrEF, unless contraindicated, to decrease hospitalizations for HF with no reduction in mortality. The best outcomes were seen in patients with a digoxin level of 0.5–1 ng/mL. However, due to the high incidence of digoxin toxicity and cardiac arrhythmias due to this drug, it should be used with caution and frequent electrolyte monitoring is recommended
- *Intravenous vasodilator therapy*: In the absence of symptomatic hypotension, IV nitroglycerin, nitroprusside or nesiritide may be considered as an addition to diuretic therapy for the rapid improvement of congestive symptoms in patients admitted with ADHF. The vasodilator in the management of acute heart failure (VMAC) study was a multicenter, randomized, double-blinded controlled trial of nesiritide, nitroglycerin and standard therapy in 489 patients hospitalized for worsening HF. Trial results showed that the combination of nesiritide plus standard therapy significantly decreased pulmonary capillary wedge pressure (PCWP) ($p < 0.001$) and dyspnea score ($p = 0.03$) at 3 hours compared with standard therapy alone. Nesiritide did not improve dyspnea compared to nitroglycerin, but did lower the PCWP more than nitroglycerin ($p = 0.03$). However, the nitroglycerin doses used in VMAC were relatively small and may account for the observed differences in PCWP.

- *Inotropic therapy*: Continuous inotropic therapy should be limited to stage D HF with NYHA class III–IV. It can also be considered rarely in ADHF refractory to diuretic and vasodilator therapy. These patients have evidence of end organ hypoperfusion. Right heart catheterization is required to aid therapy since it is initiated in patients with a cardiac index <2 L/min/m^2. Two home-based inotropes are used in the US, including the nonselective β-agonist dobutamine and the phosphodiesterase inhibitor, milrinone. Other inotropes like epinephrine or isoproterenol can also be used while an inpatient and in cardiogenic shock. The common adverse effects include hypotension, atrial and ventricular arrhythmias, and an acceleration in the decline of LV function. Once patients get to this stage, they may be evaluated for advanced HF therapies in the form of mechanical circulatory support or cardiac transplantation.
- *Device Therapy:* The benefits of device therapy in HFrEF have been well documented. There are two types of devices used in cardiomyopathy patients and it is important to understand the implant time frame and indications of these therapies.
    - *Implantable cardioverter defibrillator*: Patients with reduced LVEF are at increased risk for ventricular tachyarrhythmias leading to sudden cardiac death. Sudden death in HFrEF has been substantially decreased by aggressive guideline directed medical therapy that alters disease progression and also protects against arrhythmias. Nonetheless, patients with HFrEF remain at increased risk for sudden cardiac death due to ventricular tachyarrhythmias. The MADIT-1 and MADIT-2 trials have demonstrated survival benefit of this device in ischemic cardiomyopathy patients with LVEF ≤30%. The SCD-HEFT trial has shown similar benefit in patients with LVEF ≤ 35%, of both ischemic and nonischemic etiologies (Fig. 5.5). The survival benefit is about 1–1.5% per year based on these trials. Implantable cardioverter defibrillator is recommended in all cardiomyopathy patients for secondary prevention (e.g. after aborted sudden cardiac death due to ventricular tachyarrhythmias)
    - *Cardiac resynchronization therapy*: Ventricular dyssynchrony is present in one-third of cardiomyopathy patients and is associated with decreased cardiac work efficiency. It is usually present in patients with a QRS duration >120 ms. Cardiac resynchronization therapy is designed to resynchronize LV contraction and improve cardiac function. The device requires the placement of right atrial, right ventricular and LV (placed epicardially in the coronary sinus) leads. The device can be placed with or without ICD therapy through the right ventricular lead. Several randomized clinical trials (i.e. COMPANION, CARE-HF and MADIT-CRT) have shown significant improvement in survival, HF hospitalization and symptoms in NYHA II to ambulatory IV patients with LVEF ≤35%, when compared with guideline-directed medical therapy (Fig. 5.6).

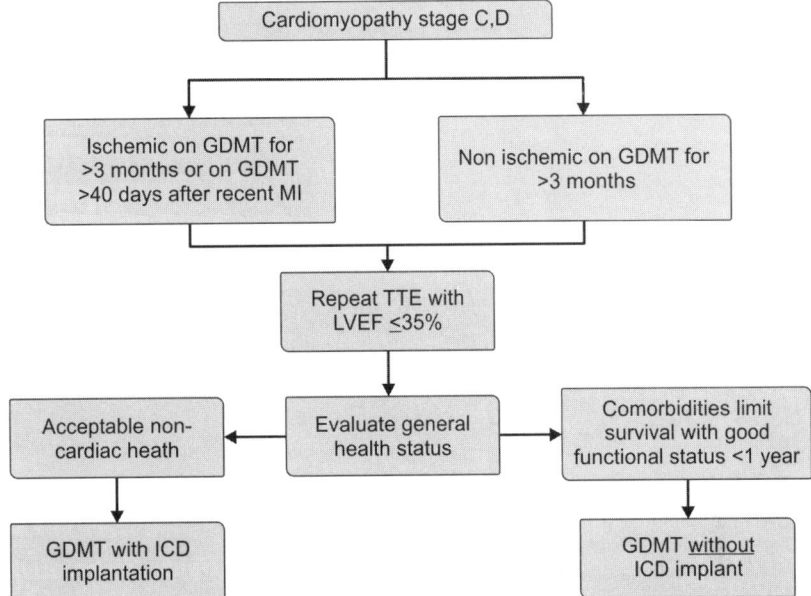

Fig. 5.5: Outline for consideration of ICD therapy as primary prevention (ICD can be single chamber, dual chamber or in conjunction with CRT therapy).

GDMT, guideline directed medical therapy; TTE, transthoracic echocardiography; ICD, internal cardioverter defibrillator; LVEF, left ventricular ejection fraction; MI, myocardial infarction; CRT, cardiac resynchronization therapy.

Source: Reprinted with permission from Russo AM, Stainback RF, Bailey SR, Epstein AE, Heidenreich PA, Jessup M, et al. ACCF/HRS/AHA/ASE/HFSA/SCAI/SCCT/SCMR 2013 appropriate use criteria for implantable cardioverter-defibrillators and cardiac resynchronization therapy. J Am Coll Cardiol. 2013;61:1318-68, Elsevier.

- *Management of stage D HF:* A subset of patients with chronic HF will continue to progress and develop persistently severe symptoms despite maximum guideline-directed medical therapy. Various terminologies have been used to describe this group of patients who are classified with ACC/AHA stage D HF, including "advanced HF," "end-stage HF" and "refractory HF." Once patients develop this stage of HF, they might be eligible for specialized, advanced treatment strategies, such as mechanical circulatory support, procedures to facilitate fluid removal, continuous inotropic infusions, or cardiac transplantation or other innovative or experimental surgical procedures, or for end-of-life care, such as hospice (Fig. 5.7). Detailed management of this group is beyond the scope of this chapter.
    - *Ventricular-assist devices:* These can be considered in stage D HF patients with acute or chronic end organ hypoperfusion. These devices are meant to extract blood from the venous system and pump it into the aorta. The devices can work in pulsatile or continuous flow fashion; can support the LV or both ventricles depending on type of device used. Left ventricular assist devices are the most commonly

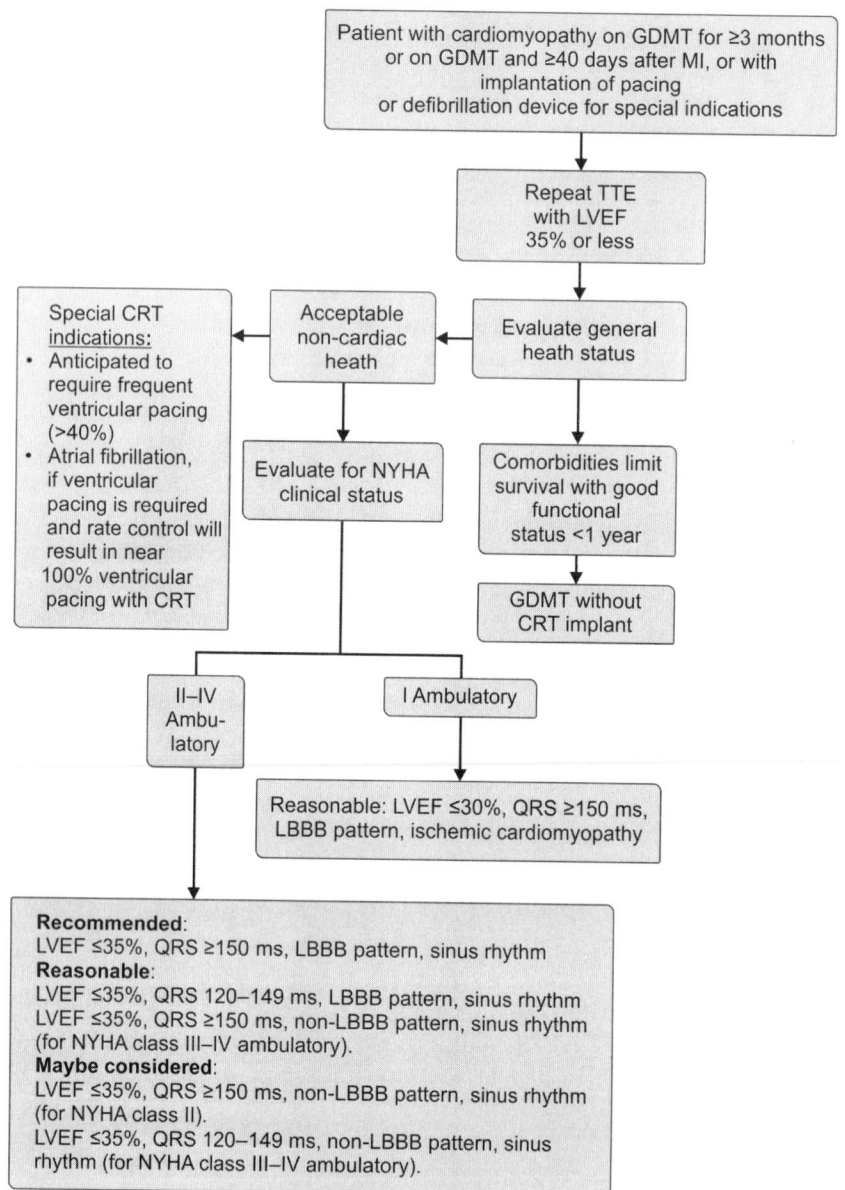

Fig. 5.6: Indications for CRT implantation

GDMT, guideline directed medical therapy; MI, myocardial infarction; TTE, transthoracic echocardiography; CRT, cardiac resynchronization therapy; NYHA, New York Heart Association; LVEF, left ventricular ejection fraction; LBBB, left bundle branch block.

Source: Reprinted with permission from Russo AM, Stainback RF, Bailey SR, Epstein AE, Heidenreich PA, Jessup M, et al. ACCF/HRS/AHA/ASE/HFSA/SCAI/SCCT/SCMR 2013 appropriate use criteria for implantable cardioverter-defibrillators and cardiac resynchronization therapy. J Am Coll Cardiol. 2013;61:1318-68, Elsevier.

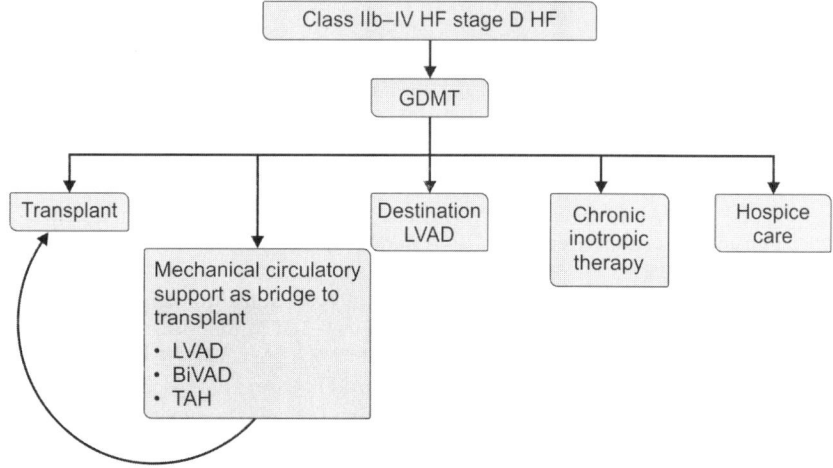

Fig. 5.7: Management of patients with stage D heart failure.

LVAD, left ventricular assist device; BiVAD, Bi ventricular assist device; TAH, Total artificial heart; GDMT, Guideline directed medical therapy.

Source: Reprinted with permission from Lindenfeld J, Albert NM, Boehmer JP, Collins SP, Ezekowitz JA, Givertz MM, et al. Executive Summary: HFSA 2010 comprehensive heart failure practice guideline. J Card Fail. 2010;16:475-539Lindenfeld, Elsevier.

used devices for LV dysfunction and stage D HF. In most situations, it can be used as a "bridge" to transplant; however, since the favorable results of REMATCH and INTrEPID trials in terms of improved survival, this device is also referred to as "destination" therapy and is being implanted worldwide in stage D HF patients.

- *Heart transplantation*: This is the definitive treatment for end-stage HF. As hemodynamic status deteriorates in a patient with stage D HF, metabolic, cellular and nutritional health is compromised. Heart transplantation early in the course is associated with excellent results, whereas later transplantation is less successful. Survival following heart transplantation is 85%, 70% and 50% at 1, 5 and 10 years, respectively.

SUGGESTED READING

1. Ammar KA, Jacobsen SJ, Mahoney DW, Ammar KA, Jacobsen SJ, Mahoney DW, et al. Prevalence and prognostic significance of heart failure stages: application of the American College of Cardiology/American Heart Association heart failure staging criteria in the community. Circulation. 2007;115:1563-70.
2. Braunwald E. Heart failure. J Am Coll Cardiol HF. 2013;1:1-20.
3. Braunwald E, Ross J Jr, Sonnenblick EH. Mechanisms of contraction of the normal and failing heart. N Engl J Med. 1967;277:794-800, 853-63, 910-20, 962-71, 1012-22.
4. Holland R, Rechel B, Stepien K, Harvey I, Brooksby I. Patients' self-assessed functional status in heart failure by New York Heart Association class: a prognostic predictor of hospitalizations, quality of life and death. J Card Fail. 2010;16:150-6.

5. Lindenfeld J, Albert NM, Boehmer JP, Collins SP, Ezekowitz JA, Givertz MM, et al. Executive Summary: HFSA 2010 comprehensive heart failure practice guideline. J Card Fail. 2010;16:475-539.
6. Owen AA, Spinale FG. Myocardial basis for heart failure: role of the cardiac interstitium. In: Mann DL (Ed). Heart Failure: A Companion to Braunwald's Heart Disease, 2nd edition. Philadelphia, PA: Elsevier; 2010. pp. 73-84.
7. Russo AM, Stainback RF, Bailey SR, Epstein AE, Heidenreich PA, Jessup M, et al. ACCF/HRS/AHA/ ASE/HFSA/SCAI/SCCT/SCMR 2013 appropriate use criteria for implantable cardioverter-defibrillators and cardiac resynchronization therapy. J Am Coll Cardiol. 2013;61:1318-68.
8. Task force for the diagnosis and treatment of acute and chronic heart failure. ESC guidelines for the diagnosis and treatment of acute and chronic heart failure 2012. Eur Heart J. 2012;33:1787-847.
9. Yancy CW, Jessup M, Bozkurt B, Butler J, Donald E, Casey DE, et al. 2013 ACCF/AHA Guideline for the management of heart failure: Executive summary: a report of the American College of Cardiology Foundation/American Heart Association Task Force on practice guidelines. J Am Coll Cardiol. 2013;62(16):1495-539.

Heart Failure with Preserved Ejection Fraction

Chapter 6

Ravinder Kumar

INTRODUCTION

Heart failure with preserved ejection fraction (HFpEF) is a clinical syndrome of heart failure (HF) with near normal or normal left ventricular (LV) ejection fraction (EF), previously referred to as diastolic HF. Its prevalence has been increasing over the last two decades and has surpassed the prevalence of patients with HF with reduced EF (HFrEF). More than half of patients with HF have preserved LVEF. Morbidity and mortality in HFpEF are comparable to that observed in patients with HFrEF, yet no effective treatment has been identified. Patients with HFpEF were previously assumed to have a better prognosis compared to those with HFrEF. However, more recent data suggest that mortality rates and rate of rehospitalization are not significantly different between the two groups. In contrast to the improvements in survival in patients with HFrEF, mortality from HFpEF has remained unchanged. Heart failure with preserved ejection fraction is a very heterogeneous disorder, which in part is the reason for the lack of success of several clinical trials.

This chapter provides an overview of the definition, epidemiology, pathophysiology, assessment and management of HFpEF.

DEFINITION OF HEART FAILURE

Heart failure is a complex clinical syndrome that results from any structural or functional impairment of ventricular filling or ejection of blood. The common clinical manifestations of HF are dyspnea, fatigue and fluid retention.

The clinical syndrome of HF may result from disorders of the pericardium, myocardium, endocardium, heart valves or great vessels or from certain metabolic abnormalities, but most patients with HF have symptoms due to impaired LV myocardial function. Heart failure may be associated with a wide spectrum of LV functional abnormalities, which may range from patients with normal LV size and preserved LVEF to those with severe dilatation and/or markedly reduced LVEF. In most patients, systolic and diastolic dysfunctions coexist irrespective of LVEF. Left ventricular ejection fraction is considered important in the classification of patients with HF because of differing patient demographics, comorbid conditions, prognosis, response to therapies and also because most clinical trials selected patients based on LVEF.

Heart failure with reduced ejection fraction is defined as the clinical diagnosis of HF and LVEF <50% and HFpEF is defined as the clinical diagnosis of HF with LVEF ≥50%. Heart failure with preserved ejection fraction is as prevalent as HFrEF. Nearly all patients with systolic dysfunction have some degree of concomitant diastolic dysfunction. The syndrome typically involves a small LV size, dyspnea, chronotropic incompetence, decreased contractile reserve and atrial enlargement.

EPIDEMIOLOGY

Heart failure with preserved ejection fraction represents about one-half of the HF burden. The incidence is increasing and has surpassed the incidence of HFrEF. The prevalence of HFpEF, relative to HFrEF, is rising at a rate of approximately 1% per year, thereby turning HFpEF into the more prevalent HF phenotype over the next decade. Yet, in contrast to HFrEF, no improvements in outcome have been noticed over last 10-20 years. The Acute Decompensated Heart Failure (ADHERE) National Registry database showed that, compared with HFrEF, patients with HFpEF are older, more likely women, and more likely to have hypertension, but less likely to have had a myocardial infarction. Other cardiovascular (CV) comorbidities are also common including obesity, coronary artery disease, diabetes mellitus, atrial fibrillation, hyperlipidemia and obstructive sleep apnea. In the Digitalis Investigation Group (DIG) study and in a community-based HF surveillance study, compared with patients with HFrEF, HFpEF patients more likely died of non-CV causes, whereas deaths due to coronary artery disease were less frequent. Although survival has improved over time for patients with HFrEF, it has not changed for patients with HFpEF.

Diastolic dysfunction may be a manifestation of systemic disease, as there is a high association of noncardiac death with HFpEF. The irbesartan in heart failure with preserved ejection fraction study (I-PRESERVE) demonstrated that diabetes mellitus, chronic obstructive pulmonary disease and renal dysfunction were independent predictors of mortality. Among patients with HFpEF who died, a large proportion of deaths were noncardiac. The most common cause of death in HFpEF was cardiac at 60% (with 26% from sudden death, 14% from HF, 5% from myocardial infarction and 9% from stroke); however, 30% died of noncardiac causes that included renal, respiratory and infectious causes.

CLINICAL FEATURES (DEMOGRAPHIC FEATURES AND COMORBID CONDITIONS)

Patients with HFpEF are generally older than 65 years, and are predominantly women (in the range of 50-70%). Hypertension is present in most patients. Obesity, diabetes mellitus and atrial fibrillation are other common comorbidities. Patients with HFpEF present with signs and symptoms that are similar to HFrEF (i.e. dyspnea on exertion, orthopnea, paroxysmal nocturnal dyspnea, leg edema and weight gain).

Acute decompensation of HF may be related to dietary or medication noncompliance, uncontrolled hypertension, ischemia or atrial arrhythmias. Patients with HFpEF are dependent on atrial contraction for filling and thus are at risk of development of HF with the onset of atrial fibrillation.

STAGES OF HEART FAILURE

The American College of Cardiology and the American Heart Association have categorized HF into four stages: stage A is defined as high risk for HF without structural heart disease or symptoms of HF; stage B is defined as structural heart disease without signs or symptoms of HF; stage C is defined as symptomatic HF; and stage D is HF refractory to treatment. This is discussed in more detail in Chapter on 5: Heart Failure with Reduced Ejection Fraction.

ASSESSMENT OF DIASTOLIC DYSFUNCTION

The assessment of diastolic function includes characterization of LV stiffness, relaxation and pressure changes and is difficult to measure. Invasive measurements of the rate of LV pressure decline, LV relaxation time constant and stiffness modulus can characterize diastolic function.

Echocardiography is useful in assessing diastolic dysfunction (Fig. 6.1). In diastole, there are four phases: isovolumic relaxation, early filling, diastasis and atrial contraction. Two of the four phases are measured from the LV filling pattern of velocities: the early (E) and late or atrial (A) contraction velocities. The E/A ratio is used as an estimate of the relaxation pattern of the ventricle. Tissue Doppler imaging can be used to measure myocardial motion, specifically the amount the mitral annulus recoils toward the base during early diastole (referred to as e'). The LV filling pressures can be estimated by the E/e' ratio. A normal E/e' is <8, and suggests normal LV relaxation and filling pressures. The presence of elevated filling pressures is supported by E/e' of >15, E/A reversal with Valsalva maneuver, systolic < diastolic pulmonary venous inflow velocity ratio, prolonged atrial reversal duration in the pulmonary venous inflow profile, left atrial enlargement and the presence of pulmonary hypertension (when due to elevated LV filling pressure, also known as World Health Organization type 2 pulmonary hypertension).

Diastolic dysfunction is categorized by Doppler echocardiography into as follows (Fig. 6.2):
- Grade I (Mild): Defined as impaired relaxation without evidence of increased filling pressures. Reversal of the normal E/A ratio on mitral inflow Doppler is present
- Grade II (Moderate): Defined as impaired relaxation associated with moderate elevation of filling pressures. A "pseudo-normal" mitral inflow Doppler pattern is seen
- Grade III (Severe): Defined as advanced reduction in compliance. The restrictive filling mitral inflow Doppler is reversible when imaging is performed during a Valsalva maneuver

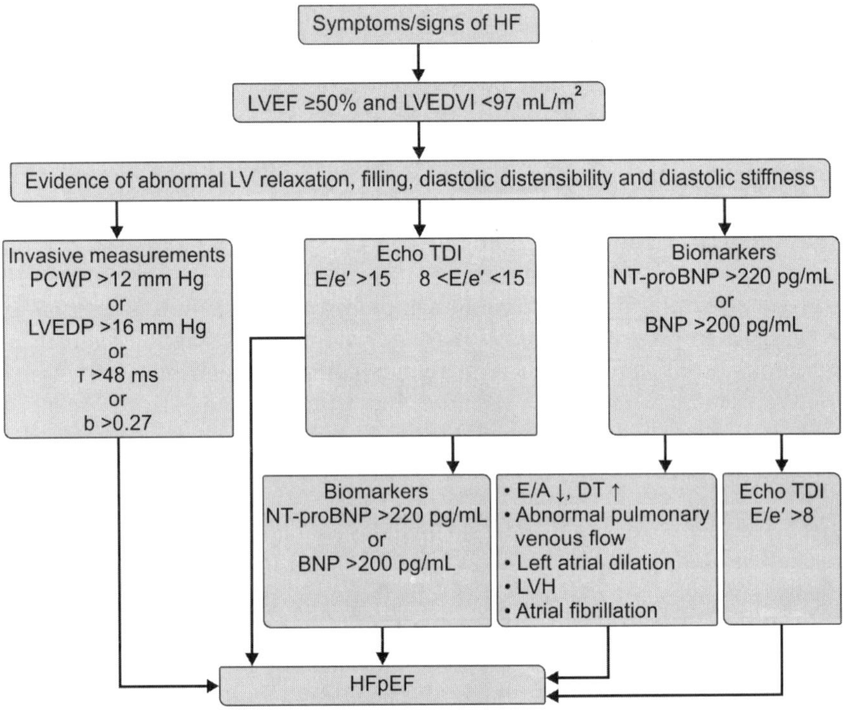

```
                    Symptoms/signs of HF
                              ↓
              LVEF ≥50% and LVEDVI <97 mL/m²
                              ↓
  Evidence of abnormal LV relaxation, filling, diastolic distensibility and diastolic stiffness
         ↓                    ↓                              ↓
  Invasive measurements    Echo TDI                      Biomarkers
  PCWP >12 mm Hg        E/e' >15   8 <E/e' <15        NT-proBNP >220 pg/mL
        or                                                    or
  LVEDP >16 mm Hg                                       BNP >200 pg/mL
        or
     τ >48 ms
        or
     b >0.27

                  Biomarkers          • E/A ↓, DT ↑         Echo TDI
              NT-proBNP >220 pg/mL    • Abnormal pulmonary   E/e' >8
                    or                  venous flow
              BNP >200 pg/mL          • Left atrial dilation
                                      • LVH
                                      • Atrial fibrillation

                              HFpEF
```

Fig. 6.1: Diagnostic algorithm for the diagnosis of HFpEF

HF, heart failure; TDI, tissue Doppler imaging; DT, deceleration time; E/A, ratio of early to late diastolic peak mitral inflow velocities; LVEF, left ventricular ejection fraction; LVEDVI, left ventricular end-diastolic volume index; LVEDP, left ventricular end-diastolic pressure; LVH, left ventricular hypertrophy; PCWP, pulmonary capillary wedge pressure; τ, time constant of isovolumic relaxation; b, left ventricular passive stiffness; BNP, brain natriuretic peptide; NT-proBNP, N-terminal proBNP.

Source: Adapted from Paulus WJ, Tschöpe C, Sanderson JE, Rusconi C, Flachskampf FA, Rademakers FE, et al. How to diagnose diastolic heart failure: a consensus statement on the diagnosis of heart failure with normal left ventricular ejection fraction by the Heart Failure and Echocardiography Associations of the European Society of Cardiology. Eur Heart J. 2007;28(20):2539-50 and reprinted *with permission* from the Oxford University Press.

- Grade IV (Severe): This is also defined as advanced reduction in compliance. However, the restrictive filling pattern is fixed and does not reverse when imaging is performed during a Valsalva maneuver.

Other imaging modalities that have been used for assessment of diastolic function are echocardiographic strain rate imaging and cardiac magnetic resonance imaging.

PATHOPHYSIOLOGY

Diastolic filling of the LV is biphasic, with rapid filling in early diastole, and late filling determined by atrial contraction, left atrial pressure and LV chamber stiffness. Diastolic dysfunction refers to the abnormal mechanical properties of the myocardium and includes abnormal LV diastolic distensibility, impaired filling and slow or delayed relaxation. In diastolic

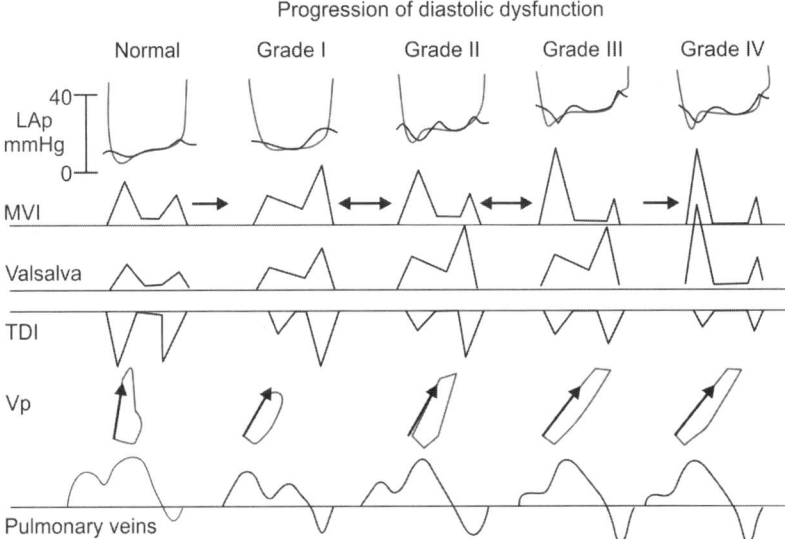

Fig. 6.2: The progression of left ventricular diastolic dysfunction can be readily assessed using a combination of Doppler echocardiographic variables. Each successive grade represents a worsening state of diastolic dysfunction

LAp, left atrial pressure; MVI, mitral valve inflow; TDI, tissue Doppler imaging; Valsalva, response of mitral valve inflow to Valsalva maneuver; Vp, mitral inflow propagation velocity.

Source: Reprinted with permission from Ommen SR, Nishimura RA. A clinical approach to the assessment of left ventricular diastolic function by Doppler echocardiography: update 2003. Heart. 2003;89:iii18-iii23, British Medical Journal Publishing Group.

dysfunction, the LV cannot accept blood at low pressures and ventricular filling is slow or incomplete unless atrial pressure rises. Therefore, there is increased dependence on filling through atrial contraction and there are higher atrial pressures to maintain filling or cardiac output. Any mechanism that interferes with actin-myosin cross-bridge detachment or with removing calcium from the cytosol can delay relaxation. Multiple factors can increase LV stiffness, including age, increased LV wall thickness relative to cavity size (as occurs with hypertension or aortic stenosis), intracellular changes in titin or microtubules, extracellular changes in collagen (e.g. an increased amount, relative increase in collagen 1 and increased degree of collagen cross-linking) and infiltration (e.g. amyloidosis). Neurohormonal and cardiac endothelial activities also modulate ventricular stiffness and relaxation.

Human and animal studies have implicated high diastolic intracellular calcium, titin isoform shift, oxidative stress, nitric oxide synthase dysfunction and myosin-binding protein C in diastolic dysfunction. Overexpression of the stiff isoform of titin has been found in endomyocardial biopsy samples of patients with HFpEF. In patients with type 1 diabetes mellitus, advanced glycation end-products and oxidative stress has been associated with LV dysfunction. Nitric oxide is known to mediate cardiac relaxation, and cardiac oxidation leading to uncoupling of cardiac nitric oxide synthase results in diastolic dysfunction. Phosphorylation of myosin-binding protein C, a protein located in the cross-bridge zones of sarcomeres, modulates myocardial contractility and loss of this regulation leads to diastolic dysfunction.

MANAGEMENT OF HFPEF

- *Treat the presenting HF syndrome* that includes relieving venous congestion and eliminating precipitating factors (e.g. hypertension, tachyarrhythmias). However, to date there are no approved therapies available for reducing mortality or hospitalization for patients with HFpEF.
  - Systolic and diastolic blood pressure should be controlled according to published clinical practice guidelines. Use of β-blocking agents, angiotensin converting enzyme (ACE) inhibitors and angiotensin receptor blockers (ARBs) for hypertension is reasonable in HFpEF. Angiotensin receptor blockers might be considered to decrease hospitalization in HFpEF.
  - Diuretics should be used for relief of symptoms due to volume overload.
  - Coronary revascularization is reasonable for patients with coronary artery disease in whom angina or demonstrable myocardial ischemia is present despite guideline-directed medical therapy.
  - Management of atrial fibrillation according to published clinical practice guidelines for HFpEF is reasonable to improve symptomatic HF.
  - Nutritional supplementation is not recommended in HFpEF.
- *Digoxin*

In a randomized, double-blind, placebo-controlled trial, the DIG showed that digoxin did not alter the primary endpoint of HF-related hospitalization or CV mortality in patients with HF and LVEF >45%.

- Angiotensin converting enzyme *inhibitors or ARBs*

Given the high prevalence of diabetes mellitus and LV hypertrophy in patients with HFpEF, there is a compelling indication for ACE inhibitors or ARBs in many patients. However, multiple trials evaluating these agents did not reveal a survival benefit when compared to placebo. In the CHARM (candesartan in heart failure: assessment of reduction in mortality and morbidity)-preserved study, it was found that among patients with HF and LVEF > 40%, candesartan (compared with placebo) had a moderate impact in preventing admissions for HF ($p = 0.014$), yet there was no difference in rates of CV death.

In the I-PRESERVE study, patients with HF and EF $\geq$ 45% had no significant difference in outcomes between irbesartan and placebo, including the composite of all-cause mortality or hospitalization for a CV cause ($p = 0.35$), the overall rate of death ($p = 0.98$), and the rate of hospitalization for CV causes ($p = 0.44$).

The PEP-CHF (perindopril in elderly people with chronic heart failure study) showed that perindopril improved functional class ($p < 0.030$) and exercise capacity ($p = 0.011$) and decreased hospitalizations for HF ($p = 0.033$).

The Hong Kong Diastolic Heart Failure Study randomized 150 patients with HFpEF (i.e. LVEF >45%) to diuretics alone, diuretics plus irbesartan or diuretics plus ramipril. The quality of life score and 6-minute walk test improved similarly, and hospitalizations were similar in all three groups. Modest improvements in Doppler systolic and diastolic indices and N-terminal pro brain natriuretic peptide (NT-proBNP) levels were seen only in the irbesartan and ramipril groups.

- *Beta-blockers*

Beta-blockers and negatively chronotropic calcium-channel blockers are often proposed for the treatment of HFpEF based on the assumption that rate lowering and prolongation of diastole results in better LV filling and output. This concept has been challenged by studies suggesting that chronotropic incompetence may be an important mechanism contributing to exercise intolerance in HFpEF.

The SENIORS (study of effects of nebivolol intervention on outcomes and rehospitalization) trial evaluated the effect of nebivolol, a β-1 selective blocker with vasodilating properties related to nitric oxide modulation, on HF morbidity and mortality. Regardless of EF, the primary composite endpoint of all cause mortality or hospital admission for CV disease was significantly reduced with nebivolol. A post hoc subgroup analysis showed no significant influence of EF on the reduction in primary events. When a threshold LVEF of 40% was used for the subgroup analysis, there was no difference in primary outcomes between the populations with LVEF ≤40% and >40%.

The SWEDIC (Swedish Doppler echocardiographic study) showed that carvedilol resulted in improvement in the E/A ratio on Doppler echocardiography, but no significant improvement occurred in other diastolic variables, such as deceleration time of early filling velocity, isovolumic relaxation time or ratio of systolic to diastolic pulmonary venous flow velocity.

- *Aldosterone receptor blocker therapy*

The treatment of preserved cardiac function heart failure with an aldosterone antagonist trial showed that spironolactone neither reduced the primary outcome of CV death, HF hospitalization, nor surviving a cardiac arrest in patients with HFpEF. However, spironolactone did reduce the risk of repeated hospitalization for HF.

The Aldo-DHF (aldosterone receptor blockade in diastolic heart failure) trial demonstrated significant improvement of echocardiographic parameters, but there was no significant improvement in exercise capacity, symptoms or quality of life in patients treated with spironolactone.

- *Novel therapeutic agents*
  - *Phosphodiesterase-5 inhibition*

    Phosphodiesterase-5 inhibitors were thought to exert beneficial effect by inhibiting the degradation of cyclic guanosine monophosphate (cGMP) and thereby improving cardiac relaxation and LV reverse remodeling. In the RELAX (phosphodiesterase-5 inhibition to improve clinical status and exercise capacity in diastolic heart failure) study, sildenafil did not significantly improve exercise capacity and clinical status in patients with HFpEF.

- *Ranolazine*

  Ranolazine is a selective inhibitor of the late sodium channel current that is activated in HF and leads to calcium overload, impaired relaxation and pro-arrhythmic after depolarization. The RALI-DHF (ranolazine for the treatment of diastolic heart failure) showed that a ranolazine infusion significantly reduced LV end diastolic pressure from 21.3 to 19.1 mm Hg and improved hemodynamic measurements such as pulmonary capillary wedge pressure; however, there was no improvement in the relaxation parameters of rate of LV pressure decline, E/e' ratio, or NT-proBNP.

- *Ivabradine*

  Ivabradine, a sinoatrial node ionic current inhibitor, reduces heart rate when elevated. Heart rate reduction improves LV filling by prolonging diastole without significant lusitropic (i.e. relaxation) or inotropic effects. In a small, short term, double-blind, randomized trial, ivabradine improved exercise capacity, increased peak oxygen consumption and reduced exercise induced increases in E/e'.

- *Alagebrium*

  Increased LV diastolic stiffness in patients with diabetes mellitus is thought to be related to myocardial deposition of advanced glycation end products. Alagebrium, an advanced glycation end products cross-link breaker, was studied in a pilot study in 23 HFpEF patients and resulted in a reduction in LV mass and an increase in e' on tissue Doppler measurement. Alagebrium is being evaluated in a multicenter trial.

- *Angiotensin receptor-neprilysin inhibitor*

  Angiotensin receptor-neprilysin inhibitor (LCZ 696) has dual actions of inhibiting the neprilysin and angiotensin receptors. Neprilysin is an enzyme responsible for degrading natriuretic peptides and its inhibition leads to increased intracellular cGMP. LCZ 696 was tested against valsartan in 301 HFpEF patients treated for 36 months in the PARAMOUNT (prospective comparison of ARNI with ARB on management of heart failure with preserved ejection fraction) trial. N-terminal pro brain natriuretic peptide was significantly reduced at 12 weeks in the LCZ 696 group compared with the valsartan group. There were no changes in echocardiographic parameters of diastolic function.

SUMMARY

Heart failure with preserved ejection fraction is a major and growing public health problem, currently representing more than half of the patients with HF. Despite improvements in understanding of the pathophysiology, no treatment has yet been shown, convincingly, to reduce morbidity and mortality in patients with HFpEF.

SUGGESTED READING

1. Berg TJ, Snorgaard O, Faber J, Torjesen PA, Hildebrandt P, Mehlsen J, et al. Serum levels of advanced glycation end products are associated with left ventricular diastolic function in patients with type 1 diabetes. Diabetes Care. 1999;22(7):1186-90.
2. Bergstrom A, Andersson B, Edner M, Nylander E, Persson H, Dahlstrom U. Effect of carvedilol on diastolic function in patients with diastolic heart failure and preserved systolic function. Results of the Swedish Doppler-echocardiographic study (SWEDIC). Eur J Heart Fail. 2004;6(4):453-61.
3. Bursi F, Weston SA, Redfield MM, Jacobsen SJ, Pakhomov S, Nkomo VT, et al. Systolic and diastolic heart failure in the community. JAMA. 2006;296(18):2209-16.
4. Cleland JG, Tendera M, Adamus J, Freemantle N, Polonski L, Taylor J, et al. The perindopril in elderly people with chronic heart failure (PEP-CHF) study. Eur Heart J. 2006;27(19):2338-45.
5. Digitalis Investigation Group. The effect of digoxin on mortality and morbidity in patients with heart failure. N Engl J Med. 1997;336(8):525-33.
6. Dupont S, Maizel J, Mentaverri R, Chillon JM, Six I, Giummelly P, et al. The onset of left ventricular diastolic dysfunction in SHR rats is not related to hypertrophy or hypertension. Am J Physiol Heart Circ Physiol. 2012;302(7):H1524-32.
7. Edelmann F, Wachter R, Schmidt AG, Kraigher-Krainer E, Colantonio C, Kamke W, et al. Effect of spironolactone on diastolic function and exercise capacity in patients with heart failure with preserved ejection fraction: the Aldo-DHF randomized controlled trial. JAMA. 2013;309(8):781-91.
8. Flashman E, Redwood C, Moolman-Smook J, Watkins H. Cardiac myosin binding protein C: its role in physiology and disease. Circ Res. 2004;94(10):1279-89.
9. Fonarow GC, Stough WG, Abraham WT, Albert NM, Gheorghiade M, Greenberg BH, et al. Characteristics, treatments, and outcomes of patients with preserved systolic function hospitalized for heart failure: a report from the OPTIMIZE-HF Registry. J Am Coll Cardiol. 2007;50(8):768-77.
10. Henkel DM, Redfield MM, Weston SA, Gerber Y, Roger VL. Death in heart failure: a community perspective. Circ Heart Fail.. 2008;1(2):91-7.
11. Kosmala W, Holland DJ, Rojek A, Wright L, Przewlocka-Kosmala M, Marwick TH. Effect of If-channel inhibition on hemodynamic status and exercise tolerance in heart failure with preserved ejection fraction: a randomized trial. J Am Coll Cardiol. 2013;62(15):1330-8.
12. Little WC, Zile MR, Kitzman DW, Hundley WG, O'Brien TX, Degroof RC. The effect of alagebrium chloride (ALT-711), a novel glucose cross-link breaker, in the treatment of elderly patients with diastolic heart failure. J Card Fail. 2005;11(3):191-5.
13. Maier LS, Layug B, Karwatowska-Prokopczuk E, Belardinelli L, Lee S, Sander J, et al. RAnoLazIne for the treatment of diastolic heart failure in patients with preserved ejection fraction: the RALI-DHF proof-of-concept study. JACC Heart Fail. 2013;1(2):115-22.
14. Massie BM, Carson PE, McMurray JJ, Komajda M, McKelvie R, Zile MR, et al. Irbesartan in patients with heart failure and preserved ejection fraction. N Engl J Med. 2008;359(23):2456-67.
15. Nishimura RA, Tajik AJ. Evaluation of diastolic filling of left ventricle in health and disease: Doppler echocardiography is the clinician's Rosetta stone. J Am Coll Cardiol. 1997;30(1):8-18.
16. Ommen SR, Nishimura RA, Appleton CP, Miller FA, Oh JK, Redfield MM, et al. Clinical utility of Doppler echocardiography and tissue Doppler imaging in the estimation of left ventricular filling pressures: a comparative simultaneous Doppler-catheterization study. Circulation. 2000;102(15):1788-94.

17. Ommen SR, Nishimura RA. A clinical approach to the assessment of left ventricular diastolic function by Doppler echocardiography: update 2003. Heart. 2003;89:iii18-iii23.
18. Owan TE, Hodge DO, Herges RM, Jacobsen SJ, Roger VL, Redfield MM. Trends in prevalence and outcome of heart failure with preserved ejection fraction. N Engl J Med. 2006;355(3):251-9.
19. Pitt B, Pfeffer MA, Assmann SF, Boineau R, Anand IS, Claggett B, et al. Spironolactone for heart failure with preserved ejection fraction. N Engl J Med. 2014;370(15):1383-92.
20. Redfield MM, Jacobsen SJ, Burnett JC Jr, Mahoney DW, Bailey KR, Rodeheffer RJ. Burden of systolic and diastolic ventricular dysfunction in the community: appreciating the scope of the heart failure epidemic. JAMA. 2003;289(2):194-202.
21. Redfield MM, Chen HH, Borlaug BA, Semigran MJ, Lee KL, Lewis G, et al. Effect of phosphodiesterase-5 inhibition on exercise capacity and clinical status in heart failure with preserved ejection fraction: a randomized clinical trial. JAMA. 2013;309(12):1268-77.
22. Silberman GA, Fan TH, Liu H, Jiao Z, Xiao HD, Lovelock JD, et al. Uncoupled cardiac nitric oxide synthase mediates diastolic dysfunction. Circulation. 2010;121(4):519-28.
23. Solomon SD, Zile M, Pieske B, Voors A, Shah A, Kraigher-Krainer E, et al. The angiotensin receptor neprilysin inhibitor LCZ696 in heart failure with preserved ejection fraction: a phase 2 double-blind randomised controlled trial. Lancet. 2012;380(9851):1387-95.
24. van Veldhuisen DJ, Cohen-Solal A, Bohm M, Anker SD, Babalis D, Roughton M, et al. Beta-blockade with nebivolol in elderly heart failure patients with impaired and preserved left ventricular ejection fraction: data from SENIORS (Study of Effects of Nebivolol Intervention on Outcomes and Rehospitalization in Seniors with Heart Failure). J Am Coll Cardiol. 2009;53(23):2150-8.
25. van Heerebeek L, Hamdani N, Falcao-Pires I, Leite-Moreira AF, Begieneman MP, Bronzwaer JG, et al. Low myocardial protein kinase G activity in heart failure with preserved ejection fraction. Circulation. 2012;126(7):830-9.
26. Yancy CW, Lopatin M, Stevenson LW, De Marco T, Fonarow GC, Committee ASA, et al. Clinical presentation, management, and in-hospital outcomes of patients admitted with acute decompensated heart failure with preserved systolic function: a report from the Acute Decompensated Heart Failure National Registry (ADHERE) Database. J Am Coll Cardiol. 2006;47(1):76-84.
27. Yancy CW, Jessup M, Bozkurt B, Butler J, Casey DE, Jr., Drazner MH, et al. 2013 ACCF/AHA guideline for the management of heart failure: a report of the American College of Cardiology Foundation/American Heart Association Task Force on Practice Guidelines. J Am Coll Cardiol. 2013;62(16):e147-239.
28. Yusuf S, Pfeffer MA, Swedberg K, Granger CB, Held P, McMurray JJ, et al. Effects of candesartan in patients with chronic heart failure and preserved left-ventricular ejection fraction: the CHARM-Preserved Trial. Lancet. 2003;362(9386):777-81.
29. Zile MR, Gaasch WH, Anand IS, Haass M, Little WC, Miller AB, et al. Mode of death in patients with heart failure and a preserved ejection fraction: results from the irbesartan in heart failure with preserved ejection fraction study (I-Preserve) trial. Circulation. 2010;121(12):1393-405.

Hypotension and Shock

Chapter 7

Jayasheel O Eshcol

INTRODUCTION

Shock is a state of inadequate oxygen delivery or consumption to meet metabolic demand, resulting in cellular hypoxia. The clinical signs of shock are altered mental status, cyanosis, cool extremities and diminished urine output (<20 mL/hour). Hypotension is commonly found in states of shock but is neither necessary nor sufficient on its own to define shock. Hypotension is defined as a systolic blood pressure (BP) <90 mm Hg or a mean arterial pressure <70 mm Hg. However, in the setting of preexisting hypertension, there may be relative hypotension resulting in hypoperfusion; therefore, a 40 mm Hg drop in systolic BP is considered hypotensive. Hypotension is a late finding of shock. It is important to recognize normotensive patients who are in shock because in the landmark SHOCK trial this population had higher mortality rate than patients who have hypotension without shock.

PHYSIOLOGY

In shock state, there is a dysfunction at multiple levels, with poor perfusion as a result of inadequate macrocirculation, dysfunction in microcirculation and ineffective metabolism at the cellular level. Even after apparent correction at the macrocirculatory level, there can be persistent signs of poor perfusion because of the perturbed microcirculation and cellular function.

- *The macrocirculation*: Tissue perfusion is determined by cardiac output and peripheral vascular resistance, and it is useful to consider the relationship of these components according to a modification of Ohm's law: BP = CO [or SV × HR] × SVR (where BP: blood pressure, CO: cardiac output, SV: stroke volume, HR: heart rate and SVR: systemic vascular resistance). Vascular resistance is modulated by the autonomic nervous system and circulating cytokines. Cardiac output is determined by intravascular volume (preload) and cardiac performance, which in turn is contingent upon afterload, contractility and HR. An alteration in each of these factors can result in poor tissue perfusion. For example, hypovolemia or a tension pneumothorax causes shock by reducing preload. There can also be simultaneous disturbance in multiple factors, such as in septic shock where there can be low SVR, low intravascular volume and depression in myocardial contractility

- *The microcirculation*: In the setting of shock, there is significant dysfunction in capillary bed blood flow. In septic and cardiogenic shock, it has been shown that there is heterogeneity in capillary blood flow with an increased proportion of capillaries with absent or reduced blood flow. This leads to a shunt physiology with inadequate oxygen delivery. This has been shown in all vital organs, including the heart, liver and brain, and is an important mechanism of organ failure
- *Intracellular dysfunction*: Because of the poor perfusion, cellular metabolism shifts to anaerobic glycolysis, which results in lactic acidosis, which, in turn, impairs cardiac contractility. Energy-dependent ion channels fail and ions shift down concentration gradients, including sodium into the cell resulting in swelling of the cell and possibly rupture. The oxidative stress resulting from imbalance of reactive oxygen species and antioxidants results in mitochondrial damage ultimately leading to organ failure.

CLASSIFICATION

Traditionally, shock has been categorized by the Hinshaw and Cox classification into obstructive, distributive, hypovolemic and cardiogenic. The first three types of shock will be described, and then cardiogenic shock will be discussed in depth.

Obstructive shock develops when there is a mechanical process impeding the vasculature, and management must be primarily focused on the relief of the obstruction. Common causes of obstructive shock include massive pulmonary embolism, pericardial tamponade and tension pneumothorax. Rarely, cases have been described with atrial myxoma, hydrothorax or hemothorax and ascites.

Distributive shock is characterized by profound vasodilation, resulting in apparent hypovolemia and inability to maintain perfusion despite increased CO (i.e. BP is low due to low SVR according to the equation: BP = CO × SVR). This is most commonly caused by the systemic inflammatory cascade found in sepsis. Distributive shock can occur from spinal cord injury, resulting in the loss of sympathetic tone and unopposed parasympathetic tone. It is also seen in anaphylaxis, where the antigen triggers immunoglobulin E-mediated release of mast cells and basophils such as histamine and prostaglandins.

Hypovolemic shock is a result of intravascular volume loss, which can be the loss of blood or plasma. This results in compensatory mechanisms to increase SVR, HR and preservation of intravascular volume. Large amounts of blood loss may be hidden in body compartments, including the peritoneum, thorax and even the thigh. Loss of plasma can be secondary to fluid losses from the gastrointestinal tract or kidneys but can also be from fluid shifting to the interstitial space as seen in pancreatitis.

Cardiogenic shock is a state of impaired cardiac performance, hemodynamically defined as a cardiac index <1.8 L/min/m^2 (without support) and a pulmonary capillary wedge pressure >18 mm Hg. The etiology can be conceptualized as myogenic, valvular or conduction/arrhythmogenic

(Table 7.1). Up to 80% of cases are due to acute myocardial infarction (MI) causing left ventricular (LV) failure, and this is the focus of this chapter.

CARDIOGENIC SHOCK—BACKGROUND, PHYSICAL EXAMINATION AND DIAGNOSTICS

Cardiogenic shock is most commonly triggered by dysfunction of the LV usually from acute ischemia, which may be reversible. Low forward output triggers the release of catecholamines, which increase contractility at the expense of increased myocardial demand and peripheral vasoconstriction (increasing afterload), which further impairs LV function. The ejection fraction is a marker of prognosis and is severely decreased in shock (e.g. in the SHOCK trial, the average ejection fraction was 30%). In addition to systolic impairment, there is nearly always diastolic dysfunction in shock.

Primary right ventricular (RV) failure in shock is infrequent, occurring 5% of cases of post-MI cardiogenic shock. It is relatively less studied as trials generally excluded patients with RV failure. In the setting of RV failure, there is usually inadequate filling of the LV and high-end diastolic pressures that may cause the septum to bow into the LV and impair left atrial emptying and systolic function. The prognosis of RV failure is similar to that of the LV, and revascularization appears to be similarly beneficial.

Table 7.1: Etiology of cardiogenic shock

Myogenic	Valvular
1. Ischemic	• Acute or acute on chronic valve disease
• Myocardial infarction	– Critical aortic stenosis
• Mechanical complications of myocardial infarction	– Endocarditis
– Papillary muscle rupture and mitral regurgitation	– Rheumatic disease
– Free wall rupture	**Conduction/arrhythmia**
– Ventricular septal defect	• Bradycardia
2. Non-ischemic	– Heart block
• Acute heart failure	– Sinus node dysfunction
– Fulminant myocarditis	• Tachycardia
– Stress cardiomyopathy	– Ventricular tachycardia and fibrillation
– Postpartum cardiomyopathy	– Atrial fibrillation with rapid ventricular response
• Acute exacerbation of chronic heart failure	
– Dilated cardiomyopathy	
– Hypertrophic obstructive cardiomyopathy	

- The *physical examination* is crucial in the recognition of cardiogenic shock. Initial findings are increased respiratory rate and HR, followed by signs of vasoconstriction, such as pale and cool extremities and diminished pulses. With progression of shock, signs of end-organ damage develop, such as altered mental status and oliguria.

  The etiology can sometimes be discovered on examination, especially if a murmur of mitral regurgitation or ventricular septal defect is recognized or pulsus paradoxus is identified suggesting cardiac tamponade.

  It is important to determine volume status and cardiac output. The jugular venous pulsation allows assessment of the right atrial pressure, and elevated jugular venous pressure along with lung crackles and edema suggest increased filling pressures. A third heart sound is a very specific finding for heart failure, usually reflecting high LV filling pressures in a dilated LV. However, it can be physiologic in pregnancy and in children. Cardiac output is more difficult to ascertain, but the presence of hypotension with narrow pulse pressure, altered mental status and pulsus alternans (beat to beat variability in the pulse that occurs in severe LV dysfunction) is suggestive of impaired cardiac output

- *Pulmonary artery catheterization* has been used since the 1970s, but the use of these catheters in cardiogenic shock is still debated. Randomized trials have failed to show benefit in various settings. However, it can be a valuable tool in guiding management, particularly when using inotropes, vasodilators or vasopressors. Filling pressures and CO can be determined, and their response to therapeutic measures can be assessed. It should be used only when they can be placed with and interpreted with adequate expertise and kept in place for the shortest time possible to minimize complications. At a minimum a centrally placed catheter should be employed to allow the use of vasopressors and obtain measurement of central venous pressure and oxygen saturations.

- *Echocardiography* can provide much of the information that previously required a pulmonary artery catheter. Central venous and pulmonary artery pressures can be estimated noninvasively. The mitral inflow and myocardial diastolic velocity ratio (i.e. E/e') can estimate LV filling pressures

- *Management*
  - *Antithrombotic therapy*: If shock is the result of MI, aspirin and full-dose heparin should be given. While clopidogrel is typically given with ST segment elevation MI, a proportion of patients with non-ST segment elevation MI may require coronary artery bypass graft surgery (CABG), so, generally, clopidogrel is withheld until angiography is performed. Glycoprotein IIb/IIIa inhibitors may provide mortality benefit according to a substudy of the PURSUIT trial, where eptifibatide was compared with placebo. Beta-blockers and calcium channel blockers are withheld in the presence of hypotension. Additional details regarding antithrombotic therapy are discussed in chapter 3: Acute Coronary Syndromes.

- *Vasodilators*: Although counterintuitive, afterload reduction can improve cardiac performance such that BP actually increases. This should only be attempted in low-grade shock or once the patient has been stabilized on inotropes. Nitroglycerin and nitroprusside are the available agents.
    - *Nitroglycerin* can be particularly useful if there is angina. It is primarily a venodilator and reduces preload, but tachyphylaxis limits its use.
    - *Nitroprusside* is an arterial and venodilator with a very short half-life, which is very convenient for use in the intensive care unit. It reduces afterload for both the left and right ventricles and has been shown to improve pulmonary capillary wedge pressure and cardiac output similar to an inotrope. The main disadvantage is that cyanide toxicity can develop, particularly in renal failure, so patients must be monitored for confusion, nausea, hyperreflexia and lactic acidosis. Thiocyanate levels can be obtained to monitor for the development of toxic levels
- *Vasopressors*: When there is profound hypotension, it is necessary to initiate vasopressors, but the deleterious effect on cardiac performance must be recognized and consideration should be given to preferentially initiate mechanical support
    - *Dopamine* is a precursor to norepinephrine and has traditionally been the vasopressor of choice in hypotension due to its vasodilatory effect in the renal vasculature in addition to its inotropic and chronotropic effect. At doses <3 μg/kg/min, the primary effect is on dopaminergic receptors in the renal and coronary circulation, resulting in vasodilation. At doses of 3–10 μg/kg/min, it works primarily as a β1 agonist increasing HR and contractility, and at doses >10 μg/kg/min dopamine causes vasoconstriction as an α agonist. However, here is concern for risk of adverse effects of dopamine. The SOAP II trial found that in patients with shock, dopamine was associated with increased adverse effects, particularly tachyarrhythmias, and in the 280 patients with cardiogenic shock, it was associated with an increase in 28-day mortality
    - *Norepinephrine* is a catecholamine with α and β1 agonist properties. It primarily causes peripheral vasoconstriction while also increasing HR and contractility. It is the vasopressor of choice in cardiogenic shock.
- *Inotropes*: In cardiogenic shock, inotropes are utilized to temporarily stabilize patients with end-organ dysfunction due to reduced cardiac output. In the ADHERE registry, inotropes have been shown to increase mortality due to tachyarrhythmias and myocardial ischemia, but they serve an important role in the acute management of shock in patients who need immediate improvement in perfusion.
    - *Dobutamine* is the inotrope of choice in cardiogenic shock. It is a short-acting agent, which increases myocardial contractility through its effect on β1 receptors leading to increased cyclic adenosine

monophosphate production. It also has some effect on peripheral β2 receptors as well, which can result in vasodilation and hypotension at the time of initiation. The primary disadvantage of dobutamine is the increase chronotropic effect and the development of tachyphylaxis after approximately 72 hours

- *Milrinone* is another inotrope that can be used. It is a noncatecholamine phosphodiesterase-3 inhibitor that leads to systemic and pulmonary vasodilation and increased contractility without increasing HR. It is particularly useful in reducing pulmonary pressures and may improve RV function. It is not recommended in acute shock due to its long half-life and hypotensive effects, and it must be renally dosed. In the OPTIME-CHF study, when milrinone was added to standard therapy there was no significant increase in mortality rate with significantly more sustained hypotension (10.7% vs. 3.2%) and atrial arrhythmias (4.6% vs. 1.5%)
- *Levosimendan* is a recently developed agent, currently only approved for use in Europe. It increases myocardial contractility and relaxation by sensitizing myofilaments to calcium. In two trials, REVIVE-II and SURVIVE, there was no difference in mortality when compared with dobutamine, and there may be increased adverse effects.

- *Revascularization*: In patients presenting with an ST segment elevation MI (STEMI) complicated by cardiogenic shock, emergency revascularization with either percutaneous coronary intervention (PCI) or CABG is recommended in suitable patients irrespective of the time delay from MI onset. In the absence of contraindications, fibrinolytic therapy should be administered to patients with STEMI and cardiogenic shock who are unsuitable candidates for either PCI or CABG. It is reasonable to use intra-aortic balloon pump (IABP) counterpulsation for patients with cardiogenic shock after STEMI who do not quickly stabilize with pharmacological therapy. Alternative LV assist devices for circulatory support may be considered in patients with refractory cardiogenic shock.

  In the landmark SHOCK trial, coronary bypass and PCI were compared with medical therapy in 300 patients with shock due to LV failure after STEMI. There was a trend toward mortality benefit at 30 days and a statistically significant 13% reduction in mortality at 6 months, which persisted at 6 years of follow-up. This benefit was limited to patients <75 years old in subgroup analysis. When there is more multivessel disease it is currently uncertain if nonculprit vessels should be revascularized. Although fibrinolysis was not studied in this trial, it is recommended if patients present within 3 hours of symptom onset and PCI is likely to be delayed beyond 90 minutes.

  In patients with mechanical complications of acute MI (e.g. ventricular septal defect or papillary muscle rupture) presenting with shock, surgical repair and revascularization are clearly the preferred options. However, in the cases without mechanical complication, the choice of coronary bypass versus PCI is less clear. It is generally accepted that, in severe three-vessel disease, CABG should be preferred. In the SHOCK trial, patients who underwent CABG were more likely to have multivessel or left main disease and were more likely to be diabetic. Registry data suggest that patients with shock and two- or three-vessel disease may have better survival with CABG. Patients with left main coronary artery lesions presenting with shock have a high mortality rate of almost 50%. Although the numbers are small, patients in the SHOCK trial with unprotected left main PCI had lower mortality rate than when treated with bypass. Therefore, in patients with cardiogenic shock complicating acute MI, unprotected left main PCI can be considered a reasonable alternative to coronary bypass.

- *Mechanical support devices*: Temporary ventricular support devices are indicated when there is profound hemodynamic collapse despite medical therapy including vasopressors and inotropes. They are used to stabilize the patient until revascularization, myocardial recovery or long-term alternative is available such as a surgically implanted durable ventricular assist device or transplant. In severe shock complicating MI, mechanical support may be necessary to maintain perfusion while revascularization is attempted. Furthermore, even after revascularization there may be a significant portion of hibernating or stunned myocardium that requires time for recovery. All percutaneous mechanical support devices require continuous heparin and carry risks of hemolysis, infection, stroke and limb ischemia.
  - The *IABP* was first developed in 1968 and is the most studied and the most commonly used mechanical support device. It improves diastolic coronary flow and reduces afterload, and guidelines encourage its use in the setting of acute MI complicated by shock. However, due to the results of several recent studies both American and European guidelines have reduced the strength of recommendations for the use of IABP in ST segment elevation MI complicated by shock to "reasonable" from "recommended." A meta-analysis of cohort studies and a Cochrane review of all randomized trials of IABP in the setting of MI showed no benefit in mortality or LV ejection fraction at 30 days, and there is increased risk of stroke and bleeding. However, in patients who receive fibrinolytics, there was an 18% reduction in 30 days mortality. In the largest randomized trial, IABP SHOCK II, which included 600 patients, there was no benefit in mortality at 30 days or 12 months. Contraindications to its use are severe aortic regurgitation or aortic dissection.
  - *Percutaneous LV assist devices* have emerged as alternative mechanical support device to IABP. The Impella catheter (Abiomed, Danvers, MA) is an axial flow pump that is positioned in the LV across the aortic valve, and the pump (inside the catheter) moves blood from the inlet port in the LV to the outlet port in the ascending aorta. Positioning is monitored by pressure waveforms

and transthoracic echocardiography. The pump can augment CO by up to 5 L/min. When compared with the IABP in the ISAR-IABP trial, there was improvement in hemodynamics at 30 minutes, but there are no studies showing improvement in outcomes. Important contraindications are severe aortic stenosis, prosthetic aortic valve, ventricular septal defect and LV thrombus. Complications include stroke, limb ischemia, hemolysis and aortic dissection

- *Extracorporeal circulatory support* may be achieved with a centrifugal pump having an integrated motor. The TandemHeart (CardiacAssist, Inc., Pittsburgh, PA) can provide up to 5 L/min of augmentation when used with percutaneous technique. An inflow cannula is advance from the femoral vein to the left atrium via transseptal puncture. Oxygenated blood is removed from the left atrium to the pump and returned via an outflow catheter placed in the femoral artery. This results in decompression of the LV. However, this device cannot be used if there is significant aortic regurgitation or a ventricular septal defect. Adverse events include complications of septal puncture, limb ischemia, stroke and hemolysis. A disadvantage compared with the Impella is that positioning cannot be monitored by pressure waveforms, and requires imaging and/or blood gases.
- *Extracorporeal membrane oxygenation* (ECMO). In most circumstances, univentricular support (as afforded by the above options) will suffice; however, when there is respiratory and circulatory failure, or if there is profound biventricular failure such as in fulminant myocarditis, ECMO is indicated. Cannulas are placed in the femoral vessels, and both cardiac output and oxygenation can be provided. Duration of support is usually limited to hours, and it also has the risks of stroke, infection and hemolysis seen with other support devices. Furthermore, since there is no LV decompression, afterload and wall stress are actually increased.

- *Therapeutic hypothermia*: In comatose patients who were successfully resuscitated after cardiac arrest, there may be neuroprotective benefit from cooling to 32-34° for 12-24 hours. A Cochrane review of three trials found that hypothermia resulted in 54% of patients having good neurologic outcome compared with 35% who were not cooled, and there was a 35% increase in survival to discharge.
- *Ventilatory support*: In all patients with cardiogenic shock, particularly those with pulmonary edema, adequate ventilatory support is necessary. If there is altered mental status, exhaustion, accessory muscle use or inability to adequately oxygenate, positive pressure ventilation with continuous positive airway pressure or bilevel positive airway pressure must be initiated. If ventilation continues to be inadequate, endotracheal intubation is indicated. Although there is a dearth of quality data specifically in cardiogenic shock patients, lung protective ventilation is recommended with a goal of <6 mL/kg tidal volumes and plateau pressures <30 cm H_2O

- *Supportive therapy*: Coincident sepsis is common, and hemodynamics must be carefully monitored for sepsis, particularly inappropriately low SVR or high central venous oxygen saturation. A restrictive transfusion strategy is recommended, targeting hemoglobin >8 g/dL for most patients and 8–10 g/dL in patients with concern for ongoing ischemia. Appropriate stress ulcer and venous thrombosis prophylaxis are recommended (Fig. 7.1).
- Mechanical complications post-MI
  - *Ventricular septal defect* usually occurs 3–5 days after MI in patients presenting with an occluded left anterior descending artery perfusing a large territory extending to the apical inferior segment (i.e. ECG with inferior and anterior ST elevations). When patients present with shock, mortality is almost inevitable unless surgical repair is performed. Despite surgery, survival is approximately 50% at 30 days. While awaiting surgery, medical therapy is targeted at reducing left to right shunting by reducing afterload with diuretics, vasodilators and IABP.
  - *Free wall rupture* is found in 20% of patients who die from MI, but it can also present with hemopericardium and hemodynamic collapse or in a subacute fashion where a pseudoaneurysm has formed. Immediate surgery is required, but pericardiocentesis, inotropes, vasopressors and potentially ventricular assist devices should be initiated for hemodynamic support (Fig. 7.2).

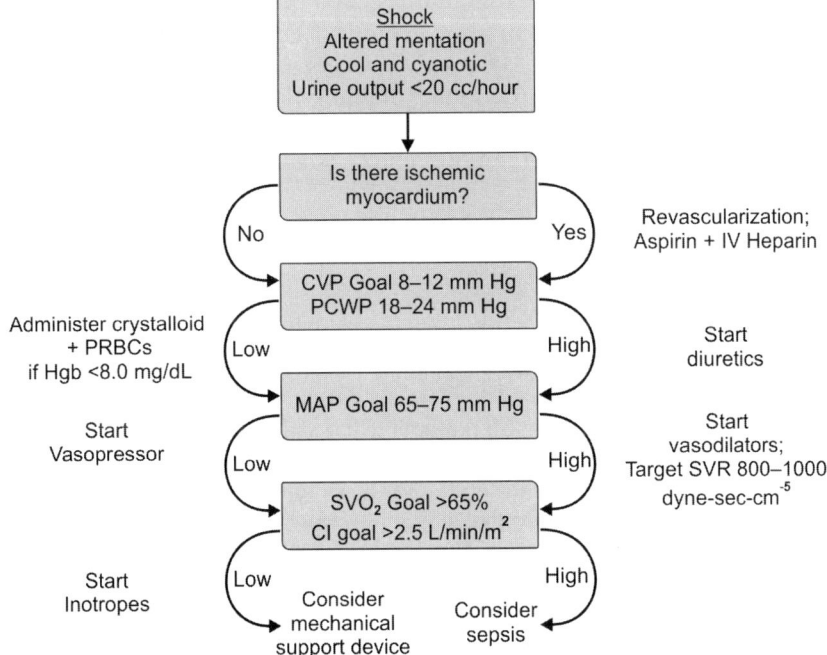

Fig. 7.1: Management of shock

PRBCs, packed red blood cells; Hgb, hemoglobin; CVP, central venous pressure; PCWP, pulmonary capillary wedge pressure; MAP, mean arterial pressure; CI, Cardiac Index; SVR, systemic vascular resistance; IV, intravenous; SVO_2, mixed venous oxygen.

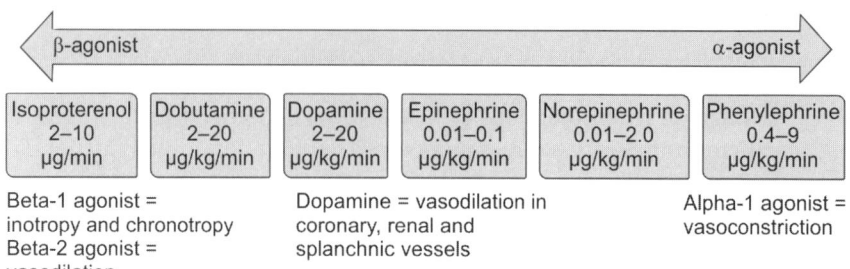

Fig. 7.2: Spectrum of vasopressor and inotrope effects

Source: Based on dose ranges in Overgaard CB, Dzavík V. Inotropes and vasopressors: review of physiology and clinical use in cardiovascular disease. Circulation. 2008;118(10):1047-56; Vincent JL, De Backer D. Circulatory shock. N Engl J Med. 2013;369(18):1726-34.

- *Acute mitral regurgitation* is usually a result of papillary muscle rupture or displacement or rupture of the chordae after an MI. If papillary muscle rupture is not present, patients can be stabilized medically and revascularized with PCI. However, in the case of papillary muscle rupture, mortality rate is 75% with medical therapy versus 50% with surgical therapy. Medical therapy involves maximal afterload reduction to promote forward flow using vasodilators and IABP if needed.
- *Arrhythmias:* Cardiogenic shock can be precipitated or further worsened by arrhythmias and prompt control is important. For bradyarrhythmias, atropine or isoproterenol is used and if needed a pacemaker is placed (see for further detail Chapter: 16 Bradyarrhythmias). For atrial tachyarrhythmias, β-blockers and calcium channel blockers can be attempted if LV function is preserved. In the setting of reduced ejection fraction or acute ischemia, cardioversion or defibrillation and antiarrhythmics, preferably amiodarone, are the treatments of choice (see for further detail Chapter 18: Tachyarrhythmias).

SUGGESTED READING

1. De Backer D, Biston P, Devriendt J, et al. Comparison of dopamine and norepinephrine in the treatment of shock. N Engl J Med. 2010;362(9):779-89.
2. Francis GS, Bartos JA, Adatya S. Inotropes. J Am Coll Cardiol. 2014;63(20):2069-78.
3. Gidwani UK, Mohanty B, Chatterjee K. The pulmonary artery catheter: a critical reappraisal. Cardiol Clin. 2013;31(4):545-65.
4. Harker M, Carville S, Henderson R, Gray H, Group GD. Key recommendations and evidence from the NICE guideline for the acute management of ST-segment-elevation myocardial infarction. Heart. 2014;100(7):536-43.
5. Hinshaw LB, Cox BG. The Fundamental Mechanisms of Shock. New York: Plenum Press; 1972.
6. Hochman JS, Sleeper LA, Webb JG, et al. Early revascularization in acute myocardial infarction complicated by cardiogenic shock. N Engl J Med. 1999;341(9):625-34.
7. Jeger R V, Radovanovic D, Hunziker PR, et al. Ten-year trends in the incidence and treatment of cardiogenic shock. Ann Intern Med. 2008;149(9):618-26.

8. O'Gara PT, Kushner FG, Ascheim DD, et al. 2013 ACCF/AHA guideline for the management of ST-elevation myocardial infarction: a report of the American College of Cardiology Foundation/American Heart Association Task Force on Practice Guidelines. Circulation. 2013;127(4):e362-425.
9. Overgaard CB, Dzavík V. Inotropes and vasopressors: review of physiology and clinical use in cardiovascular disease. Circulation. 2008;118(10):1047-56.
10. Reynolds HR, Hochman JS. Cardiogenic shock: current concepts and improving outcomes. Circulation. 2008;117(5):686-97.
11. Thiele H, Zeymer U, Neumann FJ, et al. Intraaortic balloon support for myocardial infarction with cardiogenic shock. N Engl J Med. 2012;367(14):1287-96.
12. Vincent JL, De Backer D. Circulatory shock. N Engl J Med. 2013;369(18):1726-34.
13. Werdan K, Russ M, Buerke M, Prondzinsky R, Dietz S. Coronary interventions cardiogenic shock evidence-based management of evidence-based management of cardiogenic shock after acute myocardial infarction. Interv Cardiol Rev. 2013;8(2):73-80.
14. Werdan K, Gielen S, Ebelt H, Hochman JS. Mechanical circulatory support in cardiogenic shock. Eur Heart J. 2014;35(3):156-67.

Hypertension

Chapter 8

Manish Suneja, Seth Maliske

Hypertension is a leading cause of disease burden in the United States and worldwide. An estimated 30% of adults in the United States have hypertension defined as systolic blood pressure (SBP) >140 mm Hg, diastolic blood pressure (DBP) >90 mm Hg and anyone taking antihypertensive medications. The incidence of hypertension increases with age. As our population continues to age, the number of office visits related to hypertension will continue to increase as will hypertensive-related morbidity and mortality. Hypertension increases the risk of ischemic stroke, intracerebral hemorrhage, peripheral artery disease and cardiovascular (CV) disease, including heart failure and myocardial infarction, as well as chronic kidney disease (CKD).

HEMODYNAMIC DETERMINANTS OF BLOOD PRESSURE AND THE VARIABLES AFFECTED IN SYSTEMIC HYPERTENSION

- Blood pressure (BP): Pressure is generated when the heart contracts against the resistance of the blood vessels according to the formula: MAP = CO × SVR, where
  MAP = mean arterial blood pressure, estimated by DBP + (SBP–DBP)/3, or ([2 × DBP] + SBP)/3
  CO = cardiac output
  SVR = systemic vascular resistance
- Cardiac output can be broken down as: CO = SV × HR, where
  SV = stroke volume (dependent on preload, contractility and afterload)
  HR = heart rate
- Systemic hypertension necessitates an increase in CO and/or SVR. Typically, hypertension results from an increase in SVR with normal CO, but there are exceptions:
  - In young patients with borderline hypertension, or intermittently hypertensive patients, increased CO may be the only hemodynamic disturbance (possibly due to an increased sympathetic tone). With time, CO "normalizes" and SVR increases to sustain the hypertension.
  - Even in disorders that are clearly associated with volume overload (e.g. kidney failure), the increase in CO is transient followed by an increase in SVR.

DETERMINANTS OF ARTERIAL BLOOD PRESSURE IN THE YOUNGER AS WELL AS AGED CIRCULATORY SYSTEM

Blood pressure is determined by both physical and physiological factors. Physiological factors interface with physical factors to determine BP level.
- *Physical factors*: Blood volume and arterial compliance are important physical factors that determine BP levels
  - *Blood volume* is distributed unevenly between the arterial and venous capacitance vessels sides of the vascular system. Approximately two-thirds to three-quarters of the blood volume is contained within the venous capacitance vessels; the remaining one-quarter to one-third is contained in the arterial side of the vascular tree. Arterial blood volume is determined by the difference in the blood volume ejected by the heart per unit of time (i.e. CO) and the outflow through the arterial resistance vessels into the venous capacitance vessels (i.e. the peripheral runoff). When CO and peripheral runoff are balanced, arterial blood volume and arterial pressure remain constant. If CO increases but peripheral runoff does not rise commensurately, then arterial blood volume rises and BP also increases.
  - *Arterial elasticity* is an important determinant of the rise in SBP that occurs for any given increase in blood volume. Generally speaking, arterial elasticity is inversely related to age, that is younger persons have greater arterial elasticity and with advancing age arterial elasticity declines.
  - *Arterial compliance* is determined by elastic properties of the large conduit vessels and is the change in pressure that occurs with a given change in arterial volume (i.e. $\Delta V/\Delta P$). Therefore, the greater the arterial elasticity, the smaller the rise in systolic pressure during the systolic ejection phase of the cardiac cycle. Conversely, lesser arterial elasticity causes a greater rise in SBP during the systolic ejection phase.
- *Physiological factors*: Cardiac output (i.e. the product of SV × HR) and peripheral arterial resistance, largely determined at the level of the arterioles, are the major physiological factors involved in the determination of arterial BP.

METHODS OF MEASURING BP

Accuracy of measurement begins with understanding of the three methods used to obtain a BP reading, and ensuring that the equipment to be used is accurate.
- *Mercury sphygmomanometers* use auscultation to detect blood flow through the artery and are considered to provide the gold standard of BP measurement. However, due to concerns about environmental hazards, these devices are being phased out. As a result, the mercury sphygmomanometers are being replaced with aneroid and/or oscillometric devices

- *Aneroid devices* also use auscultation to detect blood flow through the artery. Blood pressure readings on auscultation are subject to measurement error due to environmental factors (e.g. extraneous room noise), personnel factors (e.g. education, hearing ability and terminal digit preference) and device factors. Aneroid devices do not maintain stability over time and require frequent re-calibration (e.g. every 6–12 months)
- *The oscillometric method* detects vibrations in the arterial wall that occur due to blood flow and transforms the vibrations into an electrical signal, which is displayed as a digital readout of BP. However, factors other than blood flow may affect the vibrations. Thus, the oscillometric techniques will underestimate the true BP in patients with arterial stiffness or dysrhythmias. Automated upper arm devices that measure BP at the brachial artery have been shown to be reliable in clinical practice, and therefore their use is recommended over wrist or finger devices
- *Ambulatory BP monitoring* is another type of oscillometric measurement and may be done when there is the possibility of white-coat hypertension or other concerns of measurement error. White-coat hypertension (i.e. a persistent elevation in BP when measured in a clinical setting, but a normal BP when the measurement is taken at home) affects as many as one in three in the general population but is higher in the elderly and pregnant women.

Ambulatory BP monitoring records BP every 15–30 minutes (or when triggered at the patient's request) for a 24- to 48-hour period. The data are stored in the device's memory until downloaded to a computer for interpretation by the physician. The multiple recordings may provide greater diagnostic accuracy than isolated clinic measurements. However, when proper, standardized procedures are followed, the average of four duplicate clinic BP readings is as reliable as 24-hour ambulatory BP monitoring.

MEASUREMENT PROTOCOL FOR ACCURATE BLOOD PRESSURE RECORDING

- Prepare the equipment
  - Use equipment that has been (i) validated as accurate against a mercury sphygmomanometer, (ii) checked for disrepair of cuff (e.g. cracks or leaks in tubing, breaks in stitching or tears in fabric) and (iii) checked for an intact gauge (e.g. that the mercury meniscus or aneroid needle is at zero).
  - Obtain appropriate cuff size by measuring circumference of the patient's arm and choosing the cuff size that corresponds to that measurement.
- Prepare the patient
  - Confirm that the patient has not recently had nicotine or caffeine
  - Have the patient sit quietly for 5 minutes before measuring BP
  - Correctly position the patient:
    - Use a sitting or semireclining position with the back supported

- ♦ The arm should be at heart level (i.e. middle of the cuff should be at mid-sternum level)
- ♦ Legs should be uncrossed with feet flat and supported on the floor or on a foot rest (i.e. not dangling from examination table or bed)
  - Bare the upper arm of any constrictive clothing (i.e. be able to get at least one finger under a rolled-up sleeve)
  - Palpate the brachial artery and position center of cuff bladder over the brachial artery
- Take the BP measurement
  - Support the patient's arm at heart level
  - For auscultatory measurements:
    - ♦ Obtain an estimated systolic pressure by palpation prior to auscultation
    - ♦ Inflate the cuff as rapidly as possible to a maximum inflation level (e.g. 20 mm Hg above the estimated SBP)
    - ♦ Deflate the cuff slowly at a rate of 2–3 mm Hg/s
    - ♦ Note the first of two regular beats as the SBP (palpation helps avoid underestimating systolic pressure due to an auscultatory gap)
    - ♦ Use the last sound heard (also called the fifth Korotkoff sound) as the DBP
    - ♦ Continue deflation for 10 mmHg past last sound to assure sound is not a "skipped" beat
    - ♦ The measurement should be recorded as an even number and to the nearest 2 mm Hg (round upward)
  - Neither the patient nor observer should talk during the measurement
  - If two readings are measured, record the average of the readings
- *Record the measurement* and document the following:
  - The obtained BP reading
  - The patient's position (i.e. sitting, semirecumbent, lying and standing)
  - The arm used, including arm circumference and cuff size used
  - Type of device used to obtain the measurement (mercury, aneroid and automated)
  - State of the individual (e.g. anxious and relaxed)
  - Time of administration of any drugs that could affect BP
- *Frequency of measurements*
  - Office visits: BP should be recorded at 3–6 visits spaced over weeks to months. At each visit, BP is checked in each arm and repeated until two consecutive readings are within 5 mm Hg.
  - Ambulatory BP monitoring: 24-hour ambulatory BP monitoring records BP at preset intervals throughout the day and during sleep.
  - Home BP cuff: Measurements should be recorded every morning and evening for seven consecutive days to assess for an average home BP.

DIAGNOSIS AND CLASSIFICATION OF HYPERTENSION

Hypertension is defined as elevated average BP over time, preferably with a minimum of three properly performed readings on different days and should not be based on a single measurement. Blood pressure at rest is lower than BP during activities. There is a natural diurnal variation for people with usual work–sleep cycles, resulting in increased BP just before awakening continuing to be elevated in the morning while decreasing in the evening. Blood pressure also decreases in the early afternoon, and the nadir in BP occurs at 2–3 AM, during sleep. These data are routinely obtained by 24-hour ambulatory BP monitors. The decrease in BP during sleep is known as the "dip" and when absent is associated with an increased risk of CV events (e.g. strokes, myocardial infarctions and death). Several selected conditions known to attenuate or eliminate the normal nocturnal decline in BP include CKD, obesity, high sodium and/or low potassium diets and sleep-disordered breathing.

- *Hypertension as defined as per the Joint National Committee (JNC) guidelines*

  The stages of hypertension were defined in the 2003 by the JNC 7. When updated in 2013, the JNC 8 did not address these stages. Normal BP across all ages and races is <120 mm Hg SBP and <80 mm Hg DBP. Hypertensive patients are classified into stages according to the BP (Table 8.1). Prehypertension, white coat hypertension and masked hypertension are defined as follows:
  - *Prehypertension* is present when BP readings are between 120–139 mm Hg and 80–89 mm Hg. These individuals are at risk for the development of hypertension. Thus, lifestyle modification (i.e. exercise, weight loss, and salt and alcohol restriction) is recommended. Borderline or high normal BP is when the office readings are consistently between 135–140 mm Hg and 85–90 mm Hg in patients without CKD, diabetes mellitus or ischemic heart disease.
  - *White coat hypertension* (i.e. office hypertension) is present when the office BP is >140/90 mm Hg; yet, the outside of the office, the BP is <135/85 mm Hg during the daytime hours on 24-hour ambulatory BP monitor. These individuals have a slightly elevated CV risk compared with normotensives; however, there are no guidelines recommending pharmacological drug therapy.
  - *Masked hypertension* is when the office BP is normal (<140/90 mm Hg). However, outside of the office BP is elevated (>135/85 mm Hg). These

Table 8.1: Classification of hypertension

BP classification	SBP (mm Hg)	DBP (mm Hg)
Normal	<120	and <80
Prehypertension	120–139	or 80–90
Stage 1	140–159	or 90–99
Stage 2	>160	or >100

Source: Adapted from Chobanian AV, Bakris GL, Black HR, Cushman WC, Green LA, Izzo JL Jr., et al. Seventh report of the Joint National Committee on prevention, detection, evaluation, and treatment of high blood pressure. Hypertension. 2003;42:1206-52.

individuals are at a greatly increased risk of CV events, and medication treatment is advised. Nevertheless, this type of hypertension is very difficult to diagnose because ambulatory BP monitoring is not typically undertaken in patients with controlled office BP. Masked hypertension not infrequently occurs in patients with sleep apnea.

PHYSICAL EXAMINATION IN A PATIENT WITH HYPERTENSION

- *General appearance*: Inspection begins when the patient first enters the clinic. Observe the patient's behavior and gait for signs of neurologic deficits. Observe respiratory pattern for signs of dyspnea on exertion. Determine the patient body habitus. Central weight gain (apple shape) correlates with metabolic risk factors for CV disease
- *Waist measurement*: Patient should be wearing a gown and nonrestrictive briefs or underwear. The measurement should not be made over clothing. The patient should stand erect with the abdomen relaxed, the arms at the sides and feet together. The measurer faces the subject and places an inelastic tape around the subject in a horizontal plane at the level of the natural waist. The measurement should be taken at the end of a normal expiration without the tape compressing the skin
- *Respirations*: Respiration affects the level of BP, with SBP falling during inspiration. The basis for this effect is twofold. First, during inspiration, intrathoracic pressure falls, the lungs expand and pulmonary venous capacitance increases. This results in increased venous return to the right ventricle and diminished blood flow to the left ventricle. The decreased left ventricular preload contributes to the lowered SBP. Second, changes in intrathoracic pressure are directly transmitted to the intrathoracic aorta. The degree of fall in systemic BP is proportional to the fall in intrathoracic pressure. During the normal respiratory cycle, SBP falls between 5 and 10 mm Hg from the end of expiration to the end of inspiration.
- *Pulse*: Manual determination of pulse rate is integral to BP evaluation. Pulse rate, rhythm and pulse contour are evaluated. Tachycardia or bradycardia may reflect intrinsic cardiac disease, medical illness or reaction to medication. Similarly, rhythm reflects cardiac arrhythmias. The brachial pulse should be compared with the apical impulse (palpated or auscultated). Not all cardiac contractions are transmitted to the periphery (e.g. atrial fibrillation). Premature ventricular contractions result in uncoordinated ventricular contraction and diminished stroke volume. Thus, only assessing the presence of peripheral pulses may underestimate the true heart rate. Similarly, in patients with pulsus alternans, alternating weak and strong ventricular contractions result in only half of the cardiac contractions being effective. This discrepancy of peripheral and apical rate is known as pulse deficit. Pulsus bisferiens, a double peak in the pulse, is difficult to palpate but may manifest as a "split" Korotkoff sound.

Palpate the pulses in both arms and one leg. Coarctation of the aorta usually presents with equal radial but diminished femoral pulses. Rarely (<5%) of patients with coarctation of the aorta will present with unequal radial pulses
- *Pulse pressure*: In addition to the level of BP, the pulse pressure (i.e. the difference between SBP and DBP) may indicate an underlying medical condition. For example, a wide pulse pressure may be a consequence of a hyperdynamic left ventricle from fever, anxiety, anemia or thyrotoxicosis. Other causes of a wide pulse pressure include aortic insufficiency. Poorly compliant arterial vasculature, such as occurs with aging and/or diabetes mellitus, also causes wide pulse pressure. Conversely, a narrow pulse pressure may occur as a consequence of a poorly contractile left ventricle or cardiac tamponade
- *Neck*: The neck examination should focus on the thyroid and vascular pulsations. Visible and palpable pulsations around the clavicular heads may indicate aneurysmal dilatation of the aortic arch. As the ascending aorta and arch increase in diameter due to hypertensive atherosclerotic disease, the arch is displaced cephalad bringing the innominate, subclavian and carotid arteries origins near the thoracic outlet

  Venous pulsations reflect right atrial pressures. Visible venous pulsations in the neck can occur with right ventricular heart failure, pulmonary hypertension and/or tricuspid valve disease.
- *Cardiac examination*: The cardiac examination consists of inspection, palpation and auscultation. First, inspect and palpate the precordium to locate the point of maximal impulse (PMI). In healthy individuals, the PMI is located in the fifth left intercostal space of the mid-clavicular line. The location of the PMI reflects cardiac size. Downward or lateral displacement indicates cardiac enlargement. The size and quality of PMI reflect cardiac contractility. Normal contractility results in a quarter-sized tapping impulse. Impaired cardiac contractility results in an enlarged poorly palpable and sustained PMI (also referred to as a heave).
    - *Fourth heart sound (S4) gallop*: The S4 gallop is the result of the left atrium contracting and pumping blood into a stiff, noncompliant left ventricle. The gallop is heard best at the apex (over the area of the PMI) with the bell of the stethoscope. The S4 precedes the first heart sound (S1) and may be misinterpreted as a "split" S1. The S4 gallop correlates with the presence of an inverted or biphasic P wave (enlarged left atrium) on the electrocardiogram (ECG). Patients with first-degree heart block may have an audibly increased interval between S4 and S1. An S4 gallop is not considered a normal finding and is a result of left atrial contraction into a stiff, noncompliant left ventricle typically due to pressure-overload hypertrophy (i.e. hypertensive heart disease). Myocardial ischemia can also contribute to or cause ventricular stiffening.
    - *Third heart sound (S3) gallop*: The S3 gallop is the result of rapid ventricular filling in early diastole. The gallop may be misinterpreted

as a split second heart sound (S2). The S3 gallop represents volume overload and is usually an indicative of heart failure. However, the S3 gallop may be heard in children as well as in volume expanded states such as pregnancy; in these latter two situations, the S3 gallop does not indicate a failing left ventricular and is a normal variant.
   - *Murmurs*: Cardiac murmurs may shed light on the diagnosis of hypertensive heart disease. Early in the disease the ventricle develops hypertrophy with hyperdynamic ventricular contraction. The aortic valve may calcify and develop sclerosis. This combination results in an ejection click with an aortic sclerosis murmur. During late hypertensive heart disease, the left ventricle dilates. This dilatation expands the mitral valve annulus and may result in a murmur of mitral regurgitation.
- *Peripheral circulation*: Evaluate the arterial pulses to determine the presence of atherosclerotic vascular disease and coarctation of the aorta. Auscultate the carotid as well as other major arteries (e.g. femoral) for bruits. If no carotid bruits are present, gently palpate each carotid independently for delayed upstroke suggestive of aortic stenosis or collapsing downstroke suggestive of aortic insufficiency. The radial pulses should always be equal. Diminished femoral pulse with intact radial pulse suggests coarctation of the aorta. The posterior tibial artery should always be present.
- *Abdominal examination*: Inspect the abdomen (and chest) for scars suggesting coronary bypass surgery. Look for any pulsations suggesting aortic aneurysm. Auscultate the epigastric area for bruits. Percuss the epigastric area for signs of distended urinary bladder. Palpate the abdomen for pulsatile masses suggesting aneurysmal dilatation or an ectatic aorta. Patients with polycystic kidneys may also present with palpable abdominal masses.
- *Neurologic and ophthalmologic*: Hypertensive retinopathy is the most common physical examination finding associated with the hypertensive patient. Perform a funduscopic examination to look for retinal hemorrhages, cotton wool spots and papilledema. A thorough neurologic examination should be performed in all hypertensive patients to evaluate for cerebral ischemia. Most patients with essential hypertension are asymptomatic. Headache was not associated with BP in a study of 76 patients that linked 24-hour ambulatory monitoring of their BP with a symptom diary of when they did and did not experience headache.

CLUES FOR PREVIOUSLY UNCONTROLLED HYPERTENSION

It is not infrequent that clinicians encounter patients in whom they do not have prior medical records that document important historical trends in BP. Patients are also often unaware of their prior level of BP control. Nevertheless, there are relatively easily detectable clues to the prior level of BP control. Documentation of any or all of these findings (Table 8.2) would suggest that BP control has been less than optimal.

> **Table 8.2:** Clinically available clues indicative of poorly controlled hypertension.
>
> Retinopathy
> - Arteriolar narrowing, AV nicking
> - Focal and general arteriolar narrowing, arteriolar silver wiring
> - Hemorrhages, exudates, cotton wool, spots, papilledema and/or microaneurysms
>
> Cardiac examination
> - Laterally displaced and/or enlarged PMI
> - S4 gallop
> - Other signs of heart failure (e.g. JVP, edema and rales)
>
> Electrocardiogram
> - Voltage criteria for LVH
> - Inverted or biphasic P wave in precordial lead V1
>
> Volume examination/renal (heart failure or kidney dysfunction)
> - Evidence of volume overload (JVP, edema, crackles, etc.)
> - Elevated creatinine and proteinuria

AV, arteriovenous; PMI, point of maximal impulse; S4, fourth heart sound; JVP, jugular venous pressure; LVH, left ventricular hypertrophy.

LIFESTYLE FACTORS IN THE HYPERTENSIVE PATIENT CONTRIBUTING TO ELEVATED BLOOD PRESSURE

- *Obesity* is a common feature of patients with resistant hypertension, and >40% patients with resistant hypertension are obese. Accordingly, obesity is known to be associated with resistance to pharmacological BP lowering
- *Excessive dietary salt intake* has been specifically documented as being common in patients with resistant hypertension. The frequency of salt sensitivity is increased among patients who are at least 60 years of age, patients who are African American or obese, and patients with renal impairment. Approximately 75–80% of dietary sodium intake can be linked to the consumption of high sodium foods (e.g. processed meats and canned goods)
- *Heavy alcohol intake* is associated with treatment-resistant hypertension. On the contrary, alcohol reduction is associated with a significant reduction in SBP of −3.31 mm Hg and DBP of −2.04 mm Hg. Alcohol consumption should be kept to two or fewer drinks per day in men and no more than one drink per day in women.

LIFESTYLE INTERVENTIONS TO LOWER THE RISK OF DEVELOPING HYPERTENSION

Lifestyle changes in diet and exercise along with weight loss can lower BP, and some interventions have been shown to reduce CV and overall mortality. The lifestyle modifications that are best studied include the following:
- *Low sodium diet*: The JNC 8 guidelines recommend a limitation of sodium intake to no >2.4 g per day, but a further reduction of sodium intake to 1.5 g per day can result in even greater reduction in BP. The European Society of Hypertension recommends reducing sodium intake to <2 g per day.

Hypertension is rare in populations with sodium intake of <1.2 g daily. A meta-analysis of 20 trials of hypertensive patients that looked at sodium reduction for at least 6 months revealed that a reduction of 78 mmol (1.8 g) of sodium a day resulted in 5/2.6 mm Hg improvement in SBP/DBP
- *DASH diet*: The Dietary Approaches to Stop Hypertension (DASH) trial used a diet rich in fruits and vegetables to provide increased fiber and potassium along with other trace minerals. Low-fat dairy products provided increased calcium while keeping the diet low in saturated and total fat. Trial participants randomized to the DASH diet were provided meals containing four to five servings of fruit, four to five servings of vegetables, two to three servings of low-fat dairy products and <25% of calories from fat. The diet was not sodium restricted, and subjects ingested 3 g of sodium a day. Subjects ate breakfast and dinner at the research site and were given lunches and weekend meals to take home. The results were dramatic:
  - Decreased SBP/DBP of 5.5/3.0 mm Hg
  - Decreased SBP/DBP in hypertensives of 11.4/5.5 mm Hg
  - Maximal BP response occurred after only 2 weeks.
- *Decreased alcohol intake*: In a meta-analysis of 14 randomized controlled trials of reduced alcohol consumption, investigators found that alcohol reduction was associated with an average decrease in SBP/DBP of 3.3/2 mm Hg. The effect was robust and was detected even when the analysis was restricted to only high-quality, long-term studies, including either hypertensive or normotensive participants
- *Weight loss*: Numerous studies have demonstrated reductions in BP with weight loss. In a meta-analysis of 25 studies, for every kilogram of weight lost, there was a drop in SBP/DBP of 1.1/0.9 mm Hg. A second meta-analysis looked at the change in BP related to weight loss over time and found that the peak effect on BP comes soon after the weight loss and the effect attenuates over time
- *Increased physical activity*: Aerobic exercise has been shown to lower SBP/DBP by an average of 3/2 mm Hg. The effect attenuates in studies of longer duration and in studies with less stringent verification of adherence. In a study on the dose effect of exercise, greater hypotensive effect was found with 61–90 minutes compared with 30–60 minutes a week. More than 90 minutes was not more effective than 61–90 minutes. While minutes per week did influence SBP, the DBP was not affected and the frequency of exercise did not alter the BP effect. In a separate study by the same team, increased age attenuated the BP effects of exercise but gender did not.

TARGET GOALS AND TREATMENT RECOMMENDATIONS FOR HYPERTENSION BASED ON EIGHT JOINT NATIONAL COMMITTEE (JNC 8) GUIDELINES

The JNC 8 guidelines have made recommendations for treatment targets and treatment choices (Fig. 8.1):

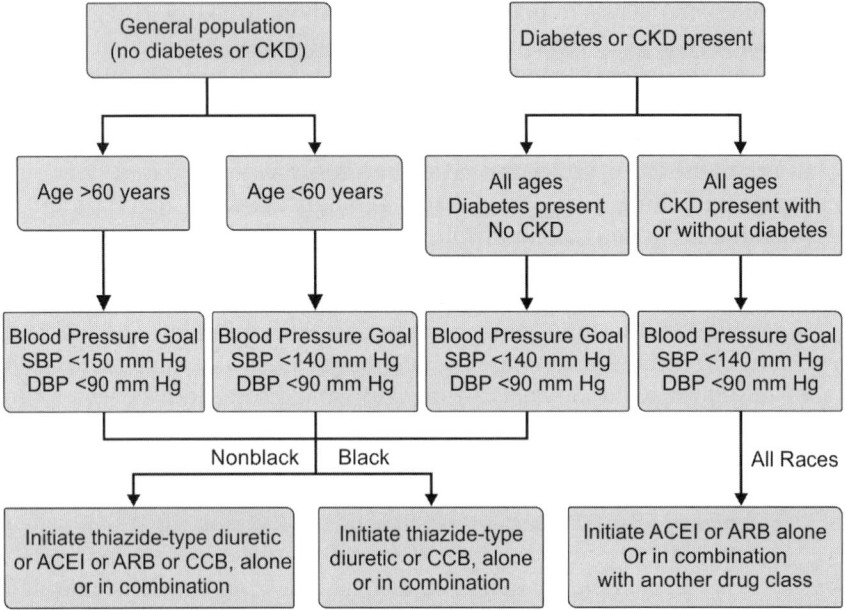

Fig. 8.1: Hypertension management algorithm.

Source: Adapted from James PA, Oparil S, Carter BL, Cushman W, Dennison-Himmelfarb C, Handler J, et al. Evidence-based guideline for the management of high blood pressure in adults: report from the panel members appointed to the eighth Joint National Committee (JNC 8). JAMA. 2014;311(5):507-20.

- In non-black populations, first-line agents include thiazide diuretics, calcium channel blockers (CCB) and angiotensin-converting enzyme inhibitors (ACE-I) or angiotensin receptor blocker (ARB)
- In black populations, first-line agents include thiazide diuretics or CCB.
- In the CKD population (black or non-black) with and without proteinuria, first-line therapy is ACE-I or ARB. This is aimed at curtailing the progression of CKD. Cardiovascular and cerebrovascular outcomes were not different between ACE-I/ARB versus β-blockers or CCB in this population
- There are no differences in recommendations for first-line therapy in the diabetic population compared with the standard, nondiabetic population
- There are no differences between ACE-I and ARB, but they should not be used together.

Primary endpoints evaluated by investigators include CV disease, cerebrovascular disease and CKD. Thiazides, CCB, ACE-I and ARBs had no statistical difference in these outcomes. Beta-blockers are no longer recommended as first-line agents for hypertension as evidence suggests this medication has an increased risk of cerebrovascular outcomes compared with the first-line agents. Alpha-blockers are also not first-line medications. In a clinical trial, the α-blocker arm was terminated early due to an increased risk for stroke and heart failure. No clinical trials have been performed to compare vasodilating agents (such as hydralazine and minoxidil), spironolactone, centrally acting agents (such as clonidine or guanfacine), aliskiren or

Table 8.3: Dosing for anti-hypertensive drugs.

	Initial daily dose, mg	Target dose, mg	Number of doses per day
ACE inhibitors			
Captopril	50	150–200	2
Enalapril	5	20	1–2
Lisinopril	10	40	1
ARBs			
Eprosartan	400	600–800	1–2
Candesartan	4	12–32	1
Losartan	50	100	1–2
Valsartan	40–80	160–320	1
Irbesartan	75	300	1
Beta-blockers			
Atenolol	25–50	100	1
Metoprolol	50	100–200	1–2
CCB			
Amlodipine	2.5	10	1
Diltiazem extended release	120–180	360	1
Nitrendipine	10	20	1–2
Thiazide-type diuretics			
Bendroflumethiazide	5	10	1
Chlorthalidone	12.5	12.5–25	1
Hydrochlorothiazide	12.5–25	25–50	1–2
Indapamide	1.25	1.25–2.5	1

ACE, angiotensin converting enzyme; ARB, angiotensin receptor blocker; CCB, calcium channel blocker.

Source: Adapted from James PA, Oparil S, Carter BL, Cushman W, Dennison-Himmelfarb C, Handler J, et al. Evidence-based guideline for the management of high blood pressure in adults: report from the panel members appointed to the eighth Joint National Committee (JNC 8). JAMA. 2014;311(5):507-20.

furosemide to the first-line agents in primary essential hypertension, and thus they are not recommended as first-line agents.

The JNC 8 guidelines provide recommendations for initial and target doses of specific medications used for the treatment of hypertension (Table 8.3).

MECHANISMS OF ACTION FOR THE PHARMACOLOGIC TREATMENT OF HYPERTENSION

- *Renin-angiotensin system antagonists*
  - ACE-I (e.g. lisinopril) impedes ACE activity and impairs the production of angiotensin II (AII). Angiotensin II stimulates renal Na^+ reabsorption and is a potent vasoconstrictor. Angiotensin II is also the predominant stimulus for the secretion of aldosterone, which promotes renal Na^+

reabsorption. These effects of AII and aldosterone collectively raise BP and may be involved in the pathogenesis of cardiac remodeling that can occur with hypertension.
  - ARBs (e.g. irbesartan) block the AT angiotensin (AT)$_1$ receptor.
  - Renin inhibitors, such as aliskiren are approved but not widely used.
- *Diuretics*
  - *Thiazide diuretics*, such as hydrochlorothiazide (HCTZ) and chlorthalidone, block the Na$^+$-Cl$^-$ cotransporter (NCC) that is expressed within the distal region of the nephron. The NCC facilitates the reabsorption of Na$^+$, Cl$^-$ and Ca^{2+} while stimulating K$^+$ secretion within the distal nephron. Despite the common misconception, the antihypertensive effect of HCTZ does not result from volume reduction per se; in fact, the mechanism of action for the antihypertensive effect of thiazide diuretics is not fully understood.
  - *Loop diuretics*, such as furosemide, inhibit Na$^+$, Cl$^-$ and K$^+$ reabsorption within the thick ascending limb of the nephron.
  - *Potassium-sparing diuretics*, such as spironolactone and amiloride, target the aldosterone-sensitive distal nephron to impair aldosterone-dependent Na$^+$ reabsorption. By blocking aldosterone activity, these diuretics also conserve potassium.
- *Alpha 1-antagonists* (e.g. prazosin) block α1 adrenoceptor-mediated vasoconstriction
- *Beta-blockers* (e.g. atenolol) impede activation of type B$_1$ adrenoceptors and thus down modulate sympathetic nervous system effects within the sino-atrial (SA) node and myocardium.
- *Calcium channel blockers*
  - Non-dihydropyridine CCBs (e.g. verapamil) bind more preferentially to L-type channels in the open state and thus more preferentially impair channel activity in the SA node to induce a mild negative inotropic effect.
  - Dihydropyridine CCBs (e.g. amlodipine) have a high affinity for L-type Ca^{2+} channels in the inactivate state and therefore preferentially bind to L-type channels in vascular smooth muscle. By preventing Ca^{2+} entry into vascular smooth muscle, these agents impede vasoconstriction.
- *Direct vasodilators* reduce arteriolar constriction. Minoxidil opens ATP-dependent K$^+$ channels. This mechanism hyperpolarizes the vascular smooth muscle cells, and in so doing, voltage-sensitive Ca^{2+} channels are closed. The mechanism of action for hydralazine is poorly understood.
- *Centrally acting drugs* (e.g. methyldopa) activate type α2 adrenoceptor activity, which attenuates sympathetic outflow.

RESISTANT HYPERTENSION

Resistant hypertension is defined by any one of the following:
- The failure to achieve BP <40/90 despite the use of three antihypertensives at adequate doses (i.e. 50% or more of the maximum recommended antihypertensive dose or highest tolerated dose) including one diuretic

- The failure to lower BP <140/90 in a patient with diabetes mellitus or CKD or
- The need for four or more BP-lowering agents to control BP
  The incidence of resistant hypertension may be as high as 10–20% of the hypertensive population. Common characteristics of those with resistant hypertension include older age, obesity, presence of obstructive sleep apnea or other sleep disordered breathing disorders, diabetes mellitus, chronic kidney disease, female sex, African American race and high consumers of sodium in diet. Many patients will have evidence of left ventricular hypertrophy on echocardiogram or ECG. Those with resistant hypertension have a greater risk of end-organ effects including heart failure, stroke, myocardial infarction and renal failure. There may be >50% increased risk of adverse CV outcomes compared with the hypertensive population that is better controlled on medications.
- *Evaluation and treatment of resistant hypertension*
  To maintain a framework for the evaluation of resistant hypertension, the following steps are recommended:
  - Establish the diagnosis of resistant hypertension as defined above with the use of ambulatory BP monitoring.
  - Determine if the patient is compliant with home medications and diet. Before one seeks out secondary causes of hypertension, screen for medication compliance and reinforce weight loss, cessation of alcohol and improved diet.
  - Evaluate effects of other prescribed and over-the-counter medications. Frequently used medications that increase BP include nonsteroidal anti-inflammatory drugs (NSAIDs), COX-2 inhibitors, weight loss agents, stimulants including nicotine and amphetamines, oral contraceptives (at least 30–35 μg), testosterone, cough suppressants and nasal sprays containing pseudoephedrine. If patients are taking certain herbal supplements, dose adjustment or elimination of these agents alone can allow for optimal BP control.
  - Optimize medication regimen and intensify as needed. Antihypertensive drugs typically complement each other; however, there are some combinations which tend to be more favorable. Diuretics are often underutilized antihypertensive agents. In the African American Study of Kidney Disease and Hypertension trial, only 60% of patients were taking diuretics. By decreasing intravascular volume and increasing natriuresis, the use of diuretics in appropriate doses may improve the efficacy of other antihypertensive agents. Hydrochlorothiazide and chlorthalidone are the main thiazide diuretics used to control BP. Although chlorthalidone and HCTZ are both once daily dosing, chlorthalidone has a longer half-life and therefore theoretically may provide more sustained BP control. However, recent data show that each is equally efficacious with no difference in CV outcomes. The effectiveness of thiazide diuretics as an antihypertensive agent is lost in CKD patients once the glomerular filtration rate drops <30 mL/min/1.73 m^2. Loop diuretics should be considered as an alternative to thiazides for further management of hypertension.

Data support the use of spironolactone as the next best agent to use in resistant hypertension after having failed maximal therapy with ACE-I, CCB and diuretics. Among patients already on a typical triple drug combination of ACE-I/ARB, CCB and a thiazide diuretic, the addition of spironolactone improves BP control. Hyperkalemia with potassium level >4.5 mmol/L is a contraindication to spironolactone use. In these cases, one should increase dose of diuretic therapy. In patients who have adverse effects from spironolactone including gynecomastia, breast tenderness and erectile dysfunction, eplerenone has been shown to provide similar reductions in BP with a better side effect profile when compared with spironolactone.

The use of other agents, such as centrally acting α agonists and direct vasodilators may have some utility in this setting.

In the setting of resistant hypertension, all healthcare providers should focus on simplifying their patients' medication regimens. One should use combination tablets and once daily dosing when possible. Also, generic medications should be used to reduce out-of-pocket costs. These efforts will improve patient compliance and ultimately allow better control of their hypertension.

EVALUATION FOR SECONDARY CAUSES OF HYPERTENSION

Resistant hypertension classically suggests the need to pursue an evaluation for secondary causes of hypertension. Yet, there are other reasons to suspect a secondary cause of hypertension. When an underlying secondary cause is identified, treatment can be drastically different than it would be for resistant or refractory hypertension. Patients should be examined for physical signs of secondary hypertensin and target organ damage (Table 8.4).

Awareness of clinical clues is the key for pursuing and evaluation and diagnosis of secondary hypertension:
- Severe hypertension at a young age (age of onset <20–30 years in absence of family history and obesity) or older age (onset >50 years)

Table 8.4: Signs and symptoms of secondary causes of hypertension

Sign or symptom	Consider
Abdominal bruit	Renovascular HTN
Heat or cold intolerance	Thyroid disease
Snoring or daytime somnolence	Sleep apnea
Headache, palpitations, pallor or perspiration	Pheochromocytoma
Decreased lower extremity blood pressure	Aortic coarctation
Truncal obesity, purple striae or goiter	Cushing's syndrome
Target organ damage	
Retinal hemorrhage	Retinal damage
Abnormal point of maximal impulse on cardiac examination	Left ventricular hypertrophy

- Hypertension refractory to medical management or, if once responsive, it becomes difficult to control
- Episode of hypertensive crisis or paroxysmal BP elevations
- Symptoms or signs related to the underlying disease (e.g. muscle weakness, episodes of tachycardia, sweating, tremor, thinning of skin and flank pain)
- Significant hypertension and unprovoked hypokalemia and metabolic alkalosis
- Loud snoring, awakening with headache and sleeping inappropriately throughout day

WHAT ARE COMMON CAUSES OF SECONDARY HYPERTENSION

- *Renal*: CKD and renal artery stenosis
  - *Renovascular hypertension* is a common cause of hypertensive crisis in elderly patients. Clinical clues that indicate renal artery stenosis include rise in serum creatinine upon starting an ACE-I or ARB, past history of coronary artery disease or peripheral vascular disease, asymmetry between kidney sizes of at least 1.5 cm on imaging and, certainly, abdominal bruits noted on physical examination. Ultrasound with Doppler studies is done as a screening test. A peripheral angiogram is done to confirm suspicion. However, it is prudent to only use this level of investigation when someone is a candidate for an invasive interventional procedure. Otherwise, medical treatment is recommended even if a diagnosis is suspected but not fully confirmed.
- *Endocrine*: Hypercortisolism, hyperaldosteronism, growth hormone excess, pheochromocytoma, hyperthyroidism, and hypothyroidism
  - *Hypertension with hypokalemia* is another clinical entity that suggests a secondary cause of hypertension. This clinical picture can be divided into three categories on the basis of serum renin and aldosterone levels.
    - *High renin and high aldosterone*: Renin-secreting tumor, renal artery stenosis and coarctation of aorta
    - *High aldosterone and low renin*: Primary hyperaldosteronism (idiopathic, adrenal source (adenoma, carcinoma, hyperplasia), or ectopic (ovarian tumor)
    - *Low aldosterone and low renin*: Hypercortisolism or state of apparent mineralocorticoid excess (e.g. ingestions of black licorice, 11 β-hydroxysteroid dehydrogenase deficiency and Liddle's syndrome)
  - *Others*: Obstructive sleep apnea, coarctation of aorta and intracranial tumors.

HOW DOES ONE DIAGNOSE AND TREAT PRIMARY HYPERALDOSTERONISM?

This entity is more common than many expect. On the basis of a series of trials, it is estimated that a hyperaldosteronism state is a contributor in

17–23% of resistant hypertension cases. Although hypokalemia makes a hyperaldosteronism state suspicious, low potassium is only present in about 50% of cases.
- Screen plasma aldosterone concentration (PAC) and plasma renin concentration
  - Spironolactone, eplerenone and amiloride should be discontinued 6 weeks before testing
- Calculate aldosterone-renin ratio (ARR)
  - ARR <20 ng/dL reliably excludes hyperaldosteronism
  - ARR >20 ng/dL is suggestive, but not diagnostic
  - Note: PAC must be >15 ng/dL for the diagnosis
- Confirmatory test with 24-hour urine collection
  - First prepare for the test by administering a 1-L normal saline intravenous bolus the night before the test as an inpatient or encourage high sodium meals day before test. This is done to expand the intravascular volume in attempt to suppress aldosterone
  - Begin the collection in the morning by first emptying the bladder and discarding that urine. This marks time 0. Then collect urine by keeping collected urine refrigerated
  - Assess urine aldosterone levels and urine sodium levels. Urine sodium >200 mEq confirms proper salt load before testing. Urine aldosterone >12 µg confirms inappropriately high urinary excretion of aldosterone in spite of high dietary salt intakes.
- Computed tomography (CT) of adrenals to evaluate for mass
  - If no mass is identified or inconclusive, consider adrenal vein sampling.
  - For a unilateral nodule, determine the suspicion for aldosterone-producing adenoma (APA) versus nonfunctioning adenoma versus carcinoma:
    - Suspect APA if age <40 years, nodule >1 cm, and if mass intensity on CT is <10 Hounsfield units
    - Suspect carcinoma if large (i.e. >4 cm), mass CT intensity is >10 Hounsfield units or with mixed attenuation
    - Nonfunctioning adenomas are more common with advancing age. If >40 years old, it is important to evaluate for a nonfunctioning adenoma
    - APA and carcinoma are treated with surgery
    - To evaluate for nonfunctioning adenoma, perform adrenal vein sampling to determine lateralization of mass. If sampling lateralizes, then treat surgically, and if no lateralization then treat medically.
  - For multinodular or if diffusely enlarged (and no nodule) then the mass is more likely to be benign
    - If patient is a surgical candidate, consider adrenal vein sampling with lateralization to determine surgical intervention.
    - If not a surgical candidate, or if patient wishes to pursue medical treatment first, one can safely forego adrenal vein sampling.
- Medical treatment
  - Aldosterone antagonist, such as spironolactone or eplerenone is recommended if no concern for carcinoma.

- Although it is important to check biochemical parameters to ascertain aldosterone excess to ultimately identify those with adrenal adenomas or carcinomas, the contribution of hyperaldosteronism to hypertension may be greater than indicated by hormone levels alone.
- Levels of aldosterone, renin, ARR and urine aldosterone are not necessarily predictive of BP response to aldosterone blockade. Spironolactone or other aldosterone blockers are therefore a cornerstone of treatment in resistant or refractory hypertension.

SUGGESTED READING

1. Chobanian AV, Bakris GL, Black HR, Cushman WC, Green LA, Izzo JL Jr., et al. Seventh report of the Joint National Committee on prevention, detection, evaluation, and treatment of high blood pressure. Hypertension. 2003;42:1206-52.
2. Dhalla IA, Gomes T, Yao Z, Nagge J, Persaud N, Hellings C, et al. Chlorthalidone versus hydrochlorothiazide for the treatment of hypertension in older adults: a population-based cohort study. Ann Intern Med. 2013;158(6):447-55.
3. Egan BM, Zhao Y, Axon RN. US trends in prevalence, awareness, treatment, and control of hypertension, 1988-2008. JAMA. 2010;303(20):2043-50.
4. Fan HQ, Li Y, Thijs L, Hansen TW, Boggia J, Kikuya M, et al. Prognostic value of isolated nocturnal hypertension on ambulatory measurement in 8711 individuals from 10 populations. J Hypertens. 2010;28(10):2036-45.
5. Gaddam KK, Nishizaka MK, Pratt-Ubunama MN, Pimenta E, Aban I, Oparil S, et al. Characterization of resistant hypertension: association between resistant hypertension, aldosterone, and persistent intravascular volume expansion. Arch Intern Med. 2008;168(11):1159-64.
6. Gus M, Fuchs FD, Pimentel M, Rosa D, Melo AG, Moreira LB. Behavior of ambulatory blood pressure surrounding episodes of headache in mildly hypertensive patients. Arch Intern Med. 2001;161(2):252-5.
7. James PA, Oparil S, Carter BL, Cushman W, Dennison-Himmelfarb C, Handler J, et al. Evidence-based guideline for the management of high blood pressure in adults: Report from the panel members appointed to the eighth Joint National Committee (JNC 8). JAMA. 2014;311(5):507-20.
8. Myat A, Redwood SR, Qureshi AC, Spertus JA, Williams B. Resistant hypertension. BMJ. 2012;345:e7473.
9. Reboldi G, Gentile G, Angeli F, Verdecchia P. Choice of ACE inhibitor combinations in hypertensive patients with type 2 diabetes: update after recent clinical trials. Vasc Health Risk Manag. 2009;5:411-27.
10. Pierdomenico SD, Cuccurullo F. Prognostic value of white-coat and masked hypertension diagnosed by ambulatory monitoring in initially untreated subjects: an updated meta-analysis. Am J Hypertens. 2011;24(1):52-8.
11. Weber MA, Schiffrin EL, White WB, Mann S, Lindholm LH, Kenerson JG, et al. Clinical practice guidelines for the management of hypertension in the community: statement by the American Society of Hypertension and the International Society of Hypertension. J Hypertens. 2014;32(1):3-15.
12. Wright JT Jr., Bakris G, Greene T, Agodoa LY, Appel LJ, Charleston J, et al. Effect of blood pressure lowering and antihypertensive drug class on progression of hypertensive kidney disease: results from the AASK trial. JAMA. 2002;288(19):2421-31.
13. Young WF Jr., Mattson C. Primary aldosteronism: diagnostic and treatment strategies. Nat Clin Pract Nephrol. 2006;2(4):198-208.

Essentials of Pulmonary Hypertension

9
Chapter

Rudhir Tandon, Sif Hansdottir

INTRODUCTION

Pulmonary hypertension (PH) is a complex disorder that causes premature disability and death for many. The subject of pulmonary hypertension has been a topic for extensive investigation over the last two decades, and many new treatment options have become available. In this chapter, we first discuss the World Health Organization (WHO) classification system of pulmonary hypertension. In this system, underlying etiologies for PH that share similar pathology, hemodynamics and management options are grouped together. We also emphasize and review the detailed work-up that is essential to correctly categorize and manage a patient with PH. Treatment strategies vary greatly and pulmonary arterial hypertension (PAH) approved drugs are only indicated for patients with WHO group-1 PAH, whereas the mainstay of treatment for other types of PH is to optimally manage the underlying etiologies. Finally, we discuss treatment guidelines and follow-up with the main focus being management of WHO group-1 PAH.

CLINICAL CLASSIFICATION AND EPIDEMIOLOGY

Pulmonary hypertension was previously classified as primary or secondary based on the presence of identified causes or risk factors. The WHO established a new clinical classification system based on similar pathological findings, hemodynamic characteristics and management in 1998. This system has subsequently undergone several revisions, most recently at the 2013 Nice World Symposium on Pulmonary Hypertension (Table 9.1).

WHO group-1 PAH encompasses a group of conditions that have been shown to respond favorably to Food and Drug Administration (FDA) approved therapies. Idiopathic PAH is a relatively rare disease. Recent epidemiologic data suggest that the prevalence of PAH may be up to 15 per million, with a prevalence of idiopathic PAH of about 6 per million. Idiopathic PAH is a diagnosis of exclusion and should only be made after a thorough diagnostic work-up has been completed to rule out other known etiologies of PH. Hereditary PAH has been reported in approximately 6–10% of patients with PAH. Pulmonary arterial hypertension can be induced by certain drugs and toxins, in particular weight loss stimulant drugs (e.g. aminorex and

Table 9.1: Classification of pulmonary hypertension (WHO)

1. Pulmonary arterial hypertension
    - 1.1 Idiopathic PAH
    - 1.2 Heritable PAH
        - 1.2.1 BMPR2
        - 1.2.2 ALK-1, ENG, SMAD-9, CAV1, KCNK3
        - 1.2.3 Unknown
    - 1.3 Drug and toxin induced
    - 1.4 Associated with
        - 1.4.1 Connective tissue diseases
        - 1.4.2 HIV infection
        - 1.4.3 Portal hypertension
        - 1.4.4 Congenital heart diseases
        - 1.4.5 Schistosomiasis

1' Pulmonary veno-occlusive disease and/or pulmonary capillary hemangiomatosis

1" Persistent pulmonary hypertension of the newborn

2. Pulmonary hypertension due to left heart disease
    - 2.1 Left ventricular systolic dysfunction
    - 2.2 Left ventricular diastolic dysfunction
    - 2.3 Valvular disease
    - 2.4 Congenital/acquired left heart inflow/outflow tract obstruction and congenital cardiomyopathies

3. Pulmonary hypertension due to lung diseases and/or hypoxia
    - 3.1 Chronic obstructive pulmonary disease
    - 3.2 Interstitial lung disease
    - 3.3 Other pulmonary diseases with mixed restrictive and obstructive pattern
    - 3.4 Sleep-disordered breathing
    - 3.5 Alveolar hypoventilation disorders
    - 3.6 Chronic exposure to high altitude
    - 3.7 Developmental lung diseases

4. Chronic thromboembolic pulmonary hypertension

5. Pulmonary hypertension with unclear multifactorial mechanisms
    - 5.1 Hematologic disorders: chronic hemolytic anemia, myeloproliferative disorders and splenectomy
    - 5.2 Systemic disorders: sarcoidosis, pulmonary histiocytosis and lymphangioleiomyomatosis
    - 5.3 Metabolic disorders: glycogen storage disease, Gaucher's disease and thyroid disorders
    - 5.4 Others: tumoral obstruction, fibrosing mediastinitis, chronic renal failure and segmental PH

WHO, World Health Organization; BMPR, bone morphogenetic protein receptor type II; CAV1, caveolin-1; ENG, endoglin.

Source: Adapted from Simonneau G, Gatzoulis MA, Adatia I. Updated clinical classification of pulmonary hypertension. J Am Coll Cardiol 2013;62:D34–41. Reprinted with permission from Elsevier Ltd.

fenfluramine), and likely with amphetamines and dasatinib. Finally, PAH can be associated with connective tissue disease, human immunodeficiency virus (HIV), portal hypertension, congenital heart diseases or schistosomiasis. Among connective tissue diseases, pulmonary arteriopathy is best established in patients with the limited cutaneous form of systemic sclerosis but can also be seen in systemic lupus erythematosus and mixed connective tissue disease. The incidence of PAH in individuals with HIV is approximately 0.5% and has not declined significantly with aggressive antiretroviral therapy. Hemodynamic studies have estimated the prevalence of PAH in 2–6% of patients with portal hypertension; however, the prevalence may be higher in patients referred for liver transplantation. It is estimated that 10% of adults with congenital heart disease have PAH. Patients with volume and pressure overload due to ventricular shunts are at higher risk of developing early PAH than patients with volume overload only (e.g. interatrial shunts).

WHO group-2 PH is the most common cause of PH and includes PH secondary to any disorder that elevates left heart filling pressures, including systolic dysfunction, diastolic dysfunction, left-sided valvular heart disease and congenital or acquired left heart inflow/outflow obstruction. The presence of PH in patients with elevated left ventricular (LV) filling pressure predicts worse outcomes and higher mortality rate. Compared with PAH, patients with PH due to left heart disease are more often older, female and with a history of systemic hypertension, and most have features of metabolic syndrome. Heart failure with preserved ejection fraction is the predominant cause of elevated left-sided filling pressures resulting in PH.

WHO group-3 PH includes patients with chronic obstructive lung disease, sleep-disordered breathing and diffuse parenchymal lung diseases, including idiopathic pulmonary fibrosis. Patients with combined pulmonary fibrosis and emphysema are particularly prone to the development of PH.

Once considered rare, chronic thromboembolic pulmonary hypertension has been shown to complicate 3.8% of acute pulmonary embolic events and is categorized as WHO group-4 PH.

Pulmonary hypertension may also occur in association with several different hematological, systemic and metabolic disorders, as outlined in WHO group-5 under unclear multifactorial mechanism.

HEMODYNAMIC CLASSIFICATION

Pulmonary hypertension is defined as a mean pulmonary artery pressure (mPAP) ≥25 mm Hg at rest. Pulmonary hypertension can be further categorized based on left heart filling pressure, as either precapillary or postcapillary. Precapillary PH is defined as mPAP ≥25 mm Hg, pulmonary artery wedge pressure (PAWP) ≤15 mm Hg and elevated pulmonary vascular resistance (PVR) (i.e. >3 Wood units). WHO groups 1, 3, 4 and 5 PH are all precapillary and are not distinguishable by hemodynamics. Higher PAWP values are indicative of left heart disease and WHO group-2 postcapillary PH. It should be noted that this classification is not absolute, and patients with well-compensated WHO group-2 PH can have a resting PAWP ≤15 mm Hg and patients with severe PAH may present with mildly elevated PAWP values. A challenge with 500 mL of fluid administered intravenously over 5–10 minutes may unmask patients with a left heart problem and a high normal PAWP at baseline and may help reduce the number of inappropriate diagnoses of PAH in this patient population.

PATHOLOGY AND PATHOGENESIS

Pulmonary hypertension develops as a result of obstructive lung vasculopathy leading to restricted flow through the pulmonary vasculature, increased PVR and ultimately right heart failure. The predominant cause of increased PVR is loss of vascular luminal cross section due to vascular remodeling produced by excessive cell proliferation and reduced rates of apoptosis, although excessive vasoconstriction plays a significant role in approximately 20% of patients. Abnormalities of three major pathways (i.e. the prostacyclin, endothelin and nitric oxide pathways) have been established as being important in the development and progression of PAH. Sustained pulmonary vasoconstriction from increased endothelin levels, decreased nitric oxide levels and/or decreased prostacyclin levels culminate in intimal hyperplasia and fibrosis, medial hypertrophy from excessive smooth muscle cell proliferation, in situ thrombosis of small pulmonary arteries and arterioles and plexiform lesions, characteristic of idiopathic and hereditary PAH (Fig. 9.1). Disordered metabolism and mitochondrial structure, inflammation, autoimmunity and dysregulation of growth factors further contribute to this proliferative, apoptosis-resistant and vasoconstrictive state, leading to macrophage-promoted remodeling and increased PVR.

GENETICS

Pulmonary arterial hypertension is inherited in <10% of cases. Mutations in bone morphogenetic protein receptor 2 (BMPR2) have been reported in approximately 75% of hereditary PAH, and 11–40% of those with idiopathic PAH. The BMPR2 is a member of the transforming growth factor-β super family, which induces apoptosis and thus its abnormality leads to excessive endothelial cell proliferation. It is inherited in an autosomal dominant pattern with incomplete penetrance and genetic anticipation. Pathogenic mutations in several other genes have been identified, including mutations in the *endoglin* gene (which expresses a protein involved in vasculogenesis), the *SMAD8* gene (which expresses an intracellular signaling molecule), the *caveolin-1* gene (which encodes a membrane protein abundant in the

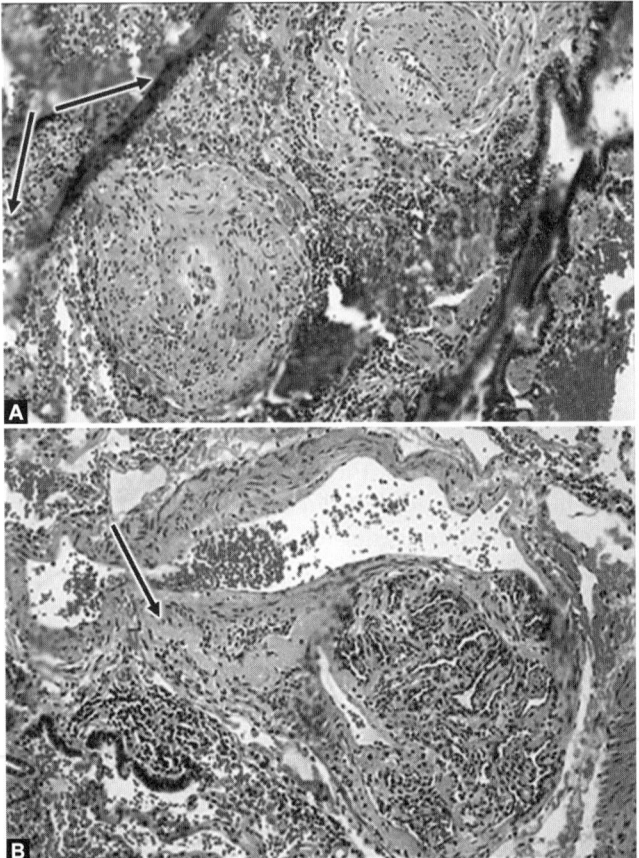

Fig. 9.1: H&E stained section (200 X) of pulmonary artery in a patient with idiopathic PAH. (A) Concentric laminar intimal fibrosis (arrows) characterized by markedly thickened intima with dramatically narrowed lumen; (B) Complex glomeruloid vascular structures (arrow) originating from pulmonary arteries (plexiform lesion), characteristic of idiopathic PAH and hereditary PAH *(For color version, see Plate 2)*

pulmonary endothelial cells) and the *KCNK3* gene (which affects potassium ion channels).

DIAGNOSIS

Pulmonary hypertension often presents with nonspecific symptoms, which can be difficult to dissociate from those caused by a known underlying pulmonary or cardiac disorder. A high index of suspicion, a meticulous history and a careful physical examination are paramount to the diagnosis of PH. Particular attention should be given to previous medical conditions, drug use (legal and illegal), risk factors for HIV or hepatitis and family history. All patients with PH should undergo a comprehensive diagnostic evaluation to clarify the etiology in order to identify underlying treatable causes and initiate appropriate therapies (Fig. 9.2).

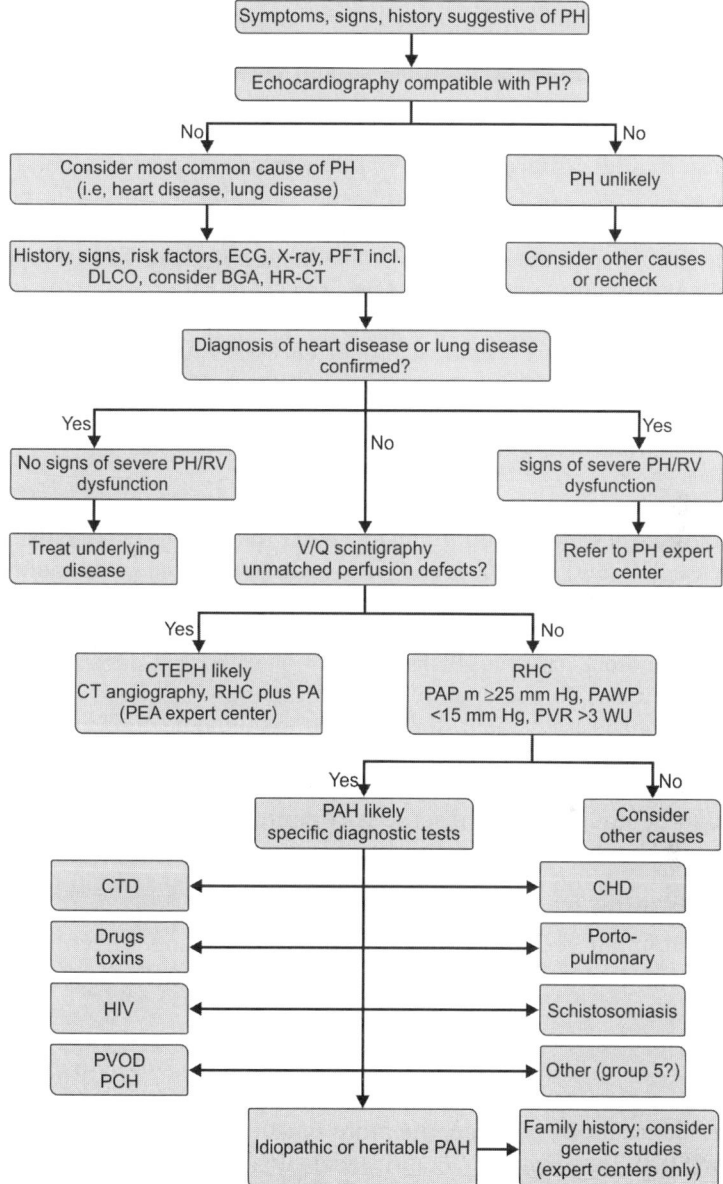

Fig. 9.2: Algorithm for evaluation of suspected pulmonary hypertension

BGA, blood gas analysis; CHD, congenital heart disease; CTD, connective tissue disease; CTEPH, chronic thromboembolic pulmonary hypertension; DLCO, diffusion capacity of the lung for carbon monoxide; ECG, electrocardiogram; HR-CT, high-resolution computed tomography; PA, pulmonary angiography; PAH, pulmonary arterial hypertension; PAPm, mean pulmonary artery pressure; PAWP, pulmonary arterial wedge pressure; PCH, pulmonary capillary hemangiomatosis; PEA, pulmonary endarterectomy; PFT, pulmonary function testing; PH, pulmonary hypertension; PVOD, pulmonary veno-occlusive disease; PVR, pulmonary vascular resistance; RHC, right heart catheter; RV, right ventricle; V/Q, ventilation/perfusion; X-ray, chest radiograph.

Source: Adapted from Hoeper MM, Bogaard HJ, Condliffe R, Frantz R, Khanna D, Kurzyna M, et al. Definitions and diagnosis of pulmonary hypertension. J Am Coll Cardiol 2013;62(25):D42-50. Reprinted *with permission* from Elsevier Ltd.

- *Clinical presentation*
  Pulmonary hypertension should be suspected in the patient with otherwise unexplained dyspnea on exertion, fatigue, weakness, syncope, chest pain and/or signs of right ventricular (RV) dysfunction, such as lower extremity edema. Physical examination findings supportive of PH include left parasternal lift, an accentuated pulmonary component of second heart sound, a pansystolic murmur of tricuspid regurgitation, a diastolic murmur of pulmonary insufficiency and an RV third heart sound. Jugular vein distension, hepatomegaly, peripheral edema, ascites and cool extremities characterize more advanced disease. The examination may also provide clues as to the underlying cause of PH. Telangiectasia, digital ulceration and sclerodactyly are seen in scleroderma. Spider nevi, testicular atrophy and palmar erythema point toward liver disease. Orthopnea or murmurs suggestive of aortic stenosis or mitral regurgitation point toward left heart disease, while inspiratory crackles may point toward interstitial lung disease.
- *Laboratory evaluation*
  Serological testing is important to detect underlying connective tissue disease, HIV and liver disease. Of note is that up to 40% of patients with idiopathic PAH may have elevated antinuclear antibodies, usually in low titer (1:80). Connective tissue diseases are diagnosed primarily on clinical and laboratory criteria. Patients with elevated antinuclear antibody and suspicious clinical features should undergo further serological and rheumatologic assessment. The HIV testing should be done in all patients with risk factors. Up to 2% of individuals with liver disease may have associated PAH, and therefore liver function tests and hepatitis serologies should be done. Thyroid disease is commonly seen in PH, and thyroid function should be checked. Biochemical markers are another noninvasive tool to assess and monitor RV dysfunction in patients. Brain natriuretic peptide (BNP) (cleaved into N-terminal (NT)-proBNP) is released from myocardium in response to wall stress. Both BNP and NT-proBNP levels have been shown to correlate with severe RV dysfunction and increased mortality.
- *Electrocardiography*
  The electrocardiogram (ECG) may demonstrate signs of RV hypertrophy, such as tall right precordial R waves, right axis deviation and RV strain. The higher the PA pressure, the more sensitive is the ECG. The ECG has insufficient sensitivity (55%) and specificity (70%) to be a screening tool for detecting significant PH.
- *Chest radiography*
  The chest radiograph is inferior to the ECG in detecting PH, but it may show central PA dilatation and pruning of peripheral blood vessels. Right atrium (RA) and RV enlargement may be seen in advanced cases. Pulmonary edema and pleural effusion are generally indicative of elevated left heart filling pressures and WHO group-2 PH.
- *Pulmonary function tests and arterial blood gases*
  Pulmonary function tests are essential to look for airflow obstruction or restrictive pulmonary pathology. Patients with PAH usually have decreased

lung diffusion capacity for carbon monoxide (40–80% of predicted typically) and mild to moderate reduction in lung volumes. Pulse oximetry should be done to look for oxygen desaturation at rest, during exercise and at night. Arterial blood gases analysis might be helpful to exclude hypoxia and acidosis as contributors to PH.

- *Echocardiography*
  Patients with suspected PH should undergo two-dimensional echocardiography with Doppler flow studies. Transthoracic echocardiography may help identify the cause of PH (e.g. valvular heart disease, LV heart failure or congenital heart disease) and the severity of disease (RV function and estimation of RV systolic pressure). Echocardiographic findings of severe PAH are featured in Figure 9.3. The estimation of systolic PAP is based on the peak velocity of the jet of tricuspid regurgitation using a simplified Bernoulli equation [since the RV/RA pressure gradient is calculated from the equation: 4 × (tricuspid regurgitation velocity)^2] and then adding the estimated RA pressure. In the absence of other major risk factors for PH, such as left heart disease or advanced lung disease, an estimated RV systolic pressure of >35–40 mm Hg requires further evaluation in a patient with unexplained dyspnea.

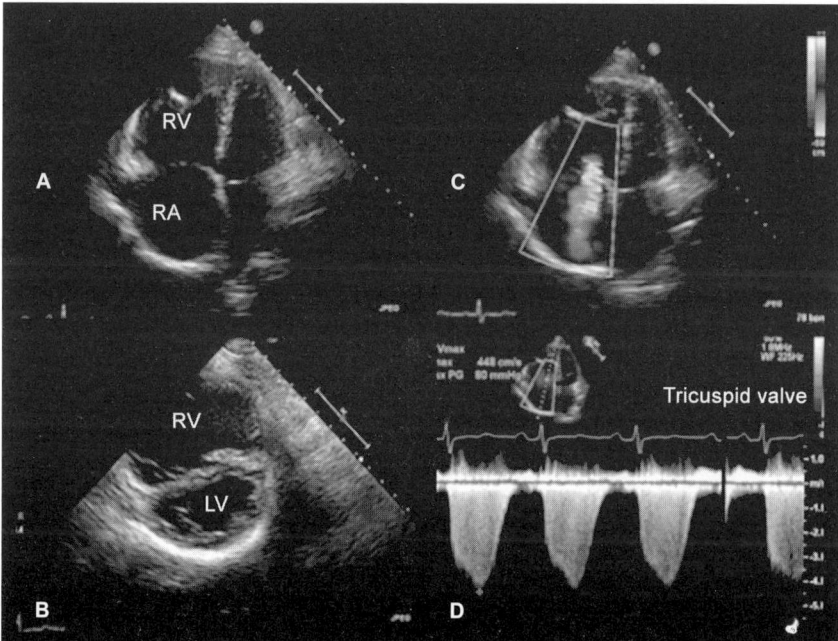

Fig. 9.3: Echocardiographic images of a patient with severe pulmonary arterial hypertension. (A) The four-chamber view shows marked enlargement of the right atrium (RA) and right ventricle (RV) as a result of elevated pulmonary artery pressures; (B) Short axis view at the level of the mitral chordae shows dilation of the RV chamber and flattened interventricular septum and "D-shaped" left ventricle (LV), suggestive of pressure overload in the RV; (C) Four-chamber view with color Doppler showing tricuspid regurgitation; (D) The continuous wave Doppler measures a peak velocity of 448 cm/s across the tricuspid valve, predicting a RV/RA peak gradient of 80 mm Hg, consistent with severe pulmonary hypertension

- *Right heart catheterization*
  Right heart catheterization (RHC) is mandatory to establish diagnosis of PH to assess the severity of hemodynamic dysfunction and to test the vasoreactivity of the pulmonary circulation. The following variables must be recorded during a diagnostic RHC: PAP (systolic, diastolic and mean), PAWP, RA pressure, RV pressure and cardiac output (CO). Patients should be screened for a left to right shunt by measuring oxygen saturation in the superior vena cava and pulmonary artery. Further sampling should be performed in patients with an increase in oxygen saturation by >7% (i.e. "step up") or if PA oxygen saturation is >75% to identify the location of a potential shunt. In patients with idiopathic PAH, pulmonary vasoreactivity testing with inhaled nitric oxide (10–20 ppm) for identification of calcium channel blocker (CCB) responders is recommended. Intravenous (IV) epoprostenol (2–12 ng/kg/min), IV adenosine (50–350 µg/min) or inhaled iloprost (5 µg) can be used as alternatives. A positive responder is defined as a reduction of mean PAP ≥10 mm Hg to reach an absolute value of mean PAP ≤40 mm Hg with an increased or unchanged CO.
- *Ventilation/perfusion lung scanning*
  Ventilation/perfusion lung scanning remains the screening method of choice for WHO group-4 chronic thromboembolic PH, as it has a higher sensitivity than computed tomography angiography. A normal or low probability ventilation/perfusion scan effectively excludes chronic thromboembolic PH. High-resolution computed tomographic scanning of the chest is useful to exclude occult interstitial lung disease or mediastinal fibrosis when the PFTs and chest radiograph are nondiagnostic.
- *Cardiac magnetic resonance imaging*
  Cardiac magnetic resonance imaging (MRI) may be used to evaluate RV morphology and function in addition to assessing the presence and severity of congenital heart disease (e.g. atrial or ventricular septal defects). A decreased stroke volume, an increased RV end-diastolic volume and a decreased LV end-diastolic volume measured at baseline are associated with a poor prognosis.

TREATMENT

Prior to 1995, there were no FDA approved therapies available for idiopathic PAH, and the median survival from diagnosis was 2.8 years. As a result of advances in management, patients without hemodynamic evidence of RV dysfunction may survive for >10 years with median survival rates of 87.8%, 76.8% and 62.8% at 1, 2 and 3 years. Treatment decisions should be based on known prognostic indicators. A multiparameter approach may include a combination of WHO functional class, cardiopulmonary exercise capacity (6-minute walk test or cardiopulmonary exercise testing), biomarkers and hemodynamic parameters, mainly RA pressure, PVR and cardiac index.

Treatment goals include improving symptoms, enhancing functional capacity and hemodynamic improvement. Another important goal is to prevent or at least delay progression of the disease. The ultimate goal is to improve survival. An evidence-based treatment algorithm based on a consensus statement is presented (Fig. 9.4). As treatments have been evaluated primarily in idiopathic PAH, hereditary PAH and PAH associated with connective tissue diseases or anorexigen use, extrapolation of these recommendations to other PAH subgroups should be done with caution.

- *General treatment measures*

  Patients with PAH require advice about general activities of daily living and need to adapt to the uncertainty associated with a serious chronic life-threatening disease. Patients should be encouraged to do low-level graded aerobic exercise, such as walking within symptom limits. Supervised exercise rehabilitation helps improve functional capacity and decrease fatigue. Patients are advised to avoid heavy physical exertion or isometric exercise (e.g. straining against a fixed resistance), as this may evoke exertional syncope. Exposure to high altitudes may contribute to hypoxic pulmonary vasoconstriction, and patients may require oxygen on commercial aircraft. In-flight oxygen administration should be considered for WHO functional classes III and IV patients and those with arterial blood oxygen pressure consistently <60 mm Hg. A sodium-restricted diet (i.e. <2,400 mg per day) is advised and is particularly important to manage volume status in patients with RV failure. Influenza and pneumococcal immunizations are advised.

  Pregnancy is associated with 30–50% mortality in patients with PAH, and therefore the general recommendation is to avoid or terminate pregnancy early in women with PAH. Progesterone-only preparations, such as medroxyprogesterone acetate and etonogestrel are effective approaches to contraception and avoid potential issues of estrogens.

- *Supportive therapy*
  - *Oral anticoagulants*: On the basis of observational studies, anticoagulation has favorable effects in patients with idiopathic PAH, hereditary PAH and PAH associated with anorexigens. The potential benefits of oral anticoagulation should be weighed against the risks in patients with other forms of PAH, especially when there is an increased risk of bleeding such as portopulmonary hypertension with esophageal varices. Warfarin anticoagulation in idiopathic PAH patients should be titrated to an international normalized ratio (INR) of 1.5–2.5. Of note is that the target INR for patients with chronic thromboembolic PH is between 2.0 and 3.0.
  - *Diuretics*: Decompensated right heart failure leads to fluid retention, elevated central venous pressure, hepatic congestion, ascites and peripheral edema. Diuretics in PAH, although not rigorously studied, appear to improve symptoms in volume-overloaded patients with right heart failure. Serum electrolytes and renal function need to be closely monitored.
  - *Oxygen*: Hypoxemia is a potent pulmonary vasoconstrictor, and experts recommend oxygen supplementation to maintain oxygen saturation

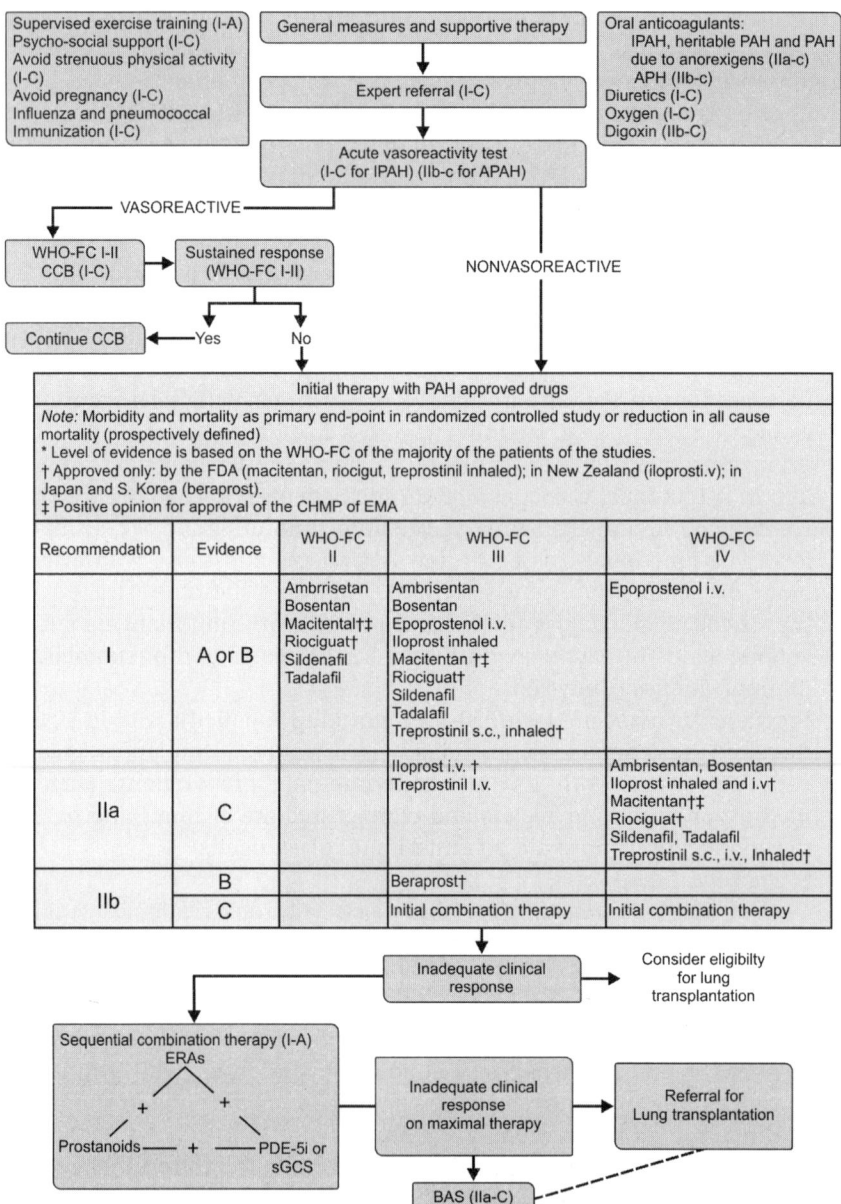

Fig. 9.4: Algorithm for the treatment of pulmonary arterial hypertension

APAH, associated pulmonary arterial hypertension; BAS, balloon atrial septostomy; CCB, calcium channel blockers; ERA, endothelin receptor antagonist; sGCS, soluble guanylate cyclase stimulators; IPAH, idiopathic pulmonary arterial hypertension; iv, intravenous; PDE-5i, phosphodiesterase type-5 inhibitor; sc, subcutaneous; WHO-FC, World Health Organization functional class.

Source: From Galie N, Corris PA, Frost A, Girgis RE, Granton J, Jing ZC, et al. Updated treatment algorithm of pulmonary arterial hypertension. J Am Coll Cardiol. 2013;62:D60-72. Reprinted *with permission* from Elsevier Ltd.

>90% or arterial blood oxygen pressure ≥8 kPA (60 mm Hg). Ambulatory oxygen should be considered when there is symptomatic benefit and correctable desaturation during exercise or at night.
- *Digoxin*: There are no data on long-term treatment with digoxin in PAH. A single dose of IV digoxin has been shown to cause a moderate increase in CO in patients with PH and RV failure.
- *Calcium channel blockers and vasoreactivity testing*: Smooth muscle cell hypertrophy, hyperplasia and vasoconstriction contribute to the pathogenesis of idiopathic PAH and hence the potential role of CCBs. Studies have shown 95% 5-year survival in patients with idiopathic PAH who have an acute vasodilator response to CCBs. For this reason, acute vasoreactivity testing is recommended in patients with idiopathic PAH to identify subjects who may respond favorably to long-term treatment with high doses of CCBs. Long-acting nifedipine, diltiazem or amlodipine are the most commonly used CCBs. The choice of CCB is based on the patient's heart rate at baseline, with a relative bradycardia favoring nifedipine or amlodipine and a relative tachycardia favoring diltiazem. Because of its potential negative inotropic effects, verapamil should be avoided. If the patient does not show an adequate response, defined as being in WHO functional class I or II and with a marked hemodynamic improvement, alternative or additional PAH therapy should be instituted.

- PAH approved drugs
  - *Prostanoids*: In patients with PAH, prostacyclin synthase is reduced, resulting in inadequate production of prostacyclin I_2, a vasodilator with antiproliferative effects. Currently, there are three commercially available prostanoids–epoprostenol (IV), treprostinil (IV, subcutaneous, inhaled and orally administered) and iloprost (inhaled). Treatment with prostanoids is initiated at a low dose and gradually increased based on side effects. Side effects are due to vasodilatory properties and include headache, jaw pain, flushing, nausea, diarrhea, skin rash and musculoskeletal pain. Intravenous epoprostenol has been shown to improve survival in idiopathic PAH. Both iloprost and treprostinil have been shown to improve symptoms, functional capacity and hemodynamics. Epoprostenol has a short half-life (3–5 minutes) and must be delivered by continuous IV infusion. Treprostinil is a more stable prostanoid with an elimination half-life of about 4.5 hours. Patients receiving IV and subcutaneous treatments must learn techniques of sterile preparation of the medication, operation of the ambulatory infusion pump and, in the case of IV delivery, care of a central venous catheter.

    A phase III clinical trial was recently completed on selexipag, a selective oral prostacyclin receptor agonist. Unlike prostacyclin I_2 analogs, selexipag does not activate other prostanoid receptors and, therefore, may have less gastrointestinal side effects. Selexipag is not currently FDA approved for PAH.

- *Endothelin receptor antagonists*: Endothelin-1 exerts vasoconstrictor and mitogenic effects by binding to two distinct receptor isoforms in the pulmonary vascular smooth muscle cells, endothelin-A and endothelin-B receptors. Activation of the endothelin system has been demonstrated in the plasma and lung tissue of PAH patients. Drugs in this class include bosentan, ambrisentan and macitentan. Endothelin receptor antagonists have been shown to improve symptoms, exercise capacity and time to clinical worsening. Common side effects include potential hepatotoxicity (in particular, bosentan), anemia, edema, potential risk of testicular atrophy, male infertility and teratogenicity.
- *Phosphodiesterase type-5 (PDE-5) inhibitors*: Inhibition of the cyclic-GMP-degrading enzyme PDE-5 results in vasodilatation through the nitric oxide/cyclic-GMP pathway. The pulmonary vasculature contains substantial amounts of PDE-5 and PDE-5 inhibitors, such as sildenafil and tadalafil, which enhance or prolong the effects of the vasodilating nucleotide cyclic-GMP. Phosphodiesterase type-5 inhibitors improve exercise capacity in patients with PAH. Side effects of PDE-5 inhibitors include headache, flushing, dyspepsia and epistaxis.
- *Soluble guanylate cyclase (sGC) stimulators*: While PDE-5 inhibitors slow cyclic-guanosine monophosphate (GMP) degradation, sGC stimulators enhance cyclic-GMP production independent of nitric oxide availability. Riociguat has a dual mode of action, acting synergistically with endogenous nitric oxide as well as directly stimulating sGC, thus increasing cyclic-GMP and promoting preferential perfusion of the well-ventilated regions of the lung. Riociguat has been found to have positive effects on pulmonary hemodynamics, WHO functional class, exercise capacity and time to clinical worsening in patients with PAH. Major side effects include headache, dyspepsia, gastritis, nausea, vomiting and diarrhea, hypotension, syncope, and rarely, bleeding and hemoptysis.

  It should be noted that riociguat is not only FDA approved for PAH but also for WHO group-4 PH due to chronic thromboembolic disease. However, thromboembolectomy remains the main and potentially curative therapy for these patients. Riociguat should be considered in inoperable patients with PH due to chronic thromboembolic disease or persistent or recurrent PH after pulmonary endarterectomy.
- *Combination therapy*: The term combination therapy describes the simultaneous use of more than one PAH-specific class of drugs (e.g. prostanoids, endothelin receptor antagonists, PDE-5 inhibitors or sGC stimulators). Combination therapy is an attractive option, as separate signaling pathways known to be involved in the pathogenesis are being targeted. Since PDE-5 inhibitors and sGC stimulators both work on the nitric oxide pathway, they should not be used in combination. The experience using combination therapy is growing, and several

clinical trials have been published that include patients treated with more than one FDA approved drug. A meta-analysis suggested that combination therapy reduced risk of clinical worsening and improved hemodynamics. It is unclear at this time whether certain combination therapies are more efficacious than others or whether to combine up front (treatment naïve patients) or add sequentially. Multiple randomized controlled trials of combination therapy are currently ongoing.
- Invasive therapies
Despite maximal medical therapy, many patients experience progressive decline, largely related to intractable right heart failure. It is in these patients that interventional and surgical therapeutic options should be considered, including lung or combined heart and lung transplantation and atrial septostomy.
  - *Lung transplantation*: Transplantation remains an invasive therapy of choice for eligible PAH patients in WHO functional class III or IV whose conditions deteriorate despite maximal pulmonary vasodilator therapy. The current survival following lung transplantation is 52–75% at 5 years and 45-66% at 10 years. Double lung transplantation is the recommended option for PAH. Combined heart and lung transplantation is generally reserved for idiopathic PAH patients with intractable right heart failure, PH in the setting of complex congenital heart disease and PH with concomitant advanced left heart disease. Lung transplantation is associated with significant shortcomings, including the need for lifelong immunosuppression and morbidity associated with increased risk for infection and allograft rejection. It should only be performed in carefully selected individuals in whom the benefits are believed to outweigh the risks.
  - *Balloon atrial septostomy*: Atrial septostomy creates a right to left interatrial shunt, decreasing right heart filling pressures and improving right heart function and left heart filling. While the created shunt decreases systemic arterial oxygen saturation, it is anticipated that the improved CO will result in overall augmentation of systemic oxygen delivery. A careful preprocedure risk assessment is essential. Predictors of procedure-related failure or death include a mean right atrial pressure of >20 mm Hg, a PVR index of >55 Wood units/m^2, oxygen saturation at rest of <85% on room air and a predicted 1-year survival of <40%. Balloon atrial septostomy is recommended only for patients who are in WHO functional class IV and have right heart failure refractory to medical therapy and transplantation is not an option.
  - *Extracorporeal membrane oxygenation (ECMO)*: Preoperative ECMO is a risk factor for poor outcome and was previously considered a contraindication to lung transplantation. Recent reports indicate that ECMO may be used in selected awake end-stage PH patients for bridging to lung transplantation. A recent study showed that, although the incidence of primary graft dysfunction requiring posttransplant

Table 9.2: Future therapies for pulmonary hypertension

Pathway	Therapy
Vasodilation	Nitric oxide, nitrite
Sympathetic nervous system	Selective > non-selective β-adrenergic blockade
Renin-angiotensin-aldosterone system	Aldosterone antagonist, vasopressin receptor antagonist, catheter-guided ablation
Vascular remodeling-metabolic alterations	Dichloroacetate, ranolazine
Anti-inflammation	Rho-kinase inhibitors, rituximab, vasoactive intestinal peptide
Selective and multikinase inhibition	Tyrosine kinase inhibitors
Stem cells	Endothelial progenitor stem cells and mesenchymal stromal cells
Gene therapy	
Devices	Cardiac resynchronization, extracorporeal life support: veno-arterial, venovenous and pumpless arteriovenous extracorporeal lung assist

Source: Adapted from Gomberg-Maitland M, Bull TM, Saggar R, Barst AJ, Elgazayerly A, Fleming TR, et al. New trial designs and potential therapies for pulmonary artery hypertension. J Am Coll Cardiol. 2013;62:D82-91. Reprinted with permission from Elsevier Ltd.

ECMO was higher and the hospital stay was longer in patients receiving pretransplant ECMO, the 2-year graft survival was 74% in PH patients.

- *Therapies under investigation*
  While treatments targeting the three traditional pathways (i.e. endothelin, nitric oxide and prostacyclin) are well established, continual research into the molecular mechanisms of PAH has led to the discovery of new putative pathways and opened up the possibility of new drug targets (Table 9.2).

SUGGESTED READING

1. Barst RJ, Rubin LJ, Long WA, et al. A comparison of continuous intravenous epoprostenol (prostacyclin) with conventional therapy for primary pulmonary hypertension. The Primary Pulmonary Hypertension Study Group. N Engl J Med. 1996;334(5):296-302.
2. Channick RN, Simonneau G, Sitbon O, et al. Effects of the dual endothelin-receptor antagonist bosentan in patients with pulmonary hypertension: a randomised placebo-controlled study. Lancet. 2001;358(9288):1119-23.
3. Galie N, Olschewski H, Oudiz RJ, et al. Ambrisentan for the treatment of pulmonary arterial hypertension: results of the ambrisentan in pulmonary arterial hypertension, randomized, double-blind, placebo-controlled, multicenter, efficacy (ARIES) study 1 and 2. Circulation. 2008;117(23):3010-19.
4. Galie N, Ghofrani HA, Torbicki A, et al. Sildenafil citrate therapy for pulmonary arterial hypertension. N Engl J Med. 2005;353(20):2148-57.
5. Galie N, Brundage BH, Ghofrani HA, et al. Tadalafil therapy for pulmonary arterial hypertension. Circulation. 2009;119(22):2894-903.

6. Galie N, Corris PA, Frost A, Girgis RE, Granton J, Jing ZC, et al. Updated treatment algorithm of pulmonary arterial hypertension. J Am Coll Cardiol. 2013;62(25 Suppl):D60-72.
7. Ghofrani HA, Galie N, Grimminger F, et al. Riociguat for the treatment of pulmonary arterial hypertension. N Engl J Med. 2013;369(4):330-40.
8. Hoeper MM, Bogaard HJ, Condliffe R, Frantz R, Khanna D, Kurzyna M, et al. Definitions and diagnosis of pulmonary hypertension. J Am Coll Cardiol. 2013;62(25 Suppl):D42-50.
9. Hoeper MM, Barbera JA, Channick RN, et al. Diagnosis, assessment, and treatment of non-pulmonary arterial hypertension pulmonary hypertension. J Am Coll Cardiol. 2009;54(1 Suppl):S85-96.
10. Humbert M, Morrell NW, Archer SL, et al. Cellular and molecular pathobiology of pulmonary arterial hypertension. J Am Coll Cardiol. 2004;43(12 Suppl S):13S-24S.
11. Machado RD, Eickelberg O, Elliott CG, et al. Genetics and genomics of pulmonary arterial hypertension. J Am Coll Cardiol. 2009;54(1 Suppl):S32-42.
12. McLaughlin VV, Shillington A, Rich S. Survival in primary pulmonary hypertension: the impact of epoprostenol therapy. Circulation. 2002;106(12):1477-82.
13. Olschewski H, Simonneau G, Galie N, et al. Inhaled iloprost for severe pulmonary hypertension. N Engl J Med. 2002;347(5):322-9.
14. Pietra GG, Capron F, Stewart S, et al. Pathologic assessment of vasculopathies in pulmonary hypertension. J Am Coll Cardiol. 2004;43(12 Suppl S):25S-32S.
15. Pulido T, Adzerikho I, Channick RN, et al. Macitentan and morbidity and mortality in pulmonary arterial hypertension. N Engl J Med. 2013;369(9):809-18.
16. Simonneau G, Gatzoulis MA, Adatia I, et al. Updated clinical classification of pulmonary hypertension. J Am Coll Cardiol. 2013;62(25 Suppl):D34-41.
17. Simonneau G, Barst RJ, Galie N, et al. Continuous subcutaneous infusion of treprostinil, a prostacyclin analogue, in patients with pulmonary arterial hypertension: a double-blind, randomized, placebo-controlled trial. Am J Respir Crit Care Med. 2002;165(6):800-4.

Aortic and Mitral Valve Disease

Chapter 10

Byron F Vandenberg, Kanu Chatterjee

Patients with aortic or mitral valve disease usually present for evaluation of new symptoms, the discovery of a new murmur or evidence of valve disease found incidentally on noninvasive imaging. A careful history and physical examination provide valuable information regarding the specific valve lesion, its severity and directing the patient toward medical or surgical treatment. An understanding of the disease natural history and appropriate diagnostic testing can also help in determining therapy. In this chapter, the etiology, pathophysiology, natural history, physical examination, diagnosis and treatment are discussed for aortic stenosis (AS), aortic regurgitation (AR), mitral regurgitation (MR) and mitral stenosis (MS). In addition, special cases unique to each valve lesion are discussed.

AORTIC STENOSIS

Etiology

Aortic stenosis usually presents as calcific AS in adults of advanced age. There are similarities between the risk factors for developing calcific AS and coronary artery disease, and these include hypertension, diabetes mellitus, hyperlipidemia and smoking. The second most frequent etiology is congenital (i.e. a bicuspid aortic valve) and is more common in the younger age group. Rheumatic heart disease is a rare cause of AS in the developed world. However, worldwide, rheumatic heart disease is a leading cause of aortic valve inflammation leading to AS. Since rheumatic heart disease usually affects the mitral valve, the diagnosis of isolated rheumatic AS should be made with caution.

Pathophysiology

As the aortic valve orifice narrows, a pressure gradient develops between the left ventricle (LV) and aorta. With increasing LV pressure, there is a compensatory increase in LV wall thickness to reduce wall stress according to the law of Laplace [i.e. wall stress = (pressure × radius)/(2 × wall thickness)]. This normalization of wall stress helps maintain normal LV ejection performance. However, the sequelae of LV hypertrophy include reductions in subendocardial coronary blood flow and coronary flow reserve. Diastolic dysfunction develops as well, due to decreased distensibility of the thickened

LV wall. When LV hypertrophy is not adequate to normalize wall stress, LV ejection performance falls due to the increased afterload of wall stress.

Natural History

The rate of progression of the decrease in valve area of calcific AS is variable, ranging from <0.1 to 0.3 cm^2 per year. Survival is nearly normal as long as the patient is asymptomatic, although there is a <1% per year risk of sudden death in asymptomatic patients with AS. Once the patient develops symptoms of angina, syncope or dyspnea, mortality increases.

Dyspnea and other symptoms of heart failure (e.g. orthopnea and paroxysmal nocturnal dyspnea) occur in about 50% of patients with AS and is related to both systolic and diastolic dysfunctions as described above.

Angina is the presenting symptom in about 35% of patients with AS and may occur in the absence of obstructive coronary artery disease, presumably related to the increased myocardial oxygen consumption from the increased wall stress and decreased coronary flow reserve.

Syncope with exertion is the presenting symptom in about 15% of patients with AS and is likely related to the inability to maintain adequate stroke volume during the fall in peripheral resistance with exercise. In addition, an elevated LV pressure may lead to a vasodepressor response.

Physical Examination

On auscultation, the first heart sound is normal but the second heart sound is often soft and single since the stenotic valve neither opens nor closes, leaving only the pulmonic component of the second heart sound audible. A paradoxically split second heart sound suggests an underlying left bundle branch block. The presence of a fourth heart sound suggests reduced LV compliance in the presence of LV hypertrophy. The murmur of AS is described as a grade ≥3/6 late-peaking systolic murmur heard best in the aortic area radiating to the carotid arteries. However, the intensity of the murmur does not correlate with disease severity since the murmur intensity may decrease as aortic flow diminishes. As AS progresses, palpation of the carotid artery demonstrates a delay in upstroke ("pulsus tardus") and a decrease in the pulse amplitude ("pulsus parvus"). However, the carotid upstroke may be normal in elderly patients because of aging effects on the vasculature. Palpation of the apical beat may demonstrate an increase in force and duration with a normal location.

Diagnosis

The electrocardiogram (ECG) may demonstrate LV hypertrophy, and the chest X-ray may demonstrate cardiomegaly from LV hypertrophy.

Transthoracic echocardiography (TTE) is indicated in patients with signs or symptoms of AS to estimate the transvalvular gradient and aortic valve area and categorize disease severity (Table 10.1). Gradients are estimated from Doppler determined velocities using the modified Bernoulli equation (i.e. ΔP

Table 10.1: Classification of aortic stenosis severity

Parameters	Mild	Moderate	Severe	Very severe	Low gradient/ low flow, severe, LVEF <50%	Low gradient, severe, LVEF ≥ 50%**
Aortic jet velocity (m/s)	2.0–2.9	3.0–3.9	≥4.0	≥5.0	<4.0*	<4.0
Mean gradient (mm Hg)	<20	20–39	≥40	≥60	<40	<40
Aortic valve area (cm²)	>1.5	1.0–1.5	≤1.0		≤1.0*	≤1.0
Indexed aortic valve area (cm²/m²)	>0.85	0.59–0.85	≤0.6			≤0.6
Doppler velocity ratio	>0.50	0.25–0.50	<0.25			

*Dobutamine stress echo demonstrates aortic valve area <1.0 cm² with aortic maximum velocity ≥4 m/s at any flow rate.

**With LV stroke volume indexed for body surface area <35 mL/m².

LVEF, left ventricular ejection fraction

Source: From Nishimura RA, Otto CM, Bonow RO, Carabello BA, Erwin JP, Guyton RA, et al. 2014 AHA/ACC guideline for the management of patients with valvular heart disease. J Am Coll Cardiol. 2014;63(22):e57-185; Vahanian A, Alfieri O, Andreotti F, Antunes MJ, Baron-Esquivias G, Baumgartner H, et al.; Joint Task Force on the Management of Valvular Heart Disease of the European Society of Cardiology (ESC); the European Association for Cardio-Thoracic Surgery (EACTS). Guidelines on the management of valvular heart disease (version 2012). Eur Heart J. 2012;33:2451-96.

$= 4v^2$, where ΔP is the pressure gradient and v is the velocity). In addition, the two-dimensional echocardiogram can evaluate LV hypertrophy, systolic and diastolic LV function and aortic valve appearance. Repeat TTE is appropriate when there is a change in symptom or clinical status. Surveillance TTE is recommended every 6–12 months for severe AS, every 1–2 years for moderate AS and every 3–5 years for mild AS.

Cardiac catheterization provides invasive estimation of the aortic valve from simultaneous measurements of LV pressure, aortic pressure and cardiac output. The area is calculated with the Gorlin equation [i.e. valve area = cardiac output/(44.3 × √transvalvular pressure gradient)].

Exercise testing is reasonable to assess physiological changes with exercise and to confirm the absence of symptoms in asymptomatic patients with severe AS (i.e. aortic peak velocity ≥4.0 m/sec or mean pressure gradient ≥40 mmHg). However, exercise testing should not be performed in patients with symptomatic severe AS.

Treatment

There is no effective medical therapy for AS, and aortic valve replacement is the only long-term therapy that affects outcome (Table 10.2). However, hypertension should be treated to guideline directed target goals. Statins do not prevent progression of AS. While asymptomatic patients have a good prognosis, once symptoms develop, valve replacement improves survival. Thus, the onset of symptoms is important to recognize because it impacts the natural history of the disease.

In patients who are at excessive operative risk with valve replacement, transcutaneous aortic valve replacement is an option. In this procedure, a stented valve is delivered into the aortic annulus percutaneously or transapically after the calcified valve is opened by prior balloon dilatation.

Percutaneous aortic balloon dilation may be considered as a bridge to surgical aortic valve replacement or transcutaneous aortic valve replacement in patients with severe symptomatic AS, needing urgent relief of valve obstruction.

Table 10.2: Indications for aortic valve replacement in patients with aortic stenosis

Recommended
Symptomatic patients with severe high-gradient AS who have symptoms by history or on exercise testing
Asymptomatic patients with severe AS and LVEF <50%
Severe AS when undergoing other cardiac surgery
Reasonable
Asymptomatic patients with very severe AS and low surgical risk
Asymptomatic patients with severe AS and decreased exercise tolerance or an exercise fall in BP
Symptomatic patients with low-flow/low-gradient severe AS with reduced LVEF with a low-dose dobutamine stress study that shows an aortic velocity >4.0 m/s (or mean pressure gradient >40 mm Hg) with a valve area <1.0 cm^2 at any dobutamine dose
Symptomatic patients who have low-flow/low-gradient severe AS who are normotensive and have an LVEF >50% if clinical, hemodynamic and anatomic data support valve obstruction as the most likely cause of symptoms
Patients with moderate AS (aortic velocity 3.0–3.9 m/s) who are undergoing other cardiac surgery
Consider
Asymptomatic patients with severe AS and rapid disease progression and low surgical risk

AS, aortic stenosis; LVEF, left ventricular ejection fraction; BP, blood pressure

Source: From Nishimura RA, Otto CM, Bonow RO, Carabello BA, Erwin JP, Guyton RA, et al. 2014 AHA/ACC guideline for the management of patients with valvular heart disease. J Am Coll Cardiol. 2014;63(22):e57-185; Vahanian A, Alfieri O, Andreotti F, Antunes MJ, Baron-Esquivias G, Baumgartner H, et al.; Joint Task Force on the Management of Valvular Heart Disease of the European Society of Cardiology (ESC); the European Association for Cardio-Thoracic Surgery (EACTS). Guidelines on the management of valvular heart disease (version 2012). Eur Heart J. 2012;33:2451-96.

Special Cases

Some patients with severe AS may present with *severe LV dysfunction and a low forward flow state*. Since valve area calculations are based on forward flow, the true severity of AS may not be correctly determined by a gradient measurement alone in patients with LV ejection fraction (EF) <50%. In patients with left ventricular ejection fraction (LVEF) <50%, calculated valve area ≤1.0 cm^2 but mean gradient <40 mm Hg (or peak aortic velocity <4.0 m/s), increasing forward flow with a low-dose dobutamine Doppler echocardiography study may be useful to distinguish patients with true severe AS (i.e. a fixed valve area ≤1.0 cm^2 but peak velocity increases to >4.0 m/s with dobutamine) versus patients with underlying cardiomyopathy unrelated to AS and moderate AS (i.e. an increase in valve area and only a modest change in gradient despite increased flow). The lack of contractile reserve (i.e. the inability to increase stroke volume by >20%) predicts a subgroup of patients with a very poor prognosis with either medical or surgical therapy.

There are patients with severe AS presenting with *low gradient and a normal LVEF*. In these patients, the low forward flow state is attributed to a low stroke volume due to a small LV end-diastolic volume indexed for body surface area (i.e. <35 mL/m^2). However, severe AS is unlikely if peak velocity is <3.0 m/s or mean gradient is <20 mm Hg.

AORTIC REGURGITATION

Etiology

Aortic regurgitation is due to abnormalities of the leaflets (e.g. rheumatic heart disease, endocarditis and bicuspid valve) or aortic root dilatation (e.g. hypertension and Marfan's syndrome) or both (e.g. aortopathy associated with bicuspid valve). The most common causes of chronic AR in developed countries are bicuspid aortic valve and calcific valve disease. Rheumatic heart disease is the leading cause in many developing countries.

Pathophysiology

The regurgitation of blood into the LV during diastole results in reduced total forward flow. However, an increase in end-diastolic volume with normal LVEF results in a compensatory increase in total and forward stroke volume. The increased total stroke volume increases pulse pressure and systolic pressure. With increased wall stress, there is compensatory LV hypertrophy and eventually LV dysfunction.

Natural History

Aortic regurgitation is generally well tolerated since the disease is slowly progressive; however, prognosis worsens when symptoms develop. Symptoms of heart failure are common in AR and are related to both diastolic and systolic dysfunction. Angina is a relatively rare symptom and likely related to

Table 10.3: Peripheral physical examination findings of aortic regurgitation	
Sign	Description
Quincke's pulse	Traction on the nailbed causes systolic erythema and diastolic blanching
Hill's	Augmentation of systolic blood pressure by >40 mm Hg above brachial blood pressure
Duroziez's	Systolic and diastolic turbulent sound when the stethoscope bell is pressed over the femoral artery
Pistol shot	Sound heard when stethoscope is placed over the femoral artery
Corrigan's pulse	Brisk upstroke and collapse of carotid pulse
De Musset's	Head bob with each cycle

Source: From Carabello B. Aortic valve disease. In: Chatterjee K (Ed). Cardiology: An illustrated text. New Delhi, India: Jaypee Brothers; 2013. pp. 986-99.

reduced myocardial perfusion from low diastolic blood pressure (BP), as well as reduced coronary flow reserve from underlying LV hypertrophy. Syncope is also a rare symptom and related to cerebral hypoperfusion in the presence of low diastolic BP.

Physical Examination

The apical beat is typically forceful and displaced inferiorly and laterally. The diastolic murmur is heard best at the left lower sternal border while the patient is sitting up and leaning forward. The murmur may be associated with a diastolic mitral rumble (i.e. the Austin Flint murmur) due to partial closure and vibration of the mitral valve by the regurgitant jet. The widened pulse pressure and increased total stroke volume lead to the presence of peripheral signs (Table 10.3).

Diagnosis

Transthoracic echocardiography is useful in the visualization of the aortic valve and root and therefore provides insight into the etiology of the AR. The width of the AR jet on Doppler helps determine the regurgitation severity. Diastolic flow reversal in the aortic arch or more distally can help identify patients with severe AR. Measurements of LV size and function can be obtained with a two-dimensional echocardiography. More sophisticated methods using Doppler can estimate the regurgitant volume.

In patients with uncertain symptomatic state, exercise testing is useful to quantitate exercise tolerance and functional capacity.

Cardiac magnetic resonance imaging is recommended for the assessment of AR severity, as well as LV volumes and function in patients with significant AR but with suboptimal TTE images or in patients with discordance between clinical assessment and severity of AR by echocardiography.

Cardiac catheterization is recommended when there is discordance between clinical assessment and echocardiography, when cardiac magnetic resonance imaging is not available or if there are contraindications to magnetic resonance imaging. At cardiac catheterization, elevated LV filling pressures are expected and aortography provides visualization of the regurgitant blood flow from the aorta to the LV, as well as the coronary artery anatomy.

Treatment

Medical management of asymptomatic patients with AR and normal LV systolic function is controversial since reproducible evidence that vasodilator therapy improves outcome is lacking. However, the goal of therapy is to maintain normal BP and treat systolic BP >140 mm Hg, preferably with a dihydropyridine calcium channel blocker or angiotensin-converting enzyme inhibitor/angiotensin receptor blocker. Beta-blockers may be less effective since the reduction in heart rate is associated with a higher stroke volume, which may contribute to an elevation of the systolic BP.

When patients with severe AR become symptomatic, valve repair or replacement is recommended (Table 10.4). While medical therapy is not a substitute for surgery, it may alleviate symptoms in patients who are considered to be at very high risk for surgery.

Symptomatic patients with normal LVEF have a better long-term postoperative survival than those with decreased LVEF (i.e. optimal outcomes are obtained when surgery is performed before LVEF decreases <50%). In addition, preoperative symptomatic status predicts postoperative outcome:

Table 10.4: Indications for aortic valve replacement in patients with aortic regurgitation

Recommended

Symptomatic patients with severe AR regardless of LV systolic function

Asymptomatic patients with chronic severe AR and LV systolic dysfunction (LVEF <50%)

Patients with severe AR while undergoing cardiac surgery for other indications

Reasonable

Asymptomatic patients with severe AR with normal LV systolic function (LVEF >50%) but with severe LV dilation (LVESD >50 mm* or indexed LVESD 25 mm/m^2)

Patients with moderate AR who are undergoing other cardiac surgery

Consider

Asymptomatic patients with severe AR and normal LV systolic function (LVEF >50%) but with progressive severe LV dilation (LVEDD >65 mm) if surgical risk is low (particularly in the setting progressive LV enlargement)

*The European Society of Cardiology guidelines also consider LVEDD >70 mm as a criteria for LV dilatation.
AVR, aortic valve replacement; AR, aortic regurgitation; LV, left ventricular; LVEF, left ventricular ejection fraction; LVESD, left ventricular end-systolic dimension; LVEDD, left ventricular end-diastolic dimension
Source: From Nishimura RA, Otto CM, Bonow RO, Carabello BA, Erwin JP, Guyton RA, et al. 2014 AHA/ACC guideline for the management of patients with valvular heart disease. J Am Coll Cardiol. 2014;63(22):e57-185; Vahanian A, Alfieri O, Andreotti F, Antunes MJ, Baron-Esquivias G, Baumgartner H, et al.; Joint Task Force on the Management of Valvular Heart Disease of the European Society of Cardiology (ESC); the European Association for Cardio-Thoracic Surgery (EACTS). Guidelines on the management of valvular heart disease (version 2012). Eur Heart. J 2012;33:2451-96.

patients with New York Heart Association functional class I or II have better survival compared with those with functional class III or IV.

Special Cases

When AR develops acutely as in leaflet damage from infective endocarditis or aorta damage from dissection, there is no time for LV enlargement, so total stroke volume and pulse pressure do not increase. The acute volume load leads to pulmonary congestion and low forward cardiac output. The mitral valve may close prematurely as the LV end-diastolic pressure rises rapidly due to filling from both the left atrium (LA) and the aorta. This results in decreased intensity of the first heart sound. The intensity of the diastolic murmur may be decreased due to the decreased diastolic pressure gradient between the aorta and LV. In patients with acute, severe AR from infective endocarditis or aortic dissection, surgery should not be delayed, especially if there is hypotension or pulmonary edema. Intra-aortic balloon counterpulsation is contraindicated in these patients since augmentation of aortic diastolic pressure will worsen the severity of the acute regurgitant volume, further increasing LV filling pressure and decreasing forward output.

Bicuspid aortic valves are frequently associated with aortic dilatation, which is more common in patients with fusion of the right and noncoronary cusp leaflets (compared with the more common fusion of the right and left coronary cusp leaflets). Transthoracic echocardiography can provide assessment of the ascending aorta in most of these patients, but, in some patients, only the sinuses can be visualized and additional imaging with magnetic resonance imaging or computerized tomography may be needed to visualize the ascending aorta above the sinotubular junction. If the aortic diameter is >4.5 cm, surveillance imaging of the ascending aorta should be performed annually. Other reasons for annual imaging are family history of aortic dissection or a rapid rate of change in aortic diameter. While there are no proven drug therapies that reduce the rate of progression of aortic dilation, control of elevated BP is recommended. Operative repair of the aortic sinus or replacement of the ascending aorta is recommended when the aortic sinus or ascending aorta diameter is >5.5 cm. Surgery is recommended with aortic dilation of 5.1–5.5 cm if there is a family history of aortic dissection or if there is rapid progression of dilation (i.e. >0.5 cm per year). If a patient is undergoing aortic valve surgery because of severe AS or AR, replacement of the ascending aorta is reasonable in patients with aortic diameter >4.5 cm.

MITRAL REGURGITATION

Etiology

Mitral regurgitation is often distinguished as primary (or "degenerative," due to leaflet pathology of the mitral valve apparatus) or secondary (or "functional," due to nonvalvular or secondary issues) (Table 10.5). While surgery may correct the cause in the case of primary MR, in secondary MR the mitral valve is usually normal, and optimal therapy therefore may be difficult to determine.

Table 10.5: Etiologies of mitral regurgitation

Primary

Leaflet	Mitral valve prolapse, infective or noninfective endocarditis, degenerative disease, rheumatic heart disease, congenital heart disease (e.g. cleft mitral valve), trauma and radiation heart disease
Chordae tendineae	Chordal rupture due to infective endocarditis or mitral valve prolapse, degenerative disease, rheumatic heart disease, mitral valve prolapse, trauma, congenital heart disease and Marfan's syndrome
Papillary muscles	Rheumatic heart disease, endomyocardial fibrosis and congenital heart disease (e.g. parachute mitral valve)

Secondary

LV enlargement	Dilated cardiomyopathy
Annular enlargement or disorder	Dilated cardiomyopathy, mitral annular calcification
Papillary muscles	Ischemic heart disease*

*The posterior papillary muscle is more susceptible to dysfunction since its perfusion is by a single source: the posterior descending artery. The anterior papillary muscle has a dual blood source: diagonal branches of the left anterior descending artery and the obtuse marginal branches of the circumflex artery.

Source: From Nishimura RA, Otto CM, Bonow RO, Carabello BA, Erwin JP, Guyton RA, et al. 2014 AHA/ACC guideline for the management of patients with valvular heart disease. J Am Coll Cardiol. 2014;63(22):e57-185; Sharma S, Dalvi BV. Mitral valve disease. In: Chatterjee K (Ed). Cardiology: An illustrated text. New Delhi, India: Jaypee Brothers; 2013. pp. 1000-17.

Pathophysiology

In MR, forward stroke volume is reduced due to regurgitation of blood from the LV to the LA in systole. To maintain normal forward stroke volume, the LV volume increases and the LVEF is usually normal to high. Myocardial dysfunction may develop but the LVEF remains normal due to the reduced afterload. Thus, LVEF is typically about 70%, and a mild reduction in LVEF or LVEF <60% may represent LV dysfunction.

Natural History

As long as MR is compensated and the patient remains asymptomatic, prognosis is relatively good. However, survival is reduced when symptoms develop. Dyspnea on exertion is related to elevated LA pressure and pulmonary hypertension. As pulmonary artery systolic pressure approaches 50 mm Hg, prognosis worsens. Palpitations suggest the presence of atrial fibrillation or ventricular ectopy. Hoarseness is rare and related to recurrent laryngeal nerve compression by the enlarged LA.

Physical Examination

The apical impulse is slightly displaced inferiorly and laterally. The second heart sound may be widely split in severe MR, due to the premature closure of the aortic valve, although the split narrows as LV function decreases. In addition, the intensity of the pulmonic component of the second heart sound increases with the development of pulmonary hypertension. The presence of a third heart sound reflects rapid filling of the LV.

The murmur of MR is usually described as blowing and high-pitched and holosystolic. However, with mitral valve prolapse, the murmur is late systolic and may be associated with a mid systolic click. It is best heard at the apex and increases with expiration.

Diagnosis

Transthoracic echocardiography provides information regarding the etiology and severity of MR. Other information provided includes LV size and function, LA size and pulmonary artery systolic pressure. Patients typically undergo transesophageal echocardiography (TEE) because of the improved definition of mitral anatomy and MR severity compared with TTE. Echocardiographic findings suggesting severe MR are a regurgitant jet area >40% of the LA area, a vena contracta (i.e. width of the regurgitant flow jet at leaflet coaptation) ≥0.7 cm, systolic flow reversal in the pulmonary vein, elevated LV early filling velocity >120 cm/s and LA enlargement.

In cases where TTE provides suboptimal imaging, cardiac magnetic resonance imaging may be of value in assessing MR severity, cardiac chamber volumes and LVEF.

Annual or semiannual TTE is recommended in asymptomatic patients with severe MR as surveillance of LV function and pulmonary artery pressure. For patients with moderate primary MR, a follow-up echo to assess for changes in MR severity is recommended every 1–2 years and every 3–5 years for mild MR.

Cardiac catheterization with left ventriculography and/or hemodynamic measurements (e.g. LV filling and pulmonary artery pressures) are indicated when clinical assessment and noninvasive imaging are discordant.

An exercise stress test may be useful in some patients to establish baseline functional capacity.

Treatment

Medical therapy of symptomatic primary severe MR is limited and includes diuretics to reduce diastolic filling pressures and standard heart failure medications if LV systolic function is reduced. The definitive treatment of primary MR is surgical correction, but patients may require medical therapy while awaiting surgery. Vasodilator therapy is not recommended as an option to surgery for normotensive, asymptomatic patients with chronic primary MR and normal LV systolic function.

Current guidelines recommend surgery for symptomatic patients with severe MR and asymptomatic patients with a dilated (i.e. LV end-systolic dimension ≥4.0 cm) and/or dysfunctional (i.e. LVEF 30–60%) LV (Table 10.6). Other reasonable indications are significant pulmonary hypertension and the development of atrial fibrillation.

Mitral repair is the preferred strategy since the patient avoids the potential complications of a prosthetic valve (see Chapter 12: Prosthetic Heart Valves), and operative risk is lower compared with replacement. Mitral

Table 10.6: Indications for mitral valve replacement/repair in patients with mitral regurgitation

Mitral repair

Recommended

In preference to MVR when surgical treatment is indicated for patients with chronic severe primary MR limited to the posterior leaflet*

In preference to MVR when surgical treatment is indicated for patients with chronic severe primary MR involving the anterior leaflet or both leaflets when a successful and durable repair can be accomplished

Concomitant MV repair or replacement is indicated in patients with chronic severe primary MR undergoing cardiac surgery for other indications

Reasonable

Asymptomatic patients with chronic severe primary MR with preserved LV function (LVEF >60% and LVESD <40 mm) in whom the likelihood of a successful and durable repair without residual MR is >95% with an expected mortality rate of <1% when performed at a Heart Valve Center of Excellence

Asymptomatic patients with chronic severe nonrheumatic primary MR and preserved LV function in whom there is a high likelihood of a successful and durable repair with (i) new onset of AF or (ii) resting pulmonary hypertension (PA systolic arterial pressure >50 mm Hg)

Patients with chronic moderate primary MR undergoing cardiac surgery for other indications

Consider

Patients with rheumatic mitral valve disease when surgical treatment is indicated if a durable and successful repair is likely or if the reliability of long-term anticoagulation management is questionable

Patients with chronic moderate secondary MR who are undergoing other cardiac surgery

Mitral valve surgery

Recommended

Symptomatic patients with chronic severe primary MR and LVEF >30%

Asymptomatic patients with chronic severe primary MR and LV dysfunction (LVEF 30–60% and/or LVESD >40 mm)

Reasonable

Patients with chronic severe secondary MR who are undergoing coronary artery bypass grafting or aortic valve replacement

Consider

Symptomatic patients with chronic severe primary MR and LVEF <30%

Severely symptomatic patients (NYHA class III/IV) with chronic severe secondary MR

Transcatheter MV repair

Consider

Severely symptomatic patients (NYHA class III/IV) with chronic severe primary MR who have a reasonable life expectancy but a prohibitive surgical risk because of severe comorbidities

*MVR should not be performed for treatment of isolated severe primary MR limited to less than one half of the posterior leaflet unless MV repair has been attempted and was unsuccessful.

MR, mitral regurgitation; MV, mitral valve; MVR, mitral valve replacement; LV, left ventricle; LVEF, left ventricular ejection fraction; LVESD, left ventricular end-systolic diameter; AF, atrial fibrillation; PA, pulmonary artery; NYHA, New York Heart Association

Source: From Nishimura RA, Otto CM, Bonow RO, Carabello BA, Erwin JP, Guyton RA, et al. 2014 AHA/ACC guideline for the management of patients with valvular heart disease. J Am Coll Cardiol. 2014;63(22):e57-185; Vahanian A, Alfieri O, Andreotti F, Antunes MJ, Baron-Esquivias G, Baumgartner H, et al.; Joint Task Force on the Management of Valvular Heart Disease of the European Society of Cardiology (ESC); the European Association for Cardio-Thoracic Surgery (EACTS). Guidelines on the management of valvular heart disease (version 2012). Eur Heart J. 2012;33:2451-96.

valve replacement with preservation of the chordal apparatus is preferred to complete removal of the apparatus since retention of the chords is associated with preserved LV function and improves survival.

Finally, transcatheter mitral valve repair using a clip device has been shown to reduce severity of MR, alleviated symptoms and lead to reverse LV remodeling, although less effective than surgical repair. This percutaneous option may be considered in inoperable patients with severely symptomatic, chronic, severe primary MR.

The treatment of secondary MR includes medications that may reverse remodeling of a dilated LV (e.g. angiotensin-converting enzyme inhibitors and β-blockers), as well as diuretics and spironolactone. Cardiac resynchronization in appropriate candidates may reduce MR severity. In the presence of ischemic-induced MR, revascularization should be considered since there is the potential for improvement in LV function.

Special Cases

Acute MR usually develops from chordal rupture, papillary muscle dysfunction, or leaflet tear or perforation. The LA pressure rises abruptly resulting in pulmonary congestion. Transthoracic echocardiography is useful in determining the etiology of acute MR. The majority of these patients require early valve repair or replacement surgery. Vasodilators may be useful in reducing regurgitation and stabilizing patients awaiting surgery; however, their use is often limited by systemic hypotension due to low forward output. Intra-aortic balloon counterpulsation may be needed to achieve hemodynamic stability until surgery can be performed.

MITRAL STENOSIS

Etiology

The predominant cause of MS is rheumatic fever. Calcific mitral valve disease and extensive calcification of the mitral apparatus may result in MS in the elderly.

Pathophysiology

In rheumatic MS, a fibrotic process involves the leaflet commissures, cusps, chordae and papillary muscles, resulting in a funnel-shaped mitral orifice. Because of the pressure gradient across the mitral valve, the LA enlarges and LA thrombi can develop in the presence of stasis of blood flow. If pulmonary hypertension is long-standing, morphologic changes can occur in the pulmonary vasculature such that the pulmonary hypertension may not reverse after the mitral valve obstruction is relieved.

Natural History

Rheumatic MS is usually a slowly progressive disease, characterized by a long latent phase between the initial rheumatic illness and the development of stenosis. In industrialized nations, symptoms are usually delayed until the fifth decade of life. However, in India, severe MS presents earlier. The rate of progressive decrement in valve area is about 0.1 cm² per year.

Symptoms result from increased LA pressure and reduced cardiac output related to the obstruction to LV filling. Dyspnea on exertion, orthopnea and paroxysmal nocturnal dyspnea are therefore common symptoms. Hemoptysis and cough reflect underlying pulmonary venous congestion. Palpitations suggest the development of atrial fibrillation. Hoarseness may result from compression of the recurrent laryngeal nerve by the LA.

Physical Examination

The first heart sound intensity may be increased due to closure of a pliable mitral valve, while a low-intensity first heart sound suggests underlying valve calcification. The second heart sound is usually split with an accentuated pulmonic component reflecting pulmonary hypertension. An opening snap occurs after the second heart sound and reflects the elevated LA pressure opening the mitral valve in diastole. As MS severity increases and LA pressure rises, the opening snap moves closer to the second heart sound. However, the opening snap may be absent if the valve is severely calcified and/or fibrotic.

The murmur of MS is described as a low-frequency diastolic rumble heard best at the apex with the stethoscope bell in the lateral position.

Diagnosis

Transthoracic echocardiography provides information on mitral valve gradient, valve area and morphology, as well as estimates of pulmonary artery systolic pressure and LV function. A valve area ≤1.5 cm² is considered to be severe MS, and this usually corresponds to a transmitral mean gradient of >5–10 mm Hg (Table 10.7). The rheumatic mitral valve demonstrates a doming appearance of the leaflets related to commissural fusion. A scoring system based on valve thickening, mobility and calcification, as well as severity of

Table 10.7: Classification of mitral stenosis severity			
	Progressive	Severe	Very severe
Valve area (cm²)	>1.5	<1.5 <1.0*	<1.0
Mean gradient (mm Hg)	≤5	>5 >10*	
Pulmonary artery systolic pressure (mm Hg)	<30	>30	

*European Society of Cardiology guideline
Source: From Nishimura RA, Otto CM, Bonow RO, Carabello BA, Erwin JP, Guyton RA, et al. 2014 AHA/ACC guideline for the management of patients with valvular heart disease. J Am Coll Cardiol. 2014;63(22):e57-185; Vahanian A, Alfieri O, Andreotti F, Antunes MJ, Baron-Esquivias G, Baumgartner H, et al.; Joint Task Force on the Management of Valvular Heart Disease of the European Society of Cardiology (ESC); the European Association for Cardio-Thoracic Surgery (EACTS). Guidelines on the management of valvular heart disease (version 2012). Eur Heart J. 2012;33:2451-96.

Table 10.8: Indications for percutaneous or surgical repair of mitral stenosis

Percutaneous mitral balloon valvuloplasty

Recommended

Symptomatic patients with severe MS (MVA <1.5 cm^2) and favorable valve morphology in the absence of contraindications

Reasonable

Asymptomatic patients with very severe MS (MVA <1.0 cm^2) and favorable valve morphology in the absence of contraindications

Consider

Asymptomatic patients with severe MS (MVA <1.5 cm^2) and favorable valve morphology who have new onset of AF in the absence of contraindications

Symptomatic patients with MVA >1.5 cm^2 if there is evidence of hemodynamically significant MS during exercise (e.g. pulmonary artery wedge pressure >25 mm Hg or mean mitral valve gradient >15 mm Hg)

Severely symptomatic patients (NYHA class III/IV) with severe MS (MVA <1.5 cm^2) who have suboptimal valve anatomy and are not candidates for surgery or at high risk for surgery

Mitral valve surgery

Recommended

Severely symptomatic patients (NYHA class III/IV) with severe MS (MVA <1.5 cm^2) who are not high risk for surgery and who are not candidates for or failed previous PMBV

Severe MS (MVA <1.5 cm^2) undergoing other cardiac surgery

Reasonable

Severely symptomatic patients (NYHA class III/IV) with severe MS (MVA <1.5 cm^2), provided there are other operative indications

Consider

Patients with moderate MS (MVA 1.6–2.0 cm^2) undergoing other cardiac surgery

Mitral valve surgery and excision of the left atrial appendage may be considered for patients with severe MS (MVA <1.5 cm^2) who have had recurrent embolic events while receiving adequate anticoagulation

MS, mitral stenosis; MVA, mitral valve area; AF, atrial fibrillation; NYHA, New York Heart Association; PMBC, percutaneous mitral balloon valvuloplasty.

Source: From Nishimura RA, Otto CM, Bonow RO, Carabello BA, Erwin JP, Guyton RA, et al. 2014 AHA/ACC guideline for the management of patients with valvular heart disease. J Am Coll Cardiol. 2014;63(22):e57-185; Vahanian A, Alfieri O, Andreotti F, Antunes MJ, Baron-Esquivias G, Baumgartner H, et al.; Joint Task Force on the Management of Valvular Heart Disease of the European Society of Cardiology (ESC); the European Association for Cardio-Thoracic Surgery (EACTS). Guidelines on the management of valvular heart disease (version 2012). Eur Heart J. 2012;33:2451-96.

subvalvular calcification, helps predict suitable candidates for percutaneous balloon mitral valvuloplasty. Transesophageal echocardiography is indicated in candidates for balloon mitral valvuloplasty to exclude LA thrombus and significant MR, which would be contraindications to the procedure (Table 10.8).

Exercise testing during Doppler echocardiography (or invasive hemodynamic assessment) is useful to evaluate the response of mean mitral gradient and pulmonary artery pressure when there is a discrepancy between clinical and resting echocardiographic findings. A rise in RV systolic pressure to >60 mmHg with exercise suggests hemodynamically significant MS.

Surveillance TTE should be performed to reevaluate asymptomatic patients for changes in valve gradient and pulmonary hypertension: every year if valve area <1.0 cm^2, every 1–2 years if valves area $\leq$1.5 cm^2 and every 3–5 years if valve area is >1.5 cm^2.

Treatment

There is a limited role for medical management in MS and sinus rhythm. Diuretics may relieve congestive symptoms.

When atrial fibrillation develops, attention is directed at rate control and anticoagulation. The risk of stroke is elevated in patients with MS and atrial fibrillation, so oral anticoagulation is recommended with a dose-adjusted vitamin K antagonist (e.g. warfarin) and a goal international normalized ratio of 2.0–3.0. For patients with AF and MS who are unsuitable for or choose not take full-dose anticoagulation, combination therapy with aspirin and clopidogrel is recommended rather than aspirin alone. In patients in sinus rhythm, indications for anticoagulation are the presence of LA thrombus or prior embolic event.

Survival is improved with relief of the obstruction compared with medical therapy alone in symptomatic patients (Table 10.8). Since pulmonary hypertension increases the risk of a surgical procedure, relief of the obstruction should be pursued before pulmonary hypertension is significant. Percutaneous balloon valvuloplasty is the preferred technique for relieving MS, through splitting of the commissures. In patients with valve anatomy unsuitable for balloon valvuloplasty, significant MR or with a LA clot, surgery may be advised instead. These surgical options include open mitral valvotomy or mitral replacement (the latter if there is significant MR as well as MS).

Special Cases

Women with MS may present initially during *pregnancy* because of the associated increase in intravascular volume and cardiac output. Percutaneous balloon mitral valvuloplasty has been performed in the second trimester.

SUGGESTED READING

1. Carabello B. In: K Chatterjee, (ed). Aortic valve disease. In: Chatterjee K (Ed). Cardiology: An Illustrated Text. New Delhi, India: Jaypee Brothers; 2013. pp. 986-99.
2. Nishimura RA, Otto CM, Bonow RO, Carabello BA, Erwin JP, Guyton RA, et al. 2014 AHA/ACC guideline for the management of patients with valvular heart disease. J Am Coll Cardiol. 2014;63(22):e57-185.
3. Sharma S, Dalvi BV. In: K Chatterjee, (ed).Mitral valve disease. In: Chatterjee K (Ed). Cardiology: An Illustrated Text. New Delhi, India: Jaypee Brothers; 2013. pp. 1000-17.
4. Vahanian A, Alfieri O, Andreotti F, Antunes MJ, Baron-Esquivias G, Baumgartner H, et al.; Joint Task Force on the Management of Valvular Heart Disease of the European Society of Cardiology (ESC); the European Association for Cardio-Thoracic Surgery (EACTS). Guidelines on the management of valvular heart disease (version 2012). Eur Heart J. 2012;33:2451-96.
5. You JJ, Singer DE, Howard PA, Lane DA, Eckman MH, Fang MC, et al. Antithrombotic therapy for atrial fibrillation: Antithrombotic therapy and prevention of thrombosis, 9th edition: American College of Chest Physicians evidence-based clinical practice guidelines. Chest. 2012;141(2)(Suppl):e531S-75S.

Infective Endocarditis

Chapter 11

Andres Vargas-Estrada

Infective endocarditis (IE) is an infection of the endothelium of the heart (including but not limited to the valves) macroscopically seen as vegetations. While IE was previously classified according to its mode of presentation (i.e. acute, subacute or chronic), it is now categorized according to the underlying cardiac condition, location, presence of intracardiac devices or mode of acquisition.

The overall incidence of IE is 3-10 per 100,000 patient-years, with a higher incidence in intravenous (IV) drug users, elderly patients and patients with prosthetics or intracardiac devices.

PREDISPOSING CONDITIONS

- *Valvular heart disease*
  - High risk: Prior endocarditis, rheumatic valvular disease, aortic valve disease, complex cyanotic lesions and valve prosthesis (1.5-3% at 12 months and 3-6% at 5 years)
  - Medium risk: Mitral valve disease (including mitral valve prolapse with mitral regurgitation or leaflet thickening) and hypertrophic cardiomyopathy
- *Increased risk of bacteremia* (since 20% of bacteremic patients develop endocarditis):
  - Intravenous drug abuse, indwelling venous catheter, poor dentition, hemodialysis, diabetes mellitus, immunosuppressed status, prolonged surgery and reoperation

ETIOLOGY AND PROGNOSIS

The three most common bacterial causes of IE are streptococci, staphylococci and enterococci, with *Streptococcus* and *Staphylococcus* accounting for 80% of cases. *Staphylococcus* has now surpassed viridans group *Streptococcus* as the leading cause of bacterial endocarditis, related to the increase in healthcare-associated cases of IE, while cases attributable to oral streptococci have decreased in industrialized countries. Patients with *Streptococcus bovis* should undergo evaluation for gastrointestinal (GI) malignancy. Enterococcal endocarditis is frequently associated with malignancy or manipulation of the genitourinary (GU) or GI tract.

With prosthetic valve endocarditis, a wide spectrum of organisms can be responsible within the first year of operation, although within the first 2 years, *Staphylococcus epidermidis* is the most common pathogen. After 1 year, microorganisms infecting prosthetic valves are similar to native valve IE.

The HACEK (*Haemophilus parainfluenzae, Haemophilus aphrophilus; Actinobacillus, Cardiobacterium, Eikenella, Kingella*) group of organisms causes large (i.e. >1 cm) vegetations, large-vessel embolism and congestive heart failure. The HACEK and fungal endocarditis should be suspected when large vegetations are present.

We are also now faced with multidrug-resistant *Streptococcus viridans* and oxacillin-resistant *Staphylococcus aureus* (community acquired as well as healthcare-associated). The development of intermediate and high-level resistance to vancomycin has also been documented. Vancomycin and aminoglycoside resistance among enterococci is also a common finding in healthcare-associated infections.

In-hospital mortality rate ranges from 15% to 20% and 1-year mortality rate is approaching 40%, although rates vary across patient subgroups. For example, mortality rate is <10% for patients with left-sided native valve IE due to oral *Streptococcus*, but it is ≥40% for patients with prosthetic valve IE due to *S. aureus*.

CLINICAL MANIFESTATIONS

Acute IE arises with marked toxicity and progresses over several days to weeks to valvular destruction and metastatic infection. Subacute IE evolves over several weeks to months with mild or modest toxicity and rarely causes metastatic infection. Factors contributing to the rate of progression include virulence of the causative organism, general health of the patient and extent of the underlying valvular disease.

- *Persistent bacteremia*
  - Fever is common (occurring in about 80% of cases), night sweats
  - Anorexia, weight loss and fatigue
- *Valvular or perivalvular infection*
  - New or worsening of a known murmur
  - Congestive heart failure (in 32.3%)
  - Conduction abnormalities
- *Systemic embolization* occurs in 15–35% of cases
  - There is an increased risk of systemic embolization in patients with large, mobile vegetations on the mitral valve and infections due to *S. aureus*. Most emboli occur within the first 2–4 weeks of antimicrobial therapy
  - Cerebral emboli (in 16.9%) present with acute stroke or transient ischemic attack but can be complicated by brain abscess or meningitis
  - Peripheral arterial emboli (in 22.6%) to the extremities present with acute onset of cold/painful extremity with reduced or absent pulse. Embolization to the spleen, kidney or bowel may present with evidence of kidney injury or signs of peritonitis

- Coronary artery emboli are rare but may mimic acute coronary syndrome
- Pulmonary (septic) embolism may occur in patients with right sided IE
- *Immune complex phenomena*
  - Arthritis
  - Glomerulonephritis
  - Elevated rheumatoid factor and erythrocyte sedimentation rate

PHYSICAL EXAMINATION

A new murmur and fever are the hallmarks (in more than 85%). Fever may be absent in elderly or immunosuppressed patients. Murmurs may be absent with right-sided, mural or intracardiac device infections. Frequent examinations are recommended to monitor for changes in known murmurs.
- *Eye*
  - Fundoscopic examination: Roth spots (which are retinal hemorrhages plus pale center and occur in ≤5% of cases), chorioretinitis or endophthalmitis
  - Conjunctiva: petechiae or hemorrhage
- *Oral*
  - Petechiae on the palate
- *Cardiovascular*
  - Valvular regurgitation with or without thrill (raising suspicion of ruptured mitral valve chord or perforated valve)
  - Decreased prosthetic valve sound
  - Pericardial rub
- *Abdomen*
  - Tender
  - Splenomegaly (in about 11% of cases)
- *Musculoskeletal*
  - Arthritis/arthralgia
  - Vertebral tenderness
- *Extremities*
  - Janeway lesions, which are septic emboli presenting as nontender, hemorrhagic macules on the palms or soles and occurring (in ≤5% of cases)
  - Osler's nodes (in 10–20%), which are a manifestation of immune complexes and presenting with tender nodules on pads of digits
  - Proximal nail bed splinter hemorrhages (in 8% of cases)
  - Petechiae (in 20–40%)
  - Clubbing (in 10–20%)
- *Central nervous system (CNS): mental status changes or focal deficits from*
  - Cerebral emboli (in 20% of cases)
  - Brain abscess (in <5%)

DIAGNOSIS

A definite diagnosis of IE is provided by pathological criteria:
- Culture or histological *demonstration of microorganisms* in a vegetation, a vegetation that has embolized, or an intracardiac abscess specimen or
- Histological examination *demonstration of active endocarditis* in a vegetation or intracardiac abscess.

In the absence of pathologic demonstration of microorganisms or active endocarditis, the diagnosis of IE is made on the basis of clinical criteria. The variability in clinical presentation of IE requires a diagnostic strategy that is both sensitive for disease detection and specific for its exclusion.

The modified Duke criteria should be used in evaluating a patient with suspected IE. This uses combinations of major and minor criteria (Table 11.1) to stratify patients with suspected IE into the following three categories: definite, possible or rejected. Definitions for the diagnosis of IE by the modified Duke criteria are as follows:
- Definitive
  - Two major criteria or
  - One major and three minor or
  - Five minor

Table 11.1: Major and minor criteria used in modified Duke criteria

Major criteria

- Positive blood culture typical microorganisms known to cause IE (i.e. viridans streptococci, *Streptococcus bovis*, HACEK group, *Staphylococcus aureus* or community-acquired enterococci in the absence of a primary focus), from two separate blood cultures or a single blood culture positive for *Coxiella burnetii* or immunoglobulin G antibody >1:800.

- Evidence of endocardial involvement documented by echocardiogram (defined as follows: oscillating intracardiac mass on valve or supporting structures, in the path of regurgitant jets, or on implanted material in the absence of an alternative anatomic explanation; or abscess; or new partial dehiscence of prosthetic valve; new valvular regurgitation (worsening or changing or preexisting murmur not sufficient)

Minor criteria

- Predisposing heart condition or intravenous drug use
- Fever, with temperature >38°C
- Vascular phenomena: septic major arterial emboli, septic pulmonary infarcts, mycotic aneurysm, intracranial hemorrhage, conjunctival hemorrhage and Janeway lesions
- Immunologic phenomena: positive rheumatoid factor, glomerulonephritis, Osler's nodes and Roth spots
- Microbiologic evidence: positive blood culture not meeting major criteria (excluding a single positive culture for coagulase-negative staphylococci and organisms that do not cause endocarditis)

IE, infective endocarditis; HACEK, *Haemophilus parainfluenzae, Haemophilus aphrophilus; Actinobacillus, Cardiobacterium, Eikenella, Kingella.*

Source: Adapted from Baddour LM, Wilson WR, Bayer AS, Fowler VG, Bolger AF, Levison ME, et al. Infective Endocarditis. Diagnosis, antimicrobial therapy, and management of complications. Circulation. 2005;111:e394-433.

- Possible
  - One major and one minor or
  - Three minor
- Rejected
  - Alternative diagnosis explaining IE or
  - Resolution of syndrome with antibiotics in ≤4 days or
  - No pathologic evidence of IE at surgery or autopsy, with antibiotic therapy ≤4 days.

Evaluation

- *Blood cultures*
  - At least two sets (aerobic and anaerobic bottles) of blood cultures should be obtained in patients at risk for IE (i.e. those with congenital or acquired valvular heart disease, previous IE, prosthetic heart valves, certain congenital or heritable heart malformations, immunodeficiency states or IV drug abuse) who have unexplained fever for >48 hours, or patients with newly diagnosed left-sided valve regurgitation before antibiotics are started. Ideally, blood cultures should be drawn >6 hours apart at peripheral sites before initiation of antimicrobial therapy in patients with chronic or subacute presentation. However, this delay is not feasible in patients presenting with severe sepsis or shock, and two or more cultures at separate times should be obtained in these patients. When three sets of blood cultures are performed, the pathogen is identified in about 90% of cases.
  - Additional serologic tests (e.g. *Bartonella*, *Coxiella burnetii* and *Brucella*) may be needed if cultures are negative (see below regarding culture negative endocarditis).
  - Repeat blood cultures (at least two sets) after appropriate antibiotics have been started every 24–48 hours until they are negative.
- *Echocardiogram*
  - Transthoracic echocardiography (TTE) is recommended in patients with suspected IE to identify vegetations, characterize hemodynamic severity of valvular lesions, assess ventricular function, pulmonary pressures and detect complications.
  - The sensitivity of TTE for the diagnosis of native valve vegetations ranges from 50% to 90%, but it is reduced in cases of small vegetations and in IE affecting intracardiac devices or prostheses. Sensitivity is only 36–69% in patients with prosthetic valve IE. Transthoracic echocardiography and/or transesophageal echocardiography (TEE) are recommended for reevaluation of patients with IE who have a change in clinical signs or symptoms (e.g. new murmur, embolism, persistent fever, heart failure, abscess or atrioventricular block) and in patients at high risk of complications (e.g. extensive infected tissue, large vegetation on initial echocardiogram or staphylococcal, enterococcal or fungal infections).
  - Transesophageal echocardiography increases the sensitivity of detecting vegetations to ≥90%. The specificity for both TTE and TEE

is >90%. However, a negative TEE should not override strong clinical evidence of endocarditis, especially in the diagnosis of prosthetic valve endocarditis.
- Transesophageal echocardiography is recommended in all patients with known or suspected IE when TTE is nondiagnostic, when complications have developed or are clinically suspected or when intracardiac device leads are present.
- Intraoperative TEE is recommended for patients undergoing valve surgery for IE.
- In addition to the recommendations above for obtaining a TEE, the following are considered "reasonable" indications for TEE:
  * Patients with possible IE with *S. aureus* bacteremia without a known source.
  * Patients with a prosthetic valve in the presence of persistent fever without bacteremia or a new murmur.
  * Patients with nosocomial *S. aureus* bacteremia with a known portal of entry from an extracardiac source, since the frequency of IE is approximately 30%.
- *Cardiac computed tomography (CT)*
  - A cardiac CT is reasonable to evaluate the morphology in the setting of suspected paravalvular infections when the anatomy cannot be clearly delineated by echocardiography.

TREATMENT

Patients with IE should be evaluated and managed by consultation with a multispecialty heart valve team, including infectious disease specialist, cardiologist, and cardiac surgeon, and in surgically managed patients, this team should also include a cardiac anesthesiologist.

- *Antibiotics*
  For pending blood culture results, empiric antibiotic therapy can be initiated till reports are obtained (Table 11.2). Epidemiologic factors can assist in choosing appropriate empiric therapy, which is especially important in the treatment of culture negative endocarditis (Table 11.3). Guidance from antibiotic sensitivity data and infectious disease consultation is indicated to target appropriate therapy. Patients with known valvular heart disease should not receive antibiotics before blood cultures are obtained for unexplained fever.
- *Anticoagulation*
  It is reasonable to temporarily discontinue anticoagulation in patients with IE who develop CNS symptoms compatible with embolism or stroke regardless of the other indications for anticoagulation. Temporary discontinuation of vitamin K antagonist (VKA) might be considered in patients receiving VKA at the time of IE diagnosis.
  Patients with prosthetic valves who receive warfarin anticoagulation and develop endocarditis should have their warfarin discontinued and replaced

Table 11.2: Treatment regimens (with dosages as recommended for patients with normal renal function)

Streptococci endocarditis

Native valve IE caused by highly penicillin-susceptible viridans group streptococci
- Aqueous crystalline penicillin G sodium 12–18 million units per 24 h continuously or in four or six equally divided doses for 4 weeks duration (this regimen is preferred in most patients >65 years or patients with impairment of eighth cranial nerve function or renal function); or
- Ceftriaxone sodium 2 g per 24 h IV or IM in one dose for 4 weeks duration; or
- Vancomycin hydrochloride 30 mg/kg per 24 h in two equally divided doses daily (not to exceed 2 g per 24 h unless serum concentrations are inappropriately low) for 4 weeks if patients are unable to tolerate penicillin or ceftriaxone. Vancomycin dosage should be adjusted to obtain peak (i.e. 1 h after infusion completed) serum concentration of 30–45 µg/mL and a trough concentration range of 10–15 µg/mL
- A 2-week regimen of aqueous crystalline penicillin G sodium or ceftriaxone sodium (dosage and route above) can be used if there is no evidence of cardiac or extracardiac abscess. However, gentamicin sulfate at a dose of 3 mg/kg per day IV or IM in one dose should be added for the entire 2 weeks. The 2-week regimen is not intended for patients with evidence of decreased renal function (i.e. creatinine clearance <20 mL/min), impaired eighth cranial nerve function or Abiotrophia, Granulicatella or Gemella infection). The gentamicin dosage should be adjusted using a nomogram for calculating daily dosing

Native valve IE caused by relatively resistant Streptococcus bovis or viridans group Streptococcus
- Aqueous crystalline penicillin G sodium 24 million units per 24 h IV continuously or in four to six equally divided doses (however, if minimum inhibitory concentration is >0.5 µg/mL, treat with a regimen recommended for enterococcal endocarditis) for 4 weeks plus gentamicin at 3 mg/kg per 24 h IV or IM in one dose (with dosing per nomogram) for 2 weeks; or
- Ceftriaxone 2 g per 24 h IV or IM for a 4-week duration plus gentamicin at 3 mg/kg per 24 h IV or IM in one dose (with dosing per nomogram) for 2 weeks; or
- Vancomycin 30 mg/kg per day divided twice daily for 4 weeks for those unable to tolerate penicillin or ceftriaxone.

Prosthetic valve endocarditis viridans group streptococci
- Above regimens for a 6-week duration of therapy

Staphylococci endocarditis

Native valve oxacillin-sensitive staphylococci endocarditis
- Nafcillin or oxacillin 12 g per 24 h in four to six equally divided doses for 6 weeks if IE left-sided or complicated right-sided (and 2 weeks for uncomplicated right-sided IE), with the optional addition of gentamicin 3 mg/kg per 24 h IV or IM in two or three equally divided doses for 3–5 days (the dose should be administered in close temporal proximity to nafcillin or oxacillin). Penicillin G 24 million units per 24 h IV in four to six equally divided doses may be used in place of nafcillin or oxacillin if the strain is penicillin susceptible (i.e. minimum inhibitory concentration of <0.1 mg/mL) and the dose does not produce β-lactamase.
- For penicillin-allergic (nonanaphylactoid type) patients, recommend cefazolin 6 g per 24 h IV in three equally divided doses for 6 weeks with the optional addition of gentamicin 3 mg/kg per 24 h IV or IM in two or three equally divided doses for 3–5 days. However, in patients with anaphylactoid type reactions to β-lactams, the recommendation is vancomycin 30 mg/kg per 24 h in two equally divided doses for 6 weeks

Native valve oxacillin-resistant staphylococci endocarditis
- Vancomycin 30 mg/kg per 24 h in two equally divided doses for 6 weeks, with adjustment of dosage to achieve 1-h serum concentration of 30–45 µg/mL and trough concentration of 10–15 µg/mL.

Prosthetic valve oxacillin-sensitive staphylococci endocarditis
- Nafcillin or oxacillin 12 g per 24 h IV in six equally divided doses plus rifampin 900 mg PO or IV per 24 h in three equally divided doses for at least 6 weeks plus gentamicin 3 mg/kg per 24 h in two or three equally divided doses for 2 weeks. Gentamicin should be administered in close proximity to nafcillin or oxacillin dosing.

Contd...

Contd...

- Penicillin G 24 million units per 24 h IV in four to six equally divided doses may be used in place of nafcillin or oxacillin if the strain is penicillin susceptible (i.e. minimum inhibitory concentration of <0.1 mg/mL) and the dose does not produce β-lactamase.

Prosthetic valve oxacillin-resistant staphylococci endocarditis
- Vancomycin 30 mg/kg per 24 h divided in two equally divided doses plus rifampin 900 mg PO or IV per 24 h in three equally divided doses for at least 6 weeks plus gentamicin 3 mg/kg per 24 h in two or three equally divided doses for 2 weeks. Adjust the vancomycin dosage to achieve a 1-h serum concentration of 30–45 µg/mL and trough concentration of 10–15 µg/mL.

Enterococcal endocarditis
Native or prosthetic valve IE with enterococcus sensitive to penicillin, gentamicin and vancomycin
- Ampicillin sodium 12 g per 24 h IV in six equally divided doses plus gentamicin 3 mg/kg per 24 h IV or IM in three equally divided doses for 4–6 weeks; or
- Aqueous crystalline penicillin G sodium 18–30 million units per 24 h IV either continuously or in six equally divided doses plus gentamicin 3 mg/kg per 24 h IV or IM in three equally divided doses for 4–6 weeks
- If penicillin or ampicillin intolerant, vancomycin 30 mg/kg per 24 h in two equally doses plus gentamicin sulfate 3 mg/kg per 24 h IV or IM in three equally divided doses for 6 weeks.

Four weeks of therapy is recommended for patients with native valve IE and symptoms of illness for <3 months and 6 weeks if the duration of symptoms is >3 months. A minimum of 6 weeks of therapy is recommended for patients with IE involving a prosthetic valve or other prosthetic cardiac material. Gentamicin dosage should be adjusted to achieve peak serum concentration of 3–4 µg/mL and a trough concentration of <1 µg/mL. However, if creatinine clearance is <50 mL/min, an infectious disease specialist should be consulted.

Native or prosthetic valve IE with enterococcus resistant to gentamicin (and susceptible to streptomycin)
- Ampicillin sodium 12 g per 24 h IV in six equally divided doses plus streptomycin sulfate 15 mg/kg per 24 h IV or IM in two equally divided doses for 4–6 weeks; or
- Aqueous crystalline penicillin G sodium 24 million units per 24 h IV either continuously or in six equally divided doses plus streptomycin sulfate 15 mg/kg per 24 h IV or IM in two equally divided doses for 4–6 weeks.

As for patients with enterococcus IE sensitive to gentamicin, 4 weeks of therapy is recommended for patients with native valve IE and symptoms of illness for <3 months and 6 weeks if the duration of symptoms is >3 months. A minimum of 6 weeks of therapy is recommended for patients with IE involving a prosthetic valve or other prosthetic cardiac material.

Native or prosthetic valve IE with enterococcus resistant to penicillin (and susceptible to gentamicin and vancomycin)
- If strain is producing β-lactamase: Ampicillin-sulbactam 12 g per 24 h in four equally divided doses plus gentamicin sulfate 3 mg/kg per 24 h IV or IM in three equally divided doses for 6 weeks. If unable to tolerate ampicillin-sulbactam, vancomycin hydrochloride 30 mg/kg per 24 h IV in two equally divided doses plus gentamicin sulfate 3 mg/kg per 24 h IV or IM in three equally divided doses for 6 weeks.
- If the strain has intrinsic penicillin resistance: Vancomycin and gentamicin in same dose as above (i.e. for ampicillin-sulbactam intolerant) and consultation with a specialist in infectious diseases is recommended.

Native or prosthetic valve IE with enterococcus resistant to penicillin, gentamicin and vancomycin
- Vancomycin resistant enterococci are often multidrug-resistant, and there are few therapeutic options. Because of the complexity of treating these patients, consultation with an infectious disease specialist is recommended.

Contd...

Contd...

> **HACEK group endocarditis (native prosthetic valve)**
> - Ceftriaxone 2 g per 24 h IV or IM in 1 dose for 4 weeks; or
> - Ampicillin-sulbactam 12 g per 24 h IV divided in four equally divided doses for a total duration of 4 weeks is recommended.
> - For patients unable to tolerate cephalosporin and ampicillin therapy, the recommendation is to use ciprofloxacin 1,000 mg per 24 h PO or 800 mg per 24 h IV in two equally divided doses for 4 weeks.
> - For patients with IE involving prosthetic valve or cardiac material, the duration of therapy should be extended to 6 weeks.
>
> **Bartonella species endocarditis**
> - Treatment with infectious diseases consultation is doxycycline 200 mg per 24 h IV or PO in two equally divided doses for 6 weeks plus gentamicin sulfate 3 mg/kg per 24 h IV or IM in three equally divided doses for 2 weeks. If patient cannot take gentamicin, substitute rifampin 600 mg per 24 h PO or IV in two equally divided doses.
>
> *Coxiella burnetii* (i.e. Q-fever) endocarditis
> - Doxycycline 100 mg orally twice a day plus hydroxychloroquine 600 mg PO day for 1.5-3 years.
>
> *Culture negative endocarditis*
> In about 10% of IE cases, blood cultures are negative, usually because patients were exposed to antibiotic agents before the diagnosis is made or because the infection is caused by fastidious microorganisms, such as *bartonella* species, *brucella* species, *Coxiella burnetii*, HACEK group bacteria or *Tropheryma whipplei* (Hoen 2013).
>
> *Native valve*
> - Treat in consultation with infectious disease specialist.
> - Ampicillin-sulbactam 12 g per 24 h IV in four equally divided doses plus gentamicin sulfate 3 mg/kg per 24 h IV or IM in three equally divided doses for a duration of 4-6 weeks.
> - If penicillin intolerant, then vancomycin 30 mg/kg per 24 h in two equally divided doses plus gentamicin sulfate (in dose above) plus ciprofloxacin 1,000 mg per 24 h PO or 800 mg per 24 h IV in two equally divided doses for 4-6 weeks.
>
> *Prosthetic valve*
> - If surgery is <1 year: Vancomycin 30 mg/ kg per 24 h in two equally divided doses plus gentamicin sulfate 3 mg/kg per 24 h IV or IM in three equally divided doses plus cefepime 6 g per 24 h IV in three equally divided doses plus rifampin 900 mg per 24 h PO or IV in three equally divided doses. Duration of therapy of gentamicin is for 2 weeks, and the duration for the other antibiotics is for 6 weeks.
> - If surgery is >1 year: The same regimen as above for native valve endocarditis with the addition of rifampin.

IE, infective endocarditis; IV, intravenous; IM, intramuscular; PO, per oral; h, hour(s) HACEK, *Haemophilus parainfluenzae, Haemophilus aphrophilus, Actinobacillus, Cardiobacterium, Eikenella, Kingella.*

Source: Adapted from Baddour LM, Wilson WR, Bayer AS, Fowler VG, Bolger AF, Levison ME, et al. Infective Endocarditis. Diagnosis, antimicrobial therapy, and management of complications. Circulation. 2005;111:e394-433.

with IV heparin. The recommendation is related to the possible need for urgent surgery. However, if there is cerebral embolization, there is potential for hemorrhagic conversion, and anticoagulation with heparin can be reversed with protamine. Aspirin therapy should also be discontinued. If there is evidence of neurologic symptoms during antibiotic therapy, all anticoagulation should be discontinued until intracranial hemorrhage is excluded by imaging.

Table 11.3: Epidemiological clues in etiological diagnosis of culture-negative endocarditis

Epidemiological feature	Common microorganism(s)
Injection drug use	*Staphylococcus aureus*, including community-acquired oxacillin-resistant strains
	Coagulase-negative staphylococci
	β-hemolytic streptococci
	Fungi
	Aerobic gram-negative bacilli, including *Pseudomonas aeruginosa*
	Polymicrobial
Indwelling cardiovascular medical devices	*S. aureus*
	Coagulase-negative staphylococci
	Fungi
	Aerobic gram-negative bacilli
	Corynebacterium sp.
Genitourinary disorders, infection, manipulation, including pregnancy, delivery and abortion	*Enterococcus* sp.
	Group B streptococci (*Streptococcus agalactiae*)
	Listeria monocytogenes
	Aerobic gram-negative bacilli
	Neisseria gonorrhoeae
Chronic skin disorders, including recurrent infections	*S. aureus*
	β-Hemolytic streptococci
Poor dental health, dental procedures	Viridans group streptococci
	Nutritionally variant streptococci
	Abiotrophia defectiva
	Granulicatella sp.
	Gemella sp.
	HACEK organisms
Alcoholism, cirrhosis	*Bartonella* sp.
	Aeromonas sp.
	Listeria sp.
	Streptococcus pneumoniae
	β-hemolytic streptococci
Burn patients	*S. aureus*
	Aerobic Gram-negative bacilli, including *P. aeruginosa*

Contd...

Contd...

Epidemiological feature	Common microorganism(s)
Fungi	
Diabetes mellitus	S. aureus
	β-hemolytic streptococci
	S pneumoniae
Early (≤1year) prosthetic valve placement	Coagulase-negative staphylococci
	S. aureus
	Aerobic gram-negative bacilli
	Fungi
	Corynebacterium sp.
	Legionella sp.
Late (>1year) prosthetic valve placement	Coagulase-negative staphylococci
	S. aureus
	Viridans group streptococci
	Enterococcus sp.
	Fungi
	Corynebacterium sp.
Dog–cat exposure	*Bartonella* sp.
	Pasteurella sp.
	Capnocytophaga sp.
Contact with contaminated milk or infected farm animals	*Brucella* sp.
	Coxiella burnetii
	Erysipelothrix sp.
Homeless, body lice	*Bartonella* sp.
AIDS	*Salmonella* sp.
	S. pneumoniae
	S. aureus
Pneumonia, meningitis	S. pneumoniae
Solid organ transplant	S. aureus
	Aspergillus fumigatus
	Enterococcus sp.
	Candida sp.
Gastrointestinal lesions	S. bovis
	Enterococcus sp.

HACEK, *Haemophilus parainfluenzae, Haemophilus aphrophilus, Actinobacillus, Cardiobacterium, Eikenella, Kingella.*

RECOMMENDATIONS FOR SURGICAL INTERVENTION

Recommended indications for early surgery (i.e. during initial hospitalization before completion of a full therapeutic course of antibiotics) include the following:
- Patients with IE who present with valve dysfunction resulting in symptoms of heart failure. In-hospital mortality rate is 21% in patients with heart failure treated with surgery versus 45% in patients treated medically
- Patients with left-sided IE caused by *S. aureus*, fungal or other highly resistant organisms
- Patients with IE complicated with heart block, annular or aortic abscess or destructive penetrating lesions
- Patients with evidence of persistent infection as manifested by persistent bacteremia or fevers lasting longer than 5–7 days after onset of appropriate antimicrobial therapy
- Patients with prosthetic valve endocarditis and relapsing infection (defined as recurrence of bacteremia after a complete course of appropriate antibiotics and subsequently negative blood cultures) without other identifiable source for portal of infection

Early surgery is "reasonable" in the following:
- Patients with IE who present with recurrent emboli or persistent vegetations despite appropriate antibiotic therapy
- Patients with native IE who exhibit mobile vegetations >10 mm in length (with or without evidence of embolic phenomenon)

An additional benefit of early surgery is the potential for successful valve repair for IE involving the mitral valve, because of the risk of infection of prosthetic materials. The aortic valve may potentially be repaired (rather than replaced) if there is a leaflet perforation. Surgery may not be necessary for patients with uncomplicated IE of prosthetic valve caused by first infection with a sensitive organism.

INFECTIVE ENDOCARDITIS PROPHYLAXIS

There are four groups of patients who should receive prophylaxis before undergoing dental procedures because they are considered to be high risk for developing IE:
- Prosthetic cardiac valves
- Prior IE
- Congenital heart disease (CHD)
  - Unrepaired cyanotic CHD including those with palliative shunts
  - Repaired CHD with prosthetic material or device either by surgery or percutaneous intervention during the first 6 months after the procedure
  - Repaired CHD with residual defect at the site or adjacent to the prosthetic device (which inhibits endothelialization)
- Cardiac transplantation patients who develop cardiac valvulopathy.

In addition, prophylactic antibiotics may be considered in patients with bicuspid aortic valves, coarctation of the aorta, severe mitral valve prolapse or hypertrophic cardiomyopathy.

Table 11.4: Antibiotic regimens for prophylaxis of infective endocarditis in adults (single dose 30–60 minutes before procedure)

Situation	Agent	Regimen
Oral	Amoxicillin	2 g
Unable to take PO medications	Ampicillin	2 g IM or IV
	Cefazolin	1 g IM or IV
	Ceftriaxone	1 g IM or IV
Allergic to PCN	Clindamycin	600 mg
	Azithromycin	500 mg
	Clarithromycin	500 mg
	Cephalexin*	2 g
Allergic to PCN and unable to take po medications	Cefazolin	1 g IM or IV
	Ceftriaxone	1 g IM or IV
	Clindamycin	600 mg IM or IV

*Cephalosporins should not be used in an individual with a history of anaphylaxis, angioedema, or urticaria with penicillins or ampicillin.

PO, per oral; IM, intramuscular; IV, intravenous; PCN, penicillin

Source: Adapted from Wilson W, Taubert KA, Gewitz M, Lockhart PB, Baddour LM, Levison M, et al. Prevention of infective endocarditis: Guidelines from the American Heart Association. Circulation. 2007;116:1736-54

All dental procedures that involve manipulation of gingival tissue, periapical region of teeth or perforation of the oral mucosa require prophylaxis. A single dose of the antibiotic of choice should be given 30–60 minutes prior to the procedure (Table 11.4). Cephalosporins should not be used in individual with a history of anaphylaxis, angioedema or urticaria with penicillin or ampicillin.

The following procedures do not require routine prophylaxis:
- Anesthetic injections through noninfective tissue
- Taking dental radiographs
- Placement or adjustment of removable orthodontic appliances
- Placement of orthodontic brackets
- Shedding of deciduous teeth
- Bleeding from trauma to lips or oral mucosa

The administration of prophylactic antibiotics solely to prevent endocarditis is not recommended for patients who undergo GI or GU tract procedures.

CARDIAC IMPLANTED ELECTRONIC DEVICE INFECTIONS

As the number of patients undergoing placement of these devices continues to increase, the number of infected devices increases. Permanent pacemaker (PPM) and implantable cardioverter defibrillator (ICD) infection incidence has ranged widely between 0.13% and 19.9% in different reports. Risk factors related to the patient characteristics include renal dysfunction, device revision, oral anticoagulation, advanced age, increased number of diseased organ systems and greater number of device or lead placements (>2 leads) and/or revisions. Early reintervention (for hematoma or lead dislodgement), fever within 24 hours before implantation and the use of preprocedural temporary pacing are risk factors related to the procedure. Negatively correlated factors for PPM/ICD infections include pectoral transvenous versus abdominal/thoracotomy, new system versus partial or complete system replacement and antibiotic prophylaxis.

The most common microorganism causing device infections is coagulase negative staphylococci (42%), followed by methicillin sensitive *S. aureus* (25%), gram-negative bacilli (9%), polymicrobial (7%), culture negative (7%) and methicillin-resistant *S. aureus* (4%).

Clinical presentations include generator pocket infection and lead or valve endocarditis. Diagnosis is best made by TEE. Management involves complete device extraction and a pathogen-directed antimicrobial regimen. Primary prophylaxis at the time of device placement is preferentially done with cefazolin 1–2 g IV once 60 minutes prior to the procedure. Prophylaxis for dental, GI or GU procedures is not routinely recommended.

Complete device removal of pacemaker or ICD system, including all leads and the generator, is indicated as part of the early management plan in patients with IE with documented infection of the device or leads. It is reasonable to remove PPM/ICD systems (leads and generator) in patients with valvular IE caused by *S. aureus* or fungi, even without evidence of device or lead infection and in patients undergoing valve surgery for valvular IE.

The duration of antibiotics should be 10–14 days after cardiac implanted electronic device (CIED) removal for pocket-site infection. Antibiotics should be given for at least 14 days after CIED removal for bloodstream infection. Duration of antimicrobial therapy should be at least 4–6 weeks for complicated infections (e.g. endocarditis or septic thrombophlebitis) or if bloodstream infection persists despite device removal and appropriate initial antimicrobial therapy.

Complete device and lead removal is recommended for all patients with:
- Definite CIED infection, as evidenced by valvular and/or lead endocarditis or sepsis
- Cardiac implanted electronic device pocket infection as evidenced by abscess formation, device erosion or chronic draining sinus without clinically evident involvement of the transvenous portion of the lead system
- Complete device and lead removal is recommended for all patients with valvular endocarditis without definitive involvement of the lead(s) and/or device
- Patients with occult staphylococcal bacteremia
- Complete device and lead removal is reasonable in patients with persistent occult gram-negative bacteremia despite appropriate antibiotic therapy.

The CIED removal is not indicated for a superficial or incisional infection without involvement of the device and/or leads. The CIED removal is not indicated for relapsing bloodstream infection due to a source other than a CIED and for which long-term suppressive antimicrobials are required.

Each patient should be evaluated carefully to determine whether there is a continued need for a new CIED. The replacement device implantation should not be ipsilateral to the extraction site. Preferred alternative locations include the contralateral side, iliac vein and epicardial implantation. When positive before extraction, blood cultures should be drawn after device removal and should be negative for at least 72 hours before a new device placement is performed. New transvenous lead placement should be delayed for at least 14 days after CIED system when there is evidence of valvular infection.

Long-term suppressive therapy should be considered for patients who have CIED infection and for those who are not candidates for complete device removal. This therapy should not be administered to patients who are candidates for infected CIED removal.

SUMMARY

The most common bacterial causes of IE are staphylococci, streptococci and enterococci, with the former two accounting for 80% of cases. The Modified Duke Criteria should be used in evaluating a patient with suspected IE. At least two sets of blood cultures should be obtained. Transthoracic echocardiography is recommended in patients with suspected IE to identify vegetations, characterize hemodynamic severity of valvular lesions, assess ventricular function, pulmonary pressures and detect complications. Empiric broad-spectrum antibiotics should be started soon after blood cultures and chosen on the basis of the clinical presentation and epidemiological clues. Early surgery is recommended for patients who present with heart failure symptoms, those with left-sided IE caused by *S. aureus* or fungal infections and those who develop heart block, annular or aortic abscess, persistent bacteremia or fevers lasting longer than 5-7 days after onset of appropriate antimicrobial therapy or recurrent emboli. A multidisciplinary team including a cardiologist, an infectious disease specialist and a cardiothoracic surgeon should be actively involved in the management of patients with IE.

SUGGESTED READING

1. Baddour LM, Wilson WR, Bayer AS, Fowler VG, Bolger AF, Levison ME, et al. Infective Endocarditis. Diagnosis, antimicrobial therapy, and management of complications. Circulation. 2005;111:e394-433.
2. Baddour LM, Epstein AE, Erickson CC, Knight BP, Levison ME, Lockhart PB, et al. Update on cardiovascular implantable electronic device infections and their management: A scientific statement from the American Heart Association. Circulation. 2010;121:458-77.
3. Gould FK, Denning DW, Elliott TS, Foweraker J, Perry JD, Prendergast BD, et al. Guidelines for the diagnosis and antibiotic treatment of endocarditis in adults: A report of the Working Party of the British Society for Antimicrobial Chemotherapy. J Antimicrob Chemother. 2012;67:269-89.

4. Habib G, Hoen B, Tornos P, Thuny F, Prendergast B, Vilacosta I, et al. Guidelines on the prevention, diagnosis, and treatment of infective endocarditis. The task force on the prevention, diagnosis, and treatment of infective endocarditis of the European Society of Cardiology. Eur Heart J. 2009;30(19):2369-413.
5. Habib G, Badano L, Tribouilloy C, Vilacosta I, Zamorano JL. Recommendations for the practice of echocardiography in infective endocarditis. Eur J Echocardiogr. 2010;11(2):202-19.
6. Hoen B, Duval X. Infective endocarditis. N Engl J Med. 2013;368(15):1425-33.
7. Klug D, Balde M, Pavin D, Hidden-Lucet F, Clementy J, Sadoul N, et al. Risk factors related to infections of implanted pacemakers and cardioverter-defibrillators. Circulation. 2007;116:1349-55.
8. Lekkerkerker JC, van Nieuwkoop C, Trines SA, van der Bom J G, Bernards A, van der elde ET, et al. Risk factors and time delay associated with cardiac device infections: Leiden device registry. Heart. 2009;95:715-20.
9. Nishimura RA, Otto CM, Bonow RO, Carabello BA, Erwin JP, Guyton RA, et al. 2014 AHA/ACC Guideline for the management of patients with valvular heart disease. J Am Coll Cardiol. 2014;63(22):e57-185.
10. Wilson W, Taubert KA, Gewitz M, Lockhart PB, Baddour LM, Levison M, et al. Prevention of infective endocarditis: Guidelines from the American Heart Association. Circulation. 2007;116:1736-54.

Prosthetic Heart Valves

Chapter 12

Byron F Vandenberg

INTRODUCTION

While the goals of valve surgery are to improve functional status and longevity, valve replacement does not provide a cure. Rather, native valve disease is exchanged for prosthetic valve disease. Optimal management of these patients includes knowledge of prostheses and current guidelines for long-term management.

TYPES OF PROSTHETIC VALVES

The ideal valve prosthesis should have excellent hemodynamics, long durability, high thromboresistance and excellent implantability. The currently available prostheses are not ideal (Fig. 12.1). Mechanical valves are durable but require chronic anticoagulation because of thrombogenicity. Biological valves do not require anticoagulation (unless there are other compelling reasons, such as atrial fibrillation) but durability is limited.

- **Mechanical valves:** Mechanical valves have three key components: occluder (i.e. the closure mechanism), housing and sewing ring. All have some degree of regurgitant flow (i.e. the washing jet) that prevents thrombus formation on the surface of the valve. The design of a mechanical valve placed in the current era has a bileaflet occluder (e.g. St. Jude Medical valve). In previous years, the design has included a cage-ball and single disc occluder design.
- **Bioprosthetic valves:** Bioprosthetic valves are considered heterograft (i.e. from porcine or bovine tissue) or homograft (i.e. human cadaver). Porcine valves may be stented with the valve tissue mounted on supportive prosthetic material or stentless in the aortic position with the valve tissue supported by the donated annulus and aortic root. Bovine pericardial valves are manufactured from shets of bovine pericardium mounted inside or outside of a supporting stent.

  The stented valve design requires a mounting platform that may be polypropylene (e.g. Carpentier–Edwards valve) or a wire backbone (e.g. Medtronic Hancock valve). Stented valves are less thrombogenic than mechanical valves and do not require long-term anticoagulation.
- **Homograft:** Homograft aortic valves are available through cooperative ventures with tissue banks. They may be chosen for patients with active

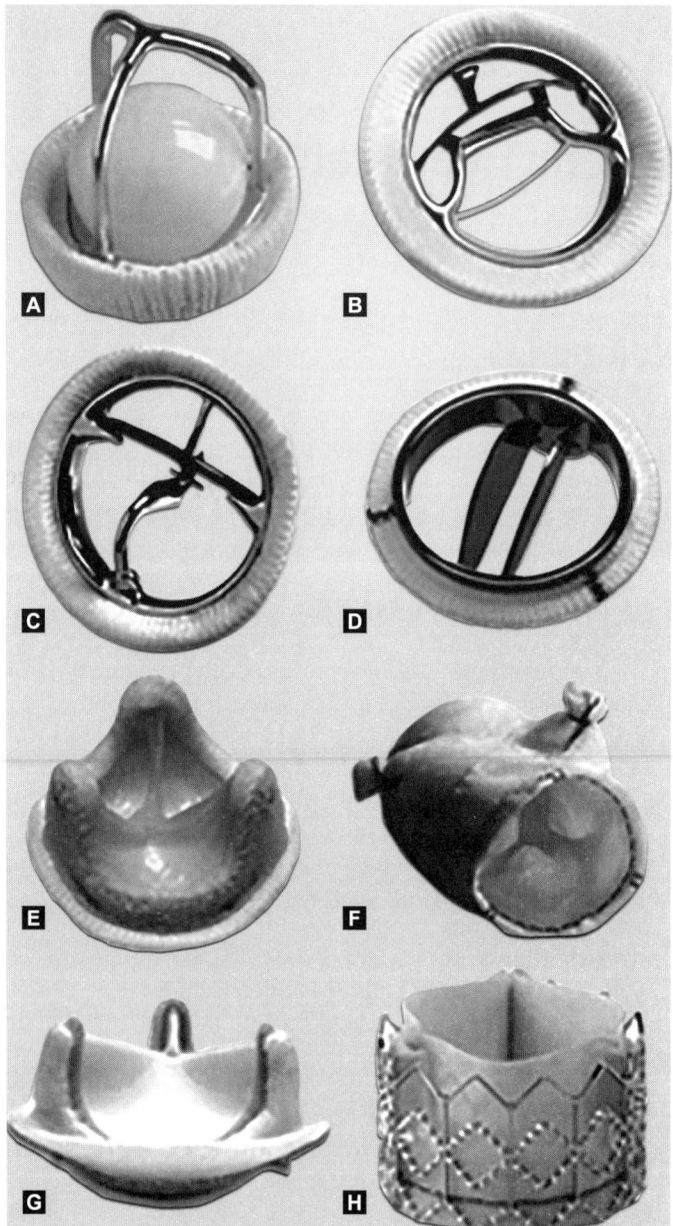

Fig. 12.1: Different models of prosthetic heart valves. (A) Starr–Edwards caged-ball valve; (B) Bjork–Shiley tilting disk valve; (C) Medtronic–Hall tilting disk valve; (D) St. Jude Medical bileaflet valve; (E) Medtronic Hancock II porcine valve; (F) Medtronic Freestyle porcine valve; (G) Carpentier-Edwards Perimount bovine pericardial valve; (H) Edwards SAPIEN transcatheter pericardial aortic valve. *(For color version, see Plate 3)*

Source: Reprinted with permission from Sun JCJ, Davidson MJ, Lamy A, Eikelboom JW. Antithrombotic management of patients with prosthetic heart valves: current evidence and future trends. Lancet. 2009;374:565-76, Davidson MJ, Lamy A, Eikelboom JW, Elsevier.

endocarditis, associated abscess or uncontrolled infection. This indication is at least partly attributed to their preincubation in antibiotics. In addition, the long-term risk of endocarditis is low. Because of limited durability, patients with homografts are more likely to undergo reoperation compared with patients undergoing replacement with a mechanical valve.

Homografts and bioprostheses have similar rates of structural valve deterioration (SVD). However, the versatility in dealing with acquired and congenital aortic root pathology by using the inclusion cylinder or full root replacement makes homografts a good second option to the Ross procedure in the young and heterografts in adults not felt to be candidates for long-term anticoagulation

- **Ross procedure (i.e. pulmonic valve autotransplantation):** In the Ross procedure, the patient's pulmonary valve and main pulmonary artery are removed and they replace the diseased aortic valve and the proximal aorta with reimplantation of the coronary arteries. Then, a pulmonary or aortic homograft is inserted into the pulmonary position. The procedure is most commonly performed in children and young adults and there is some controversy about indications in adults.

  Advantages of the procedure include: (i) the autograft may grow in children, (ii) warfarin is not required, (iii) favorable hemodynamic characteristics, (iv) low incidence of thromboembolism and (v) low endocarditis risk. Disadvantages include: (i) a complex operation that is technically demanding, (ii) in-hospital mortality of 3–5%, (iii) risk of early aortic valve failure, (iv) the homograft used to replace pulmonary valve is subject to stenosis and failure, and (v) the procedure is not recommended for patients with bicuspid valve and dilated aorta, since a bicuspid valve may be associated with degenerative changes in the pulmonary root.

  Absolute contraindications include recognized connective tissue disease (e.g. Marfan's syndrome) and chronic inflammatory disorders because of the potential involvement of the pulmonary valve/root in the disease process.

SELECTING THE OPTIMAL PROSTHESIS

An optimal valve prosthesis is characterized by excellent hemodynamics, long durability, high thromboresistance and ease of implantation. Unfortunately, none of the currently available prostheses have all these features and the selection of a prosthetic valve for the individual is determined by the relative importance of these characteristics.

Improved mortality with mechanical valves compared to porcine valves was demonstrated in early randomized trials; however, more recent randomized trials comparing contemporary mechanical and bioprosthetic aortic valves show no differences in mortality.

Nonrandomized trials demonstrate that survival rates and risk of complications are dependent on patient-related factors, such as age, left ventricular dysfunction, heart failure, coronary artery disease, coronary artery bypass grafting, arrhythmias, pulmonary hypertension and coexistent conditions, such as renal failure, lung disease, hypertension and diabetes. Thus, comparison of outcomes between mechanical and biological valves requires caution unless baseline characteristics of patients are similar. However, the choice between mechanical and bioprosthetic valves is largely related to a trade-off between the durability advantage of mechanical valves compared to lower bleeding risk of bioprostheses.

Improved life expectancy with bioprosthetic valves has been demonstrated in elderly patients undergoing aortic valve replacement compared to mechanical valves, likely related to the increased bleeding risk associated with anticoagulation use.

The selection of prosthetic heart valves for women of childbearing age is difficult. Mechanical bileaflet valves may be favored because of durability and they may be a reasonable choice for women who are compliant and committed to careful anticoagulation. However, a biological valve prosthesis may be preferred in young women who are not interested in anticoagulation or for whom close follow-up is not possible. Unfortunately, pregnancy in a woman with a bioprosthetic valve is associated with SVD and the incidence may average 24% during or shortly after the pregnancy.

The selection of the optimal prosthesis depends on a number of clinical variables, including age, ability to tolerate full dose oral anticoagulation, comorbidities, left ventricular (LV) function, body size and valve annulus size.

PROSTHESIS-PATIENT MISMATCH

Prosthesis-patient mismatch (PPM) occurs when the effective orifice area (EOA) of a normal functioning valve is too small in relation to the patient's body size and cardiac output requirements, resulting in abnormally high transvalvular gradients. Criteria for PPM have been established and are based on the EOA indexed for body surface area. The projected indexed EOA is typically determined from reference values published by echocardiography labs. Severe PPM is estimated to occur in 2–10% of patients and is defined as an EOA/m^2 ≤ 0.65 for aortic valve prostheses and ≤ 0.9 for mitral. Moderate PPM may be frequent in both the aortic (20–70%) and mitral (30–70%) positions and is defined as EOA/m^2 of ≤ 0.85 for aortic valve prostheses and ≤ 1.2 for mitral.

Prosthesis-patient mismatch in the aortic position is associated with less improvement in symptoms and functional class, less regression of LV hypertrophy and more adverse cardiac events, including mortality. Preoperative left ventricular function is predictive of a combined endpoint of increased incidence of heart failure symptoms or death related to heart failure at 3 years in patients with moderate PPM after aortic valve replacement.

PPM in the mitral position can be equated to residual mitral stenosis with similar consequences (i.e. persistence of abnormally high mitral gradients and increased left atrial and pulmonary arterial pressure). Pulmonary pressures are higher in patients with severe PPM. Unfortunately, when PPM after mitral valve replacement is predicted on the basis of projected EOA, options are limited. No alternative techniques exist to implant a larger prosthesis and durability of homografts and stentless valves are not optimal.

Management of PPM is directed at avoiding severe mismatch in patients undergoing aortic and mitral valve replacement and avoiding moderate mismatch in patients with preexisting LV dysfunction and/or severe LV hypertrophy and in patients engaging in regular and/or intense physical activity (especially younger patients).

If the projected indexed EOA predicts significant PPM in the aortic position, an alternate prosthesis or aortic root enlargement provides options. Several approaches for posterior aortic root enlargement have been described and both involve suturing a pericardial patch to the posterior root to allow enlargement of the annulus without compromising the coronary ostia. When comparing stentless valves with stented pericardial valves, studies are mixed with either reduced or equivalent rates of PPM with stentless valves.

LONG-TERM MANAGEMENT

- **Antithrombotic Therapy**
  - **General management**

    Mechanical valves are prone to thrombus formation and all such patients require warfarin therapy. For example, the lack of prophylaxis in patients with St. Jude Medical bileaflet valves is associated with a risk of embolism or thrombosis in the aortic position of 12% per year and 22% per year in the mitral position. However, even with warfarin, the thromboembolic risk is 1–2% per year. In patients with bioprosthetic valves and in sinus rhythm, the risk is 0.7% per year.

    Mitral prostheses have increased risk of thromboembolic events compared to aortic valves. In addition, the risk of a thromboembolic event is higher in the initial 3 months of implantation (before the valve is endothelialized) compared to later. Risk factors associated with an increased risk of thromboembolism include atrial fibrillation, LV dysfunction, left atrial dilation, previous history of thromboembolism and hypercoagulable condition.

    Current guidelines recommend a relatively low goal international normalized ratio (INR) of 2.0–3.0 for bileaflet or Medtronic-Hall single leaflet aortic valve prostheses, when no risk factors for thromboembolism are present. During the initial 3 months, however, a goal INR of 2.5–3.5 can be considered (because of the increased risk of thromboembolism early after valve replacement). A goal INR of 2.5–3.5 is recommended if patients with these valves have risk factors associated with increased thromboembolism. In addition, the goal INR of 2.5–3.5 is recommended in patients with Starr-Edwards cage-ball valves, single-leaflet valves (other than Medtronic-Hall) in the aortic position without risk factors and mechanical valves in the mitral position (Fig. 12.2).

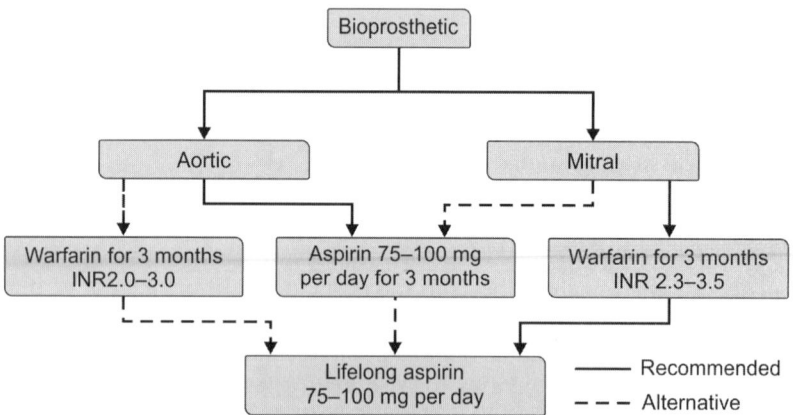

Fig. 12.2: Algorithm for antithrombotic therapy for prosthetic heart valves. Risk factors: atrial fibrillation, previous thromboembolism, left ventricular ejection fraction <35% and hypercoagulable state

Source: Reprinted with permission from Sun JCJ, Davidson MJ, Lamy A, Eikelboom JW. Antithrombotic management of patients with prosthetic heart valves: current evidence and future trends. Lancet. 2009;374:565-76, Davidson MJ, Lamy A, Eikelboom JW, Elsevier.

In those patients with a high risk of thromboembolism and in whom aspirin cannot be used, there is a suggestion of benefit for INR goals of 3.5–4.5 or to add clopidogrel to warfarin therapy. However, the higher INR goal is associated with an increased risk of bleeding.

Aspirin is recommended in a dose of 75–100 mg a day as an addition to warfarin in patients with mechanical heart valves. Turpie et al. demonstrated that the addition of 100 mg of aspirin to warfarin reduced death and embolism in patients with mechanical valves (14.3% vs. 2.8%), although bleeding risk was increased.

In patients with aortic or mitral valve bioprostheses, warfarin is indicated to achieve a goal INR of 2.0–3.0 if there are risk factors for increased risk of thromboembolism. In the absence of risk factors, warfarin for the initial 3 months after surgery is considered "reasonable" by current guidelines, although most centers use only aspirin in the aortic position. In the absence of risk factors for thromboembolism, aspirin 75–100 mg is recommended chronically.

Self-management of oral anticoagulation therapy improves survival and lowers thromboembolic risk, presumed related to a reduction in INR variability.

Pregnancy

Warfarin use during pregnancy is associated with a 20–50% rate of spontaneous abortion in the first trimester (i.e. the initial 6–12 weeks of pregnancy). The incidence of a characteristic fetal embryopathy when the fetus goes to term is approximately 4–10%. The embryopathy is characterized by nasal hypoplasia and/or stippled epiphyses. Limb hypoplasia has been reported in up to one-third of cases. The embryopathy can be prevented if warfarin is not taken during the first trimester and fetal complications are less common with warfarin doses under 5 mg per day. Frequent pregnancy tests are recommended in women taking warfarin who are attempting pregnancy.

Three anticoagulation regimens have been proposed for use in pregnant patients with mechanical valves as an alternative to warfarin:

- Continuous, intravenous dose-adjusted unfractionated heparin (UFH). While the fetal risk is lower compared to the other regimens, the maternal risks of prosthetic valve thrombosis, systemic embolization, infection, osteoporosis and heparin-induced thrombocytopenia are relatively higher
- Subcutaneous dose-adjusted UFH with the PTT at least twice control. Heparin is initiated at 17,500–20,000 U q 12 hours with PTT check at 6 hours
- Subcutaneous dose-adjusted low molecular weight heparin (LMWH) administered twice daily to maintain the anti-Xa level between 0.7 and 1.2 U per mL 4 hours after administration

The suggested dosing regimens are as follows:

- Either LMWH or UFH between 6 and 12 weeks and close to term only, with warfarin at other times
- Aggressive, dose-adjusted UFH throughout pregnancy
- Aggressive, dose-adjusted LMWH throughout pregnancy

In addition, the addition of low-dose aspirin (i.e. 75–100 mg per day) in the second and third trimesters of pregnancy is reasonable.

For women with high-risk mechanical valves (e.g. older generation valve in the mitral position or history of thromboembolism), the American College of Chest Physicians Practice Guidelines suggest the use of oral anticoagulants over heparin, in an effort to avoid maternal complications, recognizing the potential risk of fetal complications. During warfarin use in pregnancy, the INR goal is 3.0 (range 2.5–3.5).

Warfarin is relatively safe during the second and third trimesters of pregnancy, but starting 2-3 weeks before planned delivery, warfarin should be discontinued and continuous intravenous UFH given. It is reasonable to resume UFH 4 to 6 hours after delivery and begin oral warfarin in the absence of significant bleeding.

- **Noncardiac surgery:** Bridging therapy with intravenous anticoagulation may be needed in patients with mechanical valves who require interruption of warfarin therapy for noncardiac surgery, invasive procedures or dental care. However, antithrombotic therapy should not be stopped for procedures in which bleeding would be unlikely or inconsequential.

In patients with low risk of thrombosis, defined as those with a bileaflet mechanical AVR with no risk factors for increased risk of thromboembolism (i.e. atrial fibrillation, previous thromboembolism, LV dysfunction, hypercoagulable conditions, older generation thrombogenic valves, mechanical tricuspid valves or >1 mechanical valve), it is recommended that warfarin be stopped 48-72 hours before the procedure (so that the INR falls <1.5) and restarted within 24 hours after the procedure since intravenous heparin is usually unnecessary.

In patients with high risk of thrombosis (defined as those with any mechanical mitral or tricuspid valve replacement or a mechanical AVR with any risk factor for increased risk of thromboembolism), therapeutic doses of intravenous UFH should be started when the INR falls below 2.0 (typically 48 hours before surgery), stopped 4-6 hours before the procedure, restarted as early as possible after surgery as bleeding stability allows and continued (with a goal PTT of 55-70 seconds) until the INR is again therapeutic with warfarin therapy.

The use of LMWH in the perioperative period is associated with cost savings related to reduced in patient days. However, concerns about the use of LMWH in patients with mechanical valves persist and have not been adequately studied in patients with mechanical prosthetic heart valves. Close monitoring with anti-Xa assays is therefore recommended when LMWH is used in patients with mechanical valves.

In the event of emergency surgery, it is reasonable to give fresh frozen plasma to patients with mechanical valves who require interruption of warfarin. Fresh frozen plasma is preferable to high-dose vitamin K that may create a hypercoagulable state.

Prior to cardiac catheterization, in patients taking warfarin, the drug is stopped approximately 72 hours before the procedure to achieve an INR under 1.5 (unless transseptal puncture or LV puncture is planned, then the goal INR is <1.2). Following catheterization, warfarin is restarted as soon as the procedure is completed. However, if the patient has more than one risk factor for thromboembolism, heparin is started when the INR is under 2.0. Following catheterization, warfarin is restarted with an overlap of 3-5 days until the desired INR goal is achieved.

- **Echocardiography follow-up:** After valve surgery, current guidelines recommend a Doppler echocardiogram at the first postoperative visit (i.e. 2-4 weeks after discharge) if a baseline study was not obtained during hospitalization. The echocardiogram is in addition to an interval or complete history and physical examination and indicated laboratory evaluation. Routine visits annually are recommended, but with a repeat echocardiogram only if there is a change in clinical status (e.g. new murmur, concern for prosthetic valve or LV dysfunction). However, an annual echocardiogram may be considered in patients with a bioprosthetic valve after the first 5 years.

Echo parameters of interest include leaflet morphology and mobility, as well as measurement of transprosthetic gradients and EOA, estimation of the degree of regurgitation, evaluation of LV size and function and calculation of pulmonary arterial systolic pressure. Transesophageal echocardiography (TEE) can provide improved image quality and detection of cusp calcification and thickening, valvular vegetation, thrombus or pannus and reduced leaflet mobility. Mechanical valves are limited by reverberations and "shadowing" of the prosthesis. In this case, fluoroscopy may be preferred for leaflet motion assessment.

Quantitative Doppler parameters are useful in determining the intrinsic gradient of the valve, providing a comparison for subsequent studies (Table 12.1). They include as follows:

Table 12.1: Doppler parameters of prosthetic aortic and mitral valve stenosis

Parameter	Normal	Possible stenosis	Suggests significant stenosis
Aortic valve			
Peak velocity (m/s)	<3	3-4	>4
Mean gradient (mm Hg)	<20	20-35	>35
DVI	≥0.30	0.25-0.29	<0.25
EOA (cm^2)	>1.2	0.8-1.2	<0.8
Jet contour	Triangular		
Early peaking	Triangular		
Intermediate	Rounded		
Symmetrical contour			
AT (ms)	<80	80-100	>100
Mitral valve			
Peak velocity (m/s)	<1.9	1.9-2.5	≥2.5
Mean Gradient (mm Hg)	≤5	6-10	>10
EOA (cm^2)	>2.0	1.0-2.0	<1.0
PHT (ms)	<130	130-200	>200

DVI, Doppler velocity index; EOA, effective orifice area; AT, acceleration time; PHT, pressure half-time.

Source: Adapted from Zoghbi W, Chambers JB, Dumesnil JG, Foster E, Gottdiener JS, Grayburn PA, et al. Recommendations for evaluation of prosthetic valves with echocardiography and Doppler ultrasound. J Am Soc Echocardiogr. 2009;22:975-1014.

- Gradients, calculated by the Bernoulli equation. Jets may be eccentric in mechanical valves and therefore technically difficult to measure.
- EOA, calculated by continuity equation. For aortic prostheses, this includes velocity measurements in the LV outflow tract (LVOT) and across the prosthesis, as well as the LVOT diameter. For mitral prostheses, the continuity equation calculation uses stroke volume, also estimated from the LVOT velocity and diameter, in addition to the velocity measurement across the mitral prosthesis.
- Doppler velocity index, calculated from the ratio: Velocity $_{LVOT}$/Velocity $_{Prosthetic\ Valve}$. This is a dimensionless index, useful in screening for obstruction when LVOT measurements cannot be obtained.

When an elevated gradient is obtained, the differential diagnosis is:
- Pathological valve obstruction
- LVOT obstruction
- PPM
- High flow state
- Localized high gradient in presence of bileaflet mechanical valve.

PPM is suspected if the reference index EOA is low (see the previous page in this chapter–PPM for criteria used to define moderate and severe PPM). If there is no significant PPM and the DVI is normal (due to an elevated LVOT velocity), then there is probably a high flow state or LVOT obstruction. If the measured EOA is less than the reference EOA, then pathological valve obstruction or a localized high gradient associated with a bileaflet valve is suspected and fluoroscopy may help in the distinction by determining adequacy of leaflet motion. In the presence of a bileaflet mechanical valve, the smaller central orifice may give rise to a high-velocity jet that corresponds to a localized pressure drop that is largely recovered once the central flow reunites with flows originating from the two lateral orifices. A continuous wave Doppler recording includes this high-velocity jet, which leads to overestimation of gradients and underestimation of EOA compared to hemodynamics obtained at cardiac catheterization. Finally, the jet contour from the Doppler spectral recording may be helpful in discriminating prosthesis stenosis from other causes of elevated gradients since an acceleration time >100 msec suggests stenosis.

Pathologic regurgitation may be central (i.e. transvalvular) or paravavlular. In general, the criteria for grading severity of regurgitant lesions in prosthetic valves are similar to native valves largely related to the paucity of studies in patients with prosthetic valves. In the presence of mitral regurgitation, the largest diameter of the regurgitant jet emerging through the prosthesis has optimal diagnostic accuracy in comparison with other Doppler variables. However, care is needed to separate physiological from pathological regurgitation since mechanical valves have normal leakage backflow to prevent blood stasis and thrombus formation. The distinction between paravalvular and transvalvular regurgitation may require TEE.

LONG-TERM COMPLICATIONS

Thromboembolic and Bleeding Complications

When a patient has a systemic embolic event, the adequacy of anticoagulation control should be assessed. If inadequate, therapy is adjusted to maintain therapeutic goals. If anticoagulation is adequate, the dosage of antithrombotic therapy should be increased, when clinically safe, as follows:
- If the patient is not taking aspirin, add aspirin 75–100 mg per day
- If the patient is taking aspirin alone, the aspirin dose may need to be increased to 325 mg per day, clopidogrel 75 mg per day added and/or warfarin added
- If the current warfarin INR goal is 2.0–3.0, then increase the warfarin dose to achieve INR goal of 2.5–3.5
- If current warfarin INR goal is 2.5–3.5, then increase the warfarin dose to achieve INR goal of 3.5–4.5
- If the patient is taking warfarin plus aspirin 75–100 mg per day, the aspirin dose may also need to be increased to 325 mg per day if the higher dose of warfarin is not achieving the desired clinical result.

More aggressive goals for anticoagulation are expected associated risk of increased bleeding. In addition, in the presence of recent cerebral infarction, anticoagulation may need to be held to avoid hemorrhagic transformation.

Prosthetic Valve Thrombosis

Obstruction of a prosthetic valve may be caused by thrombus, pannus ingrowth or a combination of both. Prosthetic valve thrombosis has an incidence of 0.3–1.3% per patient-year with mechanical valves, but can occur early post-op after bioprosthetic valves as well, usually in the early postoperative period.

When prosthetic valve obstruction is suspected, transthoracic Doppler echocardiography is indicated to assess the hemodynamic severity of the obstruction. TEE and/or fluoroscopy may be useful to assess valve motion and/or clot burden. In the presence of obstruction, fluoroscopy demonstrates restricted leaflet motion, which may be due to thrombus or pannus. TEE and CT may be helpful in distinguishing pannus ingrowth from thrombus. Increased high-intensity transient signal due to emboli from thrombus may be detected by transcranial Doppler. Clinical history may be helpful in distinguishing thrombus from pannus ingrowth. Symptoms of obstruction are more typically gradual with pannus ingrowth. The etiology of obstruction is more likely thrombotic if anticoagulation is interrupted or subtherapeutic.

Emergency operation is reasonable for patients with a thrombosed left-sided prosthetic valve and NYHA functional class III–IV symptoms or a large clot burden. However, operative mortality approaches 15–20% with functional class IV patients.

Thrombolytic therapy is an alternative to surgery in left-sided valve thrombosis but there is a 12–15% risk of systemic embolism and a 5% risk of major bleeding. The repeat thrombosis rate is as high as 15–20%. Mortality associated with fibrinolytic therapy is 6%. Fibrinolytic therapy may be considered as a first-line therapy for patients with a thrombosed left-sided prosthetic valve, a small clot burden and NYHA functional class I–II symptoms, or if surgery is high risk or not available for patients with NYHA functional class III–IV symptoms. In cases with a large clot burden (i.e. >5–10 mm diameter), fibrinolytic therapy may be considered for patients who have NYHA functional class II–IV symptoms if emergency surgery is high risk or not available. However, fibrinolytic therapy is not effective if obstruction is due to pannus ingrowth.

Fibrinolytic therapy is also reasonable for thrombosed right-sided prosthetic heart valves with NYHA functional class III–IV symptoms or a large clot burden.

If fibrinolytic therapy is successful, it should be followed by intravenous UFH until warfarin achieves an INR of 3.0–4.0 for aortic prosthetic valves and 3.5–4.5 for mitral prosthetic valves. These patients should also receive aspirin.

Intravenous UFH is an alternative to fibrinolytic therapy and may be considered for patients with a thrombosed valve who are in NYHA functional class I–II and have a small clot burden. A trial of continuous infusion fibrinolytic therapy may be helpful if the initial UFH trial is not successful.

Bleeding Complications

The annual risk of bleeding in randomized trials is 1–3% and is more common in mechanical valves and in patients over 65 years. Bleeding is often due to excessive anticoagulation and can be managed by withholding warfarin and monitoring the level of anticoagulation with serial INR determinations. Guidelines for managing bleeding complications are provided by the American College of Chest Physicians.

Structural Valve Deterioration

Mechanical prostheses have excellent durability and SVD is rare with contemporary valves. Structural valve deterioration after bioprosthetic valve replacement begins at about 5 years for mitral position and at about 8 years for aortic position. The percent freedom from valvular deterioration and valve-related death decreases at a faster rate after 5 years compared with the first 5 years (i.e. there appears to be an almost exponential rate of decline over time). With conventional stented bioprostheses, the freedom from structural failure is 70–90% at 10 years and 50–80% at 15 years. However, certain pericardial valves have improved durability compared to porcine valves. Unfortunately, reoperation for bioprosthetic valve failure has a significantly higher mortality than the initial valve replacement.

Approximately three-quarters of porcine valve degenerative failures manifest as regurgitation, usually related to cusp tears in calcified cusps.

Pure stenosis due to calcific cuspal stiffening and tears occur in 10–15% and perforations unrelated to calcification occur in about 10–15%. Calcification is a major contributor to bioprosthesis failure to such an extent that it is considered one of the predisposing causes of cusp tears.

Premature deterioration of bioprostheses may be related to tissue fixation methods. Glutaraldehyde reduces antigenicity of heterografts; however, membrane damage may predispose to calcium crystal nucleation, contributing to subsequent calcium crystal growth. Additional mechanisms include atherosclerosis and immune rejection (due to residual antigens).

Risk factors associated with bioprosthetic SVD include the following:
- Younger patients, related to the heightened and more effective immune response in response to residual animal antigens
- Mitral position, related to higher closure pressure and increased stress on the valve
- Renal insufficiency
- Hyperparathyroidism
- Hypertension. In the aortic position, SVD of bioprostheses may be related to stress from elevated diastolic BP.
- Endocarditis: A diagnosis of infective endocarditis (IE) is based on the presence of either major or minor clinical criteria and is discussed in the chapter on IE. TEE is recommended in patients with prosthetic valve endocarditis (PVE). The incidence of PVE is about 0.3–1.2% per patient-year and accounts for 10–30% of all cases of IE.

Overall, *Staphylococcus aureus* is the most common causative organism of PVE followed by coagulase-negative *staphylococci, streptococci* and *enterococci*. However, the microbiology varies according to time of developing endocarditis after valve surgery. In patients with PVE within 1 year of surgery and no drug abuse, methicillin-resistant coagulase-negative staphylococcus was the most common organism in a recent series, followed by *S. aureus*. For late PVE, *Streptococcus viridans* and *S. aureus* were the most common organisms. However, cultures may remain negative in both early and late PVE.

In cases of early endocarditis, the infection usually involves the junction between the sewing ring and annulus, leading to perivalvular abscess, dehiscence and fistula. Surgery is frequently required in these patients. In later PVE, similar sites of infection occur in mechanical valves, but infection is more frequently located on the leaflets of patients with bioprostheses.

Echocardiographic criteria for IE include (i) an oscillating intracardiac mass on the valve, supporting structures (including implanted material) or in the path of regurgitant jet, (ii) abscess, usually manifest as echo-lucency or echo-density in the valve ring (and they may infiltrate the septum and conduction systems or result in fistula formation), (iii) new partial dehiscence of prostheses, and (iv) new valvular regurgitation.

If the initial TEE is negative and clinical suspicion persists, a repeat TEE in 7–10 days may be advisable. In addition, repeat TEE may be useful when there is a change in clinical status during antibiotic therapy (e.g. progression in heart failure symptoms, change in murmur, new atrioventricular block or arrhythmia).

Medical therapy alone is more likely to succeed in late PVE and non-staphylococcal infections. Antibiotic treatment regimens are provided in the chapter on IE.

Anticoagulation is controversial in mechanical valve endocarditis. Some authorities recommend continuation of therapy but the general advice is to discontinue all anticoagulation in patients with *S. aureus* PVE who have experienced a recent central nervous system event for at least the first 2 weeks of antibiotic therapy, to prevent hemorrhagic transformation.

In-hospital mortality of PVE is 23% in some series and predictors are old age, health care-associated infection, *S. aureus* infection and complicated endocarditis.

Indications for cardiac surgery include heart failure, valve dehiscence, abscess formation and persistent bacteremia or recurrent emboli despite appropriate antibiotics. Although mortality remains high, early surgery is recommended when the infection is due to *S. aureus* or if there is a complication of PVE. The choice of the optimal valve substitute is controversial. For the mitral position, mechanical or biologic prostheses are usually placed. In the aortic position, homografts have been utilized. However, some authors believe that the success of homografts is related to the surgeon's ability to remove infected tissue. A homograft valve may be preferred for reconstruction of the aortic root in the presence of abscess because it is easier to handle than conventional prostheses and its anterior leaflet can be used to patch the defect created by resection of abscess.

Antibiotic prophylaxis of endocarditis is recommended for dental procedures that involve manipulation of either gingival tissue or the periapical region of teeth or perforation of oral mucosa. However, prophylaxis is no longer recommended for procedures that involve the respiratory tract, unless the procedure involves incision of the respiratory tract, such as tonsillectomy and adenoidectomy. Prophylaxis is no longer recommended for gastrointestinal (GI) or genitourinary (GU) procedures, including diagnostic esophagogastroduodenoscopy or colonoscopy. However, in high-risk patients with infections of the GI or GU tract, it is reasonable to administer antibiotic therapy to prevent wound infection or sepsis. For high-risk patients undergoing elective cystoscopy or other urinary tract manipulation who have enterococcal urinary tract infection or colonization, antibiotic therapy to eradicate enterococci from the urine before the procedure is reasonable. Regimens for prophylaxis are provided in the chapter on IE.

Paravalvular Regurgitation

Small paravalvular jets are common on intraoperative TEE, occurring in 10–25% of cases. These leaks typically resolve with healing and <1% require reoperation at 1-2 years. Moderate or severe regurgitation on postoperative TEE is rare (i.e. 1-2%) and requires correction, which can be performed by repair alone in about 50% of cases. The etiology of paravalvular regurgitation is likely due to infection, dehiscence or fibrosis and calcification of the annulus leading to inadequate contact between the sewing ring and annulus.

Hemolysis

Hemolysis is usually associated with either structural deterioration or paravalvular leak and due to turbulence through the valve or between the sewing ring and native ring. A paravalvular leak may be visualized with TEE. However, the severity of hemolysis is related to the eccentricity of the jet having contact with the chamber wall, rather than the severity of the regurgitation. While subclinical hemolysis can be detected in 18–51% of patients with mechanical prosthetic valve, serious hemolysis occurs in <1% due to improvements in valve design.

The hallmark of mechanical hemolytic anemia is the presence of fragmented erythrocytes in the peripheral blood smear. Other findings include reticulocytosis, low haptoglobin levels, elevated lactic dehydrogenase, indirect hyperbilirubinemia and urinary excretion of hemosiderin. The anemia is due to the inability of the bone marrow to compensate for the shorted lifespan of the erythrocytes.

Medical management is limited but there are reports of benefit with β-adrenergic blockers, presumed related to reduced shearing forces on the erythrocytes. Pentoxifylline may reduce hemolysis by improving erythrocyte deformability. Iron, folate and erythropoietin supplementation may be necessary. Reoperation is warranted if hemolysis is severe enough to require repeated blood transfusions, or if the paravalvular leak is symptomatic. Percutaneous closure of leaks with coils or ventricular septal defect occluders has emerged as a potential option in patients who are not surgical candidates.

SUGGESTED READING

1. Baddour LM, Wilson WR, Bayer AS, Fowler VG, Bolger AF, Levison ME, et al. Infective endocarditis. Diagnosis, antimicrobial therapy and management of complications. Circulation. 2005;111:e394-433.
2. Bates SM, Greer IA, Pabinger I, Sofaer S, Hirsh J. Venous thromboembolism, thrombophilia, antithrombotic therapy, and pregnancy. American College of Chest Physicians evidence-based clinical practice guidelines (8th edition). Chest. 2008;133:844S-86S.
3. David TE, Woo A, Armstrong S, Maganti M. When is the Ross operation a good option to treat aortic valve disease? J Thorac Cardiovasc Surg. 2010;139:68-75.
4. Elkayam U, Bitar F. Valvular heart disease and pregnancy. Part II. Prosthetic valves. J Am Coll Cardiol. 2005;46:403-10.
5. Habib G, Thuny F, Avierinos JF. Prosthetic valve endocarditis: current approach and therapeutic options. Prog Cardiovasc Dis. 2008;50:274-81.
6. Habib G, Hoen B, Tornos P, Thuny F, Prendergast B, Vilacosta I, et al. Guidelines on the prevention, diagnosis, and treatment of infective endocarditis (new version 2009). The task force on the prevention, diagnosis and treatment of infective endocarditis of the European Society of Cardiology. Eur Heart J. 2009;30:2369-412.
7. Halkos ME, Puskas JD. Are all bileaflet mechanical valves equal? Curr Opin Cardiol. 2009;24:136-41.

8. Lopez J, Revilla A, Villacosta I, Villacorta E, González-Juanatey C, Gómez I, et al. Definition, clinical profile, microbiological spectrum and prognostic factors of early-onset prosthetic valve endocarditis. Eur Heart J. 2007;28:760-5.
9. Lucian GB, Santini F, Mazzucco A. Autografts, homografts, and xenografts: overview on stentless aortic valve surgery. J Cardiovasc Med. 2007;8:91-6.
10. Nishimura RA, Carabello BA, Faxon DP, Fread MD, Lytle BW, O'Gara PT, et al. ACC/AHA 2008 Guideline update in valvular heart disease: focused update on infective endocarditis. J Am Coll Cardiol. 2008;52:676-85.
11. Nishimura RA, Otto CM, Bonow RO, Carabello BA, Erwin JP, Guyton RA, et al. 2014 AHA/ACC Guideline for the management of patients with valvular heart disease. J Am Coll Cardiol. 2014;63(22):e57-185.
12. Pibarot P, Dumesnil JG. Prosthesis-patient mismatch. Definition, clinical impact and prevention. Heart. 2006;92:1022-29.
13. Pibarot P, Dumesnil JG. Prosthesis-patient mismatch in the mitral position: old concept, new evidences. J Thorac Cardiovasc Surg. 2007;133:1405-8.
14. Pibarot P, Dumesnil JG. Prosthetic heart valves: selection of the optimal prosthesis and long-term management. Circulation. 2009;119:1034-48.
15. Rahimtoola SH. Choice of prosthetic heart valve in adults. J Am Coll Cardiol. 2010;55:2413-26.
16. Roudaut R, Serri K, Lafitte S. Thrombosis of prosthetic heart valves: diagnosis and therapeutic considerations. Heart. 2007;93:137-42.
17. Salem DN, O'Gara PT, Madias C, Pauker SG. Valvular and structural heart disease. American College of Chest Physicians evidence-based clinical practice guidelines (8th edition). Chest. 2008;133:593S-629S.
18. Shapira Y, Vaturi M, Sagie A. Hemolysis associated with prosthetic heart valves: a review. Cardiol Rev. 2009;17:121-4.
19. Sun JCJ, Davidson MJ, Lamy A, Eikelboom JW. Antithrombotic management of patients with prosthetic heart valves: current evidence and future trends. Lancet. 2009;374:565-76.
20. Takkenberg JJM, Klieverik LMA, Schoof PH, Van Suylen RJ, van Herwerden LA, Zondervan PE, et al. The Ross procedure: a systematic review and meta-analysis. Circulation. 2009;119:222-8.
21. Tong AT, Roudaut R, Ozkan M, Sagie A, Shahid MSA, Pontes SC, et al. Transesophageal echocardiography improves risk assessment of thrombolysis of prosthetic valve thrombosis: results of the International PRO-TEE Registry. J Am Coll Cardiol. 2004;43:77-84.
22. Turpie A, Gent M, Laupacis A, Latour Y, Gunstensen J, Basile F, et al. A comparison of aspirin with placebo in patients treated with warfarin after heart-valve replacement. N Eng J Med. 1993;329:524-9.
23. Van Geldorp MWA, Jamieson WRE, Kappetein AP, Ye J, Fradet GJ, Eijkemans MJC, et al. Patient outcome after aortic valve replacement with mechanical or biologic prosthesis. Weighing lifetime anticoagulant related event risk against reoperation risk. J Thorac Cardiovasc Surg. 2009;137:881-6.
24. Vandenberg BF. Prosthetic heart valves. In: Chatterjee K (Ed). Cardiology: An Illustrated Textbook. New Delhi, India: Jaypee Brothers Medical Publishers; 2013. pp. 1072-97.
25. Wang A, Athan E, Pappas PA, Fowler VG, Olaison L, Paré C, et al. Contemporary clinical profile and outcome of prosthetic valve endocarditis. JAMA. 2007;297:1354-61.
26. Zogbhi W, Chambers JB, Dumesnil JG, Foster E, Gottdiener JS, Grayburn PA, et al. Recommendations for evaluation of prosthetic valves with echocardiography and Doppler ultrasound. J Am Soc Echocardiogr. 2009;22:975-1014.

Pericardial Diseases

Chapter 13

Tariq Hameed

INTRODUCTION

The pericardium is a thin covering that separates the heart from the remaining mediastinal structures and consists of a fibrous outer sac and a serous, inner, double layer sac. The inner sac has two layers. The visceral, epicardial layer covers the heart and great vessels. The parietal layer is fused to the fibrous pericardium.

The pericardial cavity between the visceral and parietal layers of the serous pericardium contains <50 cc of a plasma ultra-filtrate. The pericardium provides mechanical support, lubrication, barrier to infection and inflammation. It also secretes prostaglandin that can modulate cardiac reflexes and coronary vasomotor tone. However, cardiac function can be maintained in the complete absence of a pericardium.

ACUTE PERICARDITIS AND PERICARDIAL EFFUSION

Acute pericarditis occurs when there is acute inflammation of the pericardium. The inflammatory process may be associated with the myocardium (i.e. myopericarditis) as well as with elevated troponin or creatinine kinase-myocardial band (CK-MB) levels without any focal or global left ventricular (LV) dysfunction. However, the process may also be associated with elevated troponin or CK-MB as well as focal or global LV dysfunction (i.e. perimyocarditis).

Etiology

Pericarditis and pericardial effusion (PE) can present as isolated entity or as part of an underlying systemic disease.
- *Idiopathic*: attributed to 85–90% of cases, most of which are probably viral
- *Viral*: Echoviruses and coxsackieviruses are the most common causes. The diagnosis is made by DNA detection with PCR or *in situ* hybridization in pericardial fluid/tissue. The presence of a PE is the result of direct viral damage or immune responses
- *Bacterial*: PE may occur by direct extension from pneumonia or empyema related to organisms, such as *staphylococci, pneumococci* or *streptococci*. An infectious PE may also be caused by hematogenous spread during

bacteremia or rupture of a perivalvular abscess into the pericardial space. Pericardial fluid analysis demonstrates polymorphonuclear leukocytes, low glucose, high protein and elevated LDH. Treatment is pericardiocentesis or surgical drainage and antibiotics
- *HIV-related:* PE may be part of a generalized sero-effusive process (i.e. "capillary leak syndrome") related to enhanced cytokine expression. Other causes include congestive heart failure, Kaposi sarcoma, tuberculosis and other pulmonary infections and idiopathic
- *Tuberculous:* 1–8% of pulmonary tuberculosis cases develop PE in third-world countries. Diagnosis is by isolating organism from pericardial fluid or biopsy specimen for identifying it histologically or adenosine deaminase measurement in pericardial fluid. Treatment is multidrug antimycobacterial therapy
- *Uremic or dialysis-associated:* Treatment is intensive hemodialysis and drainage
- *Postmyocardial infarction (MI) pericarditis.*
  - Early post-MI pericarditis occurs in <7 days after presentation due to transmural necrosis with inflammation affecting the adjacent visceral and parietal pericardium, more common with ST segment elevation MI (STEMI). The incidence is estimated as 5–20% of cases, although the incidence of both early and late pericarditis is reduced due to early revascularization
  - Late pericarditis or Dressler's syndrome (1–3%) is characterized by polyserositis with pericardial or pleural effusions by autoimmune etiology due to sensitization to myocardial cells. It can be seen with both STEMI and non-STEMI.
- *Postpericardiotomy and postcardiac injury:* PE occurs days to months after cardiac surgery, thoracotomy or chest trauma and is likely due to antiheart antibodies in response to myocardial injury
- *Radiation-induced:* Acute and delayed presentations are possible. PE may present up to 20 years after therapeutic radiation exposure
- *Metastatic cancer:* Metastases to the pericardium occur from primary tumors of lung, breast, Hodgkin's and non-Hodgkin's lymphoma and leukemia
- *Autoimmune and drug-induced:* Rheumatoid arthritis, systemic lupus erythematosus, scleroderma or drugs like isoniazid and hydralazine.

Clinical Presentation

- **Symptoms**
  - **Chest pain** is described as sharp and pleuritic, substernal, radiating to the neck/trapezius ridge and/or arms, exacerbated by either inspiration, coughing or supine position. It can also be prolonged and continuous, mimicking myocardial ischemia or acute aortic dissection. The patient typically assumes an upright sitting and leaning forward position, which appears to lessen the pericardial pain
  - **Shallow breathing**, due to inspiratory chest pain

- **Systemic symptoms** of fever, malaise, myalgias, arthralgias, skin rash (which is rare) or other manifestations of systemic disease.
- **Physical examination**
  - **Pericardial friction rub** is usually described as a "scratchy" sound and heard mainly at the left sternal border. The rub should be auscultated in multiple positions, including the left lateral decubitus position, supine and sitting upright. It can have three or two or even an isolated systolic component, corresponding to atrial systole, ventricular systole and ventricular diastole
  - **Pulsus paradoxus and/or elevation of venous pressure** raises the suspicion of pericardial tamponade or constriction should be suspected.

Diagnosis (Fig. 13.1)

The diagnosis of acute pericarditis should include at least two of the following criteria:
- Characteristic pleuritic chest pain
- A pericardial friction rub
- New or increasing PE
- Electrocardiographic (ECG) changes (Figs 13.2A to D). There are some typical ECG abnormalities that are seen in over 80% of patients, especially in idiopathic, postcardiac surgery and hemorrhagic pericarditis. They are rarely seen in uremic, malignant, tuberculous or autoimmune pericarditis.
  - Stage 1 (within hours of chest pain onset): Diffuse upward concave ST segment elevation in all leads except aVR and V1 without reciprocal ST depression; PR depression may be seen in all leads except aVR or V1; PR segment elevation in aVR (referred to as the "knuckle sign"); down-sloping TP segment (referred to as "Spodick's sign").
  - Stage 2 (1-5 days after chest pain onset): Normalization of the ST segments.
  - Stage 3: T wave inversion occurring after ST segment returns to baseline.
  - Stage 4: ECG returns to normal.
- **Chest radiography.** The chest X-ray is usually normal with acute pericarditis, unless the patient has a PE that appears as cardiomegaly and clear lung fields.
- **Echocardiography.** A small PE may be appreciated in approximately 40% of acute pericarditis case; however, PE may not be present and is not needed for the diagnosis of pericarditis. Other findings may include increased pericardial brightness, pericardial thickening and abnormal septal bounce, suggesting early constriction. A PE can be trivial to large and localized, loculated or circumferential. Importantly, tamponade physiology can be seen in 3% of patients.
- **Blood tests**
  - The **troponin** level can be minimally elevated as the result of epicardial inflammation and will return to normal within 1-2 weeks. However, suspect myocardial ischemia, if there is a rapid rise and drop in serial troponin levels. Prolonged, sustained levels of marked elevation

168 Common Problems in Cardiology

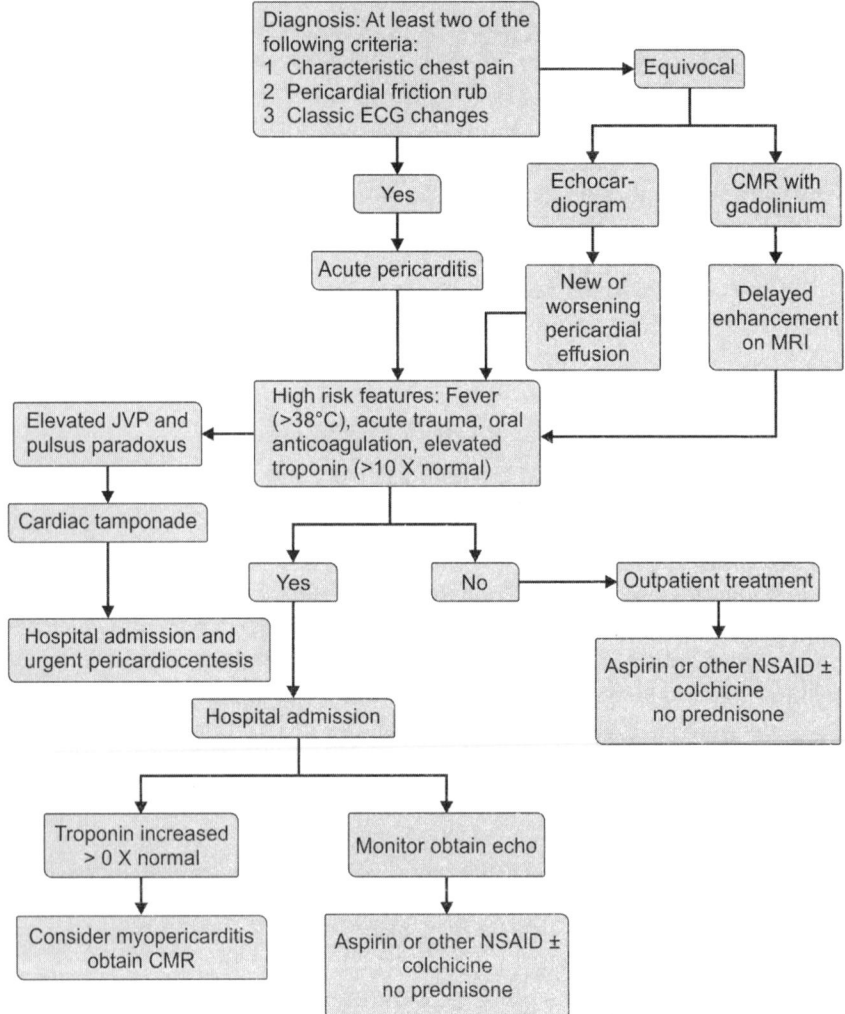

Fig. 13.1: Overview of the diagnosis and management of acute pericarditis.

Source: Reprinted from Khandaker MH, Nishimura RA. Pericardial diseases. In: Kanu Chatterjee (Ed). Cardiology: An Illustrated Textbook. New Delhi: Jaypee Brothers; 2012, *with permission.*

in troponin may suggest a concomitant myocarditis referred to as myopericarditis.
- **Viral cultures or antibody titers** are usually not clinically useful but may help clarify the etiology.
- **Markers of inflammation** such as the erythrocyte sedimentation rate (ESR) or C-reactive protein (CRP) are almost always elevated.
- **ANA and RF** should be ordered if there is suspicion for autoimmune diseases.

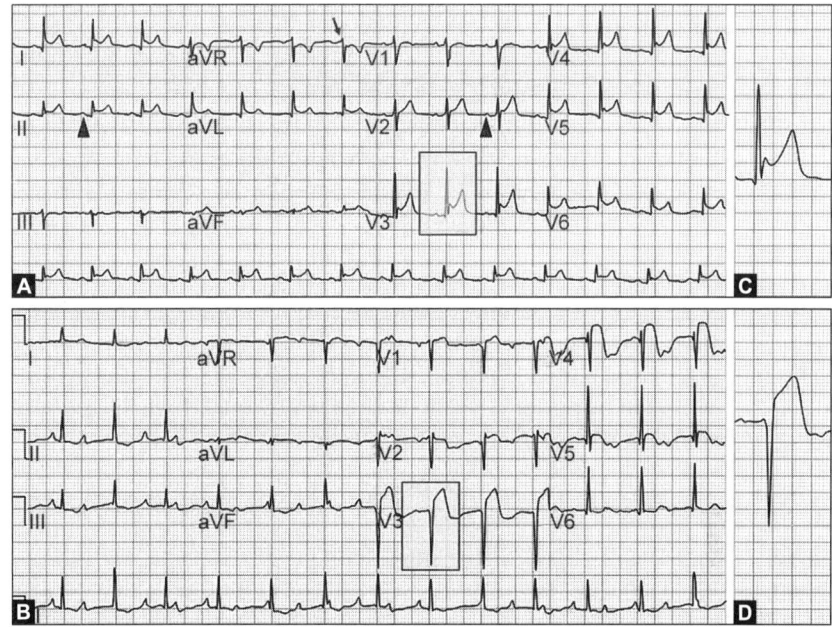

Figs 13.2A to D: Electrocardiographic abnormalities in acute pericarditis versus acute myocardial infarction. (A) Acute pericarditis reveals diffuse concave upsloping ST-segment elevation is seen in leads I, II, aVL, aVF and V2 to V6. There is also PR-segment elevation in aVR (arrow) and subtle PR segment depression in leads II and V2 (arrowheads). Reciprocal ST-segment depression is seen in aVR; (B) In acute myocardial infarction, the ST segment elevation is convex upward or "humplike". (C and D) These panels demonstrate the difference in the ST-segment elevation in acute pericarditis (panel C) and acute myocardial infarction (panel D).

Source: Reprinted from Khandaker MH, Nishimura RA. Pericardial diseases. In: Kanu Chatterjee (Ed). Cardiology: An Illustrated Textbook. New Delhi:Jaypee Brothers; 2012, *with permission.*

Treatment

The optimal treatment for an acute isolated pericarditis in a young healthy person is high-dose salicylates or nonsteroidal anti-inflammatory drugs (NSAIDs):

- **Ibuprofen** at a dose of 300–800 mg tid until the effusion disappears or if pain is no longer present, followed by gradual tapering for an additional 3 weeks. However, NSAIDs should not be used in patients who present with a concomitant myocardial infarction or known coronary artery disease because of concerns for scar thinning and rupture. Indomethacin should be avoided in elderly due to it flow reduction in coronaries
- **Aspirin** 650 mg every 6–8 hours for 2–4 weeks
- **Proton pump inhibitors** should be used in all patients on these large dosages of salicylates or NSAIDs
- **Colchicine** dosing is 0.6 mg twice a day for 1 week, followed by a taper to 0.6 mg per day for at least 6 months. It should be added to NSAID or monotherapy for the initial attack or to prevent recurrences. It significantly reduced symptoms after 72 hours and recurrence at 18 months in the

COlchicine for acute PEricarditis (COPE) trial. Colchicine should be avoided in patients with renal insufficiency, hepatobiliary disorders, blood dyscrasias and gastrointestinal motility disorders
- **Corticosteroids** should rarely be used, as it results in a higher incidence of relapsing pericarditis. But if it cannot be avoided as in case of connective tissue diseases, autoreactive or uremic pericarditis, use 60 mg PO daily for 2 days with tapering off during a week
- **Methotrexate** is ineffective
- **Pericardiectomy** should be avoided.

Patients with high-risk features should be hospitalized. High-risk features include a high fever (i.e. temperature >38°C), an immunocompromised state, concurrent oral anticoagulation, previous failure of NSAID therapy or a marked elevation of troponin (>10x upper limit normal). If high-risk features are not present, outpatient treatment is appropriate.

Prognosis

About 90% of patients with acute pericarditis, myopericarditis or perimyocarditis have normal LV function during follow-up.

CHRONIC RELAPSING/RECURRENT PERICARDITIS

Multiple, recurrent episodes of pericarditis may develop weeks to months (usually 18–20 months) after an initial episode of acute pericarditis, especially if due to idiopathic, Dressler's, autoimmune, postoperative or traumatic etiologies. The relapses may be intermittent (i.e. symptom-free intervals of >6 weeks without therapy or incessant (i.e. when weaning or discontinuation of anti-inflammatory therapy results in a relapse within <6 weeks).

Etiology

The etiology is unclear but is likely due to an autoimmune reaction activated by the initial episode. The pericardium is often thickened and fibrinous due to chronic inflammatory changes. These recurrences are frequent in patients who have received prior corticosteroid therapy for acute pericarditis.

The frequency in many clinical series varies between 8% and 80% (with an average of 24%), including pericarditis in 32%, myopericarditis in 11% and perimyocarditis in 12%.

Clinical Presentation

The typical presentation is similar to that of acute pericarditis, including chest pain in an otherwise healthy patient, treated with corticosteroids for an initial bout of acute pericarditis.

Diagnosis

The diagnostic criteria for determining the presence of pericardial inflammation are similar to acute pericarditis:

- Elevated ESR or CRP can be seen at the time of the relapse
- MRI scanning with gadolinium enhancement will show delayed gadolinium enhancement in areas of inflamed pericardium.

Treatment

The intial therapy is repeated with a second 2-week period of high-dose salicylate or NSAID with slow tapering over 3 months and/or colchicine 0.6 mg twice a day for 1 week, then taper to 0.6 mg per and continued for at least 1 year after the last episode of pericarditis.

After the second recurrence, start chronic colchicine prophylaxis (1 mg daily).

If the patient fails to respond, then prednisone should be considered (at a dose of 1-1.5 mg/kg) for at least 1 month and then tapered very slowly with 1 mg taper per month, necessitating a duration of up to 18-24 months. However, lower dose of 0.2-0.5 mg/kg of oral prednisone daily has been found to be better than 1 mg/kg daily in terms of lower recurrence rates. Following the tapering off of steroids, the salicylates or NSAIDS should be continued for at least months after the complete withdrawal of the steroids.

If the patient does not respond adequately, azathioprine (at a dose of 75-100 mg/day) or cyclophosphamide can be added, but their effectiveness is uncertain.

About 50% of patients will respond to this aggressive medical therapy, but some may need complete pericardiectomy after a steroid-free regimen for several weeks.

PERICARDIAL EFFUSION AND TAMPONADE

The development of a PE can either be idiopathic or due to a number of underlying etiologies similar to those that can cause acute pericarditis.

Its hemodynamic effects depend more on the rate of effusion accumulation rather than the total amount. An effusion can compress all four cardiac chambers with only 80 mL accumulating acutely, compromising systemic venous return and causing tamponade; however, a 2 L volume effusion accumulating slowly may result in no hemodynamic changes.

Acute tamponade may occur due to a malignancy, left ventricular rupture from a myocardial infarction, trauma, complications of invasive procedures such as cardiac catheterization and electrophysiologic procedures.

Pathophysiology

Cardiac tamponade causes increased intrapericardial pressure, which decreases myocardial transmural pressure reducing chamber diastolic compliance with a resultant decrease in stroke volume.

During inspiration, the drop in intrathoracic pressures is transmitted to the right side of the heart, resulting in an increase in systemic venous return and distention of the right ventricle (RV). Due to the high intrapericardial pressure, the free wall of the RV is not able to expand and thus the septum bulges into the left ventricle, decreasing the effective operative compliance and preload of the left ventricle with a further drop in forward stroke volume. This enhancement of ventricular interaction is the mechanism of pulsus paradoxus, which is an exaggerated drop in systemic pressure during inspiration.

Clinical Presentation

- **Symptoms:** Dyspnea (of unclear etiology as there is no pulmonary congestion), tachypnea, orthopnea
- **Physical examination**
  - Elevated jugular venous pressure (JVP), with preservation of the "x" descent, but there is blunting of the "y" descent, as the high pericardial pressure prevents early rapid diastolic filling of the RV at the time of tricuspid valve opening. Kussmaul's sign is absent. Low pressure tamponade can occur if tamponade occurs at lower level of filling pressures (i.e. <15–20 mm Hg) without JVP elevation due to hypovolemia
  - Beck's triad: Muffled heart sounds, hypotension (a hallmark of tamponade) and elevated JVP.
  - Tachycardia (which is a reflex, sympathetic response to pericardial irritation or hypotension)
  - Auscultation: Normal pulmonic sound (P2) and rarely auscultatory alternans
  - Pulsus paradoxus, defined as a drop of systolic pressure >10 mm Hg during inspiration. This sign may also be seen in constrictive pericarditis, pulmonary embolism and severe asthma/chronic obstructive lung disease. This sign may not be seen in tamponade when there is severe underlying right or left heart failure with severely elevated right or left ventricular pressure precluding compression or if there is left to right shunt.

Diagnosis

- **ECG**
  - Sinus tachycardia.
  - Widespread concave ST segment elevation and PR segment depression.
  - Low-voltage tracing and electrical alternans in massive PE
- **Echocardiography** is the diagnostic procedure of choice in a patient suspected of having pericardial tamponade
  - PE is diagnosed as an echo-free space between visceral and parietal pericardium. A separation of the two layers that is seen only in systole represents a normal or clinically insignificant amount of pericardial fluid whereas a separation that is present in both systole and diastole is associated with effusions of >50 mL. A small PE (usually <100 mL) appears <1 cm in width and is localized at posterior wall (while patient imaged in left lateral decubitus position). A moderate PE (in the range

of 100–500 mL) surrounds the heart and is 1–2 cm at its maximal width. A large effusion (>500 mL) appears >2 cm at its maximal width. A very large PE appears >2.5 cm maximal width
- Late diastolic collapse of the right atrium (RA)
- Early diastolic collapse of the RV ventricle
- Collapse of the left atrium (LA)
- Ventricular interdependence is enhancement of ventricular interaction by septal shift from right ventricle to left ventricle during inspiration (Fig. 13.3)
- Dilated inferior vena cava from the high right atrial (RA) pressure.
- Blunted initial E-velocity on the transmitral flow velocity curve due to a decrease in early rapid filling with further decrease in transmitral inflow during inspiration of ≥30% due to the blunted inspiratory filling of the left sided chambers. Also inspiration increases right-sided transtricuspid flow of >60% (from about 10% normally). These respiratory variations should not be used as a stand-alone criterion for tamponade without the presence of chamber collapse, IVC dilation or abnormal hepatic vein flows
- Expiration causes an increase in mitral E velocity and transmitral pressure gradient and reversals in the hepatic vein velocities.
- **Right heart catheterization.** Assessment of intracardiac pressures is not necessary in tamponade but may be helpful in cases of borderline diagnostic certainty. Hemodynamic findings in tamponade include the following:
  - Diastolic equalization of intracardiac pressures [i.e. intracardiac pressures within 4 mm Hg of the RA, RV, pulmonary artery (PA) and pulmonary capillary wedge pressure (PCWP)], which are raised to usually in the range of 15–20 mm Hg. These pressures are equal to pericardial sac pressures. In contrast to aortic pressure, RA pressure continues to increase significantly.
  - RA pressure shows preserved x descent with absent or attenuated y descent.

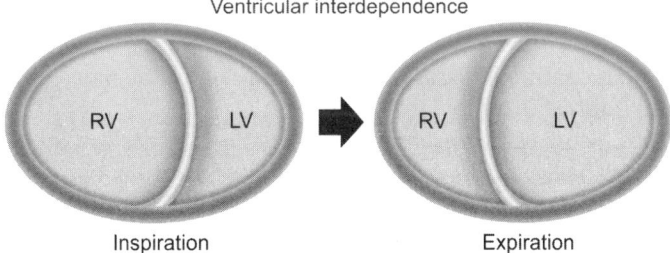

Fig. 13.3: Schematic diagram showing interventricular dependence. On inspiration (left), there is a shift of the ventricular septum toward the left ventricle; and on expiration (right), there is a shift of the ventricular septum toward the right ventricle.

Source: Reprinted from Klein AL, Abbara S, Agler DA, Appleton CP, Asher CR, Hoit B, et al. American Society of Echocardiography clinical recommendations for multimodality cardiovascular imaging of patients with pericardial disease. J Am Soc Echocardiogr. 2013;26(9):965-1012, with *permission*.

- In early tamponade, RA pressure will begin to increase, with a loss of "y" descent and a more pronounced "a" wave at the time of atrial contraction in patients who are in sinus rhythm. As cardiac tamponade progresses, aortic systolic pressure and pulse pressure decrease and pulsus paradoxus develops, as evidenced by a more pronounced decrease in pulse pressure during inspiration.
  - Hemodynamics obtained in the cardiac catheterization lab also help in differentiating cardiac tamponade from constrictive pericarditi.
- **Cardiac magnetic resonance imaging (MRI):** Magnetic resonance imaging is usually not useful to diagnose tamponade because of the time constraints and urgency usually needed to confirm the diagnosis before pericardiocentesis. However, MRI can detect loculated PE and pericardial thickening, and also differentiate simple from complex effusions and pericardial fat from pathologic thickening
- **Computed tomography (CT):** Computed tomography can help in assessing the size and distribution of a PE. In addition, CT may also differentiate among blood, exudative, chylous and serous fluid by differentiating attenuation coefficients of these substances

Treatment

Treatment with diuretics or nitrates should be avoided since they may reduce preload and provoke refractory hypotension acutely

Emergent closed pericardiocentesis

Following removal of the fluid, samples are sent for chemical and hematologic analysis as well as culture and cytology.

Pigtail catheter and negative pressure drainage are continued after the procedure for at least 24 hours until drainage completely stops or is draining <25 mL/24 hours. Drainage can be prolonged to 48–72 hours in cases of bloody PE with malignancy.

Open pericardiocentesis with pericardiotomy, pericardial window or limited pericardiectomy

This may be recommended for recurrent tamponade, loculated effusion and for tissue sampling to establish diagnosis

Resistant neoplastic processes may require intrapericardial treatment, percutaneous balloon pericardiotomy or rarely pericardiectomy.

CONSTRICTIVE PERICARDITIS

Constrictive pericarditis is pericardial compressive syndrome characterized by scarring and loss of elasticity of the pericardial sac, causing limitation of expansion of the cardiac chambers. Due to the resultant decrease in ventricular filling and an increase in diastolic pressures, constrictive pericarditis results in signs and symptoms of both left and right heart failure.

Common causes of constrictive pericarditis include idiopathic, radiation therapy, postcardiac surgery or infection (tuberculosis was common in the past and currently in developing countries). There is a subset of patients who present with constrictive pericarditis in whom no obvious etiology is evident.

Clinical Presentation

- Isolated right heart failure signs and symptoms: Peripheral edema, abdominal swelling with liver failure and secondary cirrhosis
- Left heart failure signs and symptoms: Low output state leading to decreased exercise tolerance and fatigue, recurrent pleural effusions with pulmonary venous congestion leading to exertional dyspnea, cough and orthopnea with progressive disease.

Physical Examination

- Marked elevation in JVP with a rapid "x" and "y" descent (Fig. 13.4)
- Kussmaul's sign: A rise in JVP with inspiration due to impaired diastolic filling of the right ventricle due to restriction by an inelastic pericardium.
- Distant heart sounds without significant murmur
- Pericardial knock: An early diastolic filling high-frequency sound, heard best with inspiration at the left sternal border with diaphragm, closer to the second heart sound than a typical third heart sound (S3) with LV dysfunction

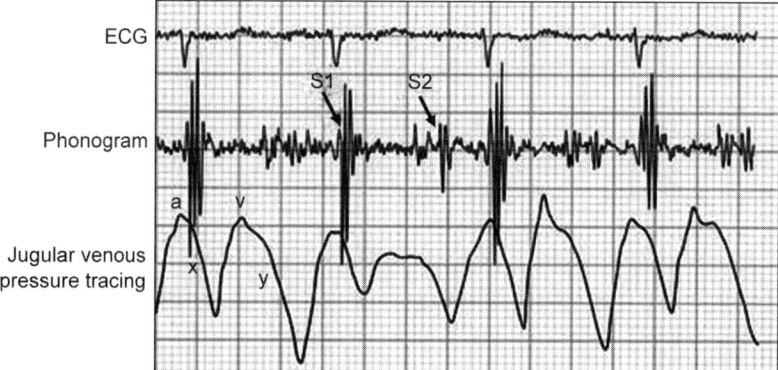

Fig. 13.4: Jugular venous pressure tracings in constrictive pericarditis. Simultaneous jugular venous pressure tracings, phonogram and electrocardiographic tracings are shown in a patient with constrictive pericarditis. The "a" wave is generated by atrial contraction and occurs just prior to S1. The "v" wave is generated by ventricular contraction. The "x" descent reflects movement of the lower portion of the right atrium toward the right ventricle during ventricular systole. The "y" descent represents the abrupt termination of the downstroke of the "v" wave during early diastole after the tricuspid valve opens and the right ventricle begins to fill passively. In a patient with constrictive pericarditis, the "a" and "v" waves are more pronounced due to contraction against higher ventricular filling pressures resulting in marked JVP elevation. Impaired diastolic filling of the right ventricle combined with enhanced longitudinal motion of the heart in constrictive pericarditis results in unusually rapid "x" and "y" descents.

Source: Reprinted from Khandaker MH, Nishimura RA. Pericardial diseases. In: Kanu Chatterjee (Ed). Cardiology: An Illustrated Textbook. New Delhi Jaypee Brothers; 2012, *with permission.*

- Emaciation with severe ascites and edema
- Dullness at both lung bases consistent with pleural effusions
- Pulsus paradoxus in one-third of patients especially when there is effusive-constrictive presentation.

Diagnosis

Constrictive pericarditis should be suspected when a patient presents with severe right heart failure in the absence of left ventricular dysfunction, valvular heart disease or pulmonary hypertension.

- **The unique pathophysiologic features** of constrictive pericarditis consist of changes during the respiratory cycle that helps in diagnosis by different modalities of testing and include:
    - **Dissociation of intrathoracic and intracardiac pressures**. In patients with a normal pericardium, there is a drop in intrathoracic pressure during inspiration. This is transmitted into the cardiac chambers so that the driving pressure from the lungs to the heart remains unchanged from expiration to inspiration. However, in patients with constrictive pericarditis, the drop in intrathoracic pressure is shielded from the intracardiac pressures. Thus, during inspiration, there will be a decrease in the driving pressure from the lungs to the heart and a decrease in filling of the LV.
    - **Enhancement of ventricular interaction**. Due to the rigid pericardium around all cardiac chambers, there is also enhancement of ventricular interaction. When there is a decrease in LV volume during inspiration, there will be a concomitant increase in right ventricular volume, causing a septal shift from RV to LV during inspiration. Conversely, during expiration, there will be an increase in LV volume, decrease in RV volume, resulting in a marked decrease in the effective operative compliance of the right ventricle. This respiratory variation in filling of the right ventricle and LV is the most specific hemodynamic feature of constrictive pericarditis. These features can be delineated by both echocardiography and cardiac catheterization.
- **Constrictive pericarditis versus restrictive cardiomyopathy:** In the modern time, the differential diagnosis is usually between that of myocardial restrictive disease versus constrictive pericarditis as after radiation therapy or open heart surgery, there may be a combination of both myocardial disease and pericardial disease. The classic findings suggesting constrictive pericarditis and to differentiate it from restrictive cardiomyopathy are:
    - Pulmonary artery systolic pressure <50 mm Hg
    - RV end-diastolic pressure (EDP) to RV systolic pressure ratio is >1/3
    - LVEDP and RVEDP are equal or nearly equal with constrictive pericarditis while LVEDP is usually higher than RVEDP in restrictive cardiomyopathy. However, the EDP may be nearly equal with restrictive cardiomyopathy if volume depleted and therefore this is a nonspecific finding.

- **Echocardiography.** Echocardiography provides an evaluation of other causes of dyspnea, such as LV systolic dysfunction, valvular disease or pulmonary hypertension. Normal LV systolic function with a dilated IVC should raise the suspicion of constrictive pericarditis. M-mode and two-dimensional echocardiography findings in constrictive pericarditis:
  - Subtle changes in septal motion. Septal "bounce" reflects the effect of increased and equalized right ventricular and left ventricular diastolic pressures.
  - Early rapid filling of the LV can be seen as a rapid expansion of the LV cavity on M-mode echocardiography
  - Enhanced interventricular interaction with a septal "shift" from the RV to the LV occurs during inspiration
  - Inferior vena cava plethora: Doppler echocardiography findings in constrictive pericarditis:
  - Inspiratory decrease in the transmitral early diastolic filling inflow (E) of 25–40%. At the onset of inspiration, the PCWP decreases more than the LV diastolic pressure resulting in a small driving pressure gradient and a diminution in the transmitral inflow (E)-velocity of 25–40% during inspiration. At the onset of expiration, the PCWP increases much more than the LV diastolic pressure creating a large driving pressure gradient, causing an increase in the transmitral inflow E velocity
  - Inspiratory increase in tricuspid valve inflow with peak E velocity increased by 40–60%
  - Hepatic flow velocities reveal an expiratory flow reversal in constriction as compared to inspiratory flow reversal in restriction
  - Pulmonary venous flow will show an increase in both systolic and diastolic velocities during expiration as compared to inspiration
  - The mitral annulus tissue (e') velocity (obtained with tissue Doppler), reflects shortening and lengthening of the myocardial fibers along a longitudinal plane during diastole, can be used to distinguish constrictive pericarditis from restrictive cardiomyopathy. In restrictive cardiomyopathy, the myocardium is diseased and this results in a diminution of the tissue Doppler mitral annulus velocity. In constrictive pericarditis, there is relatively preserved or enhanced motion of both the medial and lateral mitral annulus and thus a medial mitral annulus tissue Doppler velocity (e') of greater than 7 cm/s is suggestive of constrictive pericarditis rather than restrictive cardiomyopathy. However, the Doppler velocity profiles are diagnostic of constrictive pericarditis in only about 70–75% of patients.
- **Cardiac catheterization hemodynamic findings** (which may also be seen in restrictive cardiomyopathy, acute RV infarction or tricuspid regurgitation):
  - Severe elevation and equalization of end diastolic pressures in all four cardiac chambers
  - Early rapid filling seen as a dip and plateau or square root sign on the ventricular pressure tracing

- Increased atrial pressure with rapid "x" and "y" descent on the atrial pressure tracing.
- **Lateral chest X-ray** can show significant calcification of the pericardium in 25% of patients with constrictive pericarditis especially at atrioventricular groove
- Magnetic resonance imaging **and CT scanning** are useful in demonstrating increased pericardial thickness and calcification. However, nearly 20% of patients with surgically proven constrictive pericarditis may not have increased pericardial thickness on these imaging modalities and thus does not rule out constrictive pericarditis
- **ECG findings:** Low-voltage, generalized flattening of T waves and left atrial enlargement
- **Exploratory thoracotomy** may be needed if the diagnosis of constrictive pericarditis may still be uncertain at the end of all these diagnostic testing.

Treatment (Fig. 13.5)

Complete pericardiectomy (i.e. resection of the pericardium from phrenic nerve to phrenic nerve) is the treatment of choice although with a perioperative mortality of >5-6%. However, the procedure may result in significant improvement of symptoms in 70-80% of patients and possibly prolongation of life

The independent adverse predictors of long-term outcome by surgery include advanced age, worsening of the NYHA class at presentation, renal dysfunction, LV dysfunction/atrophy/fibrosis and prior radiation.

TRANSIENT CONSTRICTIVE PERICARDITIS

This is a condition in which there is thickening of the pericardium and constriction is mainly due to an acute inflammatory process in the pericardium along with laboratory findings of inflammation (ESR, CRP or gadolinium enhancement defects by MRI scan). Treatment involves a trial of high-dose nonsteroidal anti-inflammatory agents, salicylates or even steroids to determine whether or not resolution of the constrictive process might be possible.

EFFUSIVE CONSTRICTIVE PERICARDITIS

This is a condition in which there is both a PE and constrictive pericarditis. These patients will present with a PE and elevated filling pressures consistent with cardiac tamponade. However, once the pericardial fluid is removed, constrictive hemodynamics still persist. In these patients, a decision then needs to be made as to whether more aggressive medical therapy or surgery is required. In those patients in whom active inflammation is present, a trial of anti-inflammatory medications should be considered. In other patients, a surgical pericardiectomy is not necessary.

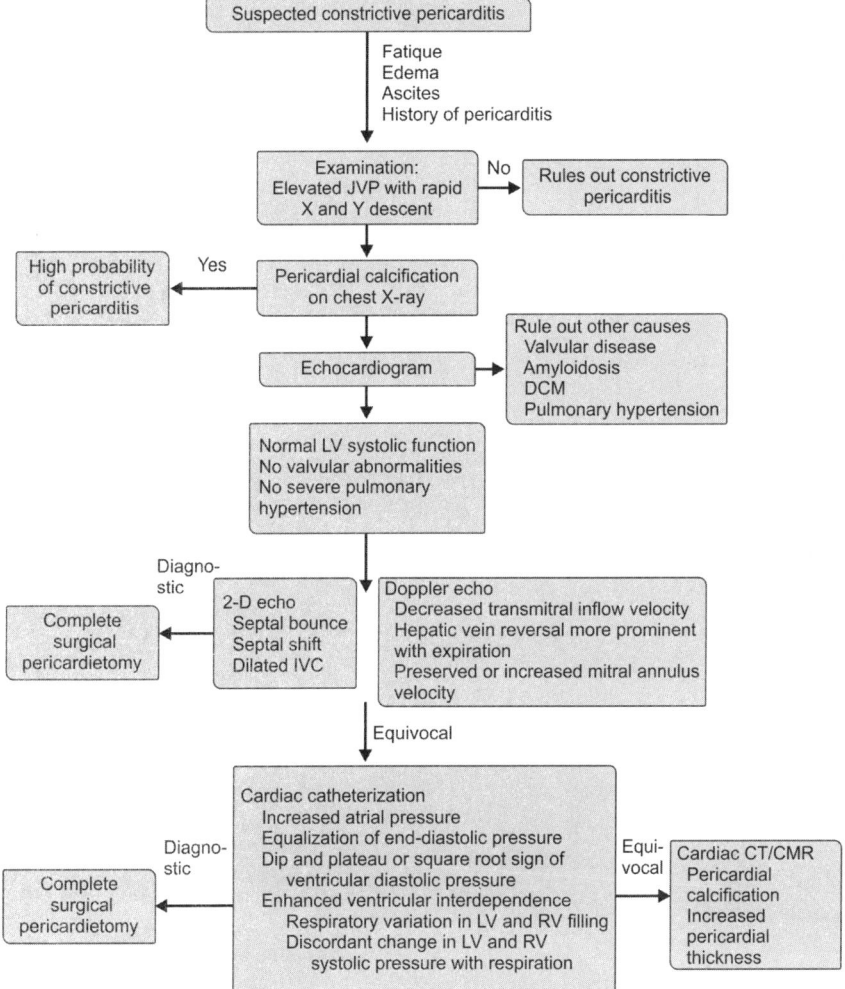

Fig. 13.5: Overview of the diagnosis and management of constrictive pericarditis.

Source: Reprinted from Khandaker MH, Nishimura RA. Pericardial diseases. In: Kanu Chatterjee (Ed). Cardiology: An Illustrated Textbook. New Dehli Jaypee Brothers; 2012, *with permission.*

SUGGESTED READING

1. Khandaker MH, Nishimura RA. Pericardial diseases. In: Kanu Chatterjee (Ed). Cardiology: An Illustrated Textbook. New Delhi: Jaypee Brothers; 2012. pp. 1489-504.
2. Klein AL, Abbara S, Agler DA, Appleton CP, Asher CR, Hoit B, et al. American Society of Echocardiography clinical recommendations for multimodality cardiovascular imaging of patients with pericardial disease. J Am Soc Echocardiogr. 2013;26(9):965-1012.
3. LeWinter M. Pericardial diseases. In: Braunwald's Heart Disease: A Textbook of Cardiovascular Medicine, 9th edition. Saunders; 2012. pp. 1651-71.

4. Maisch B, Seferović PM, Ristić AD, Erbel R, Rienmüller R, Adler Y, et al. European Society of Cardiology guidelines on the diagnosis and management of pericardial diseases. Eur Heart J. 2004; 25(7):587-610.
5. Oh JK, Seward JB, Tajik AJ. The Echo Manual, 3rd edition. Philadelphia, PA: Lippincott, Williams and Wilkins; 2007. pp. 289-309.

Syncope

14 Chapter

Olurotimi Mesubi, Alexander Mazur

INTRODUCTION

Syncope is defined as a transient loss of consciousness (LOC) due to short-lived global cerebral hypoperfusion with rapid onset, short duration and spontaneous complete recovery. Reduced cerebral perfusion secondary to a decrease in cardiac output (CO) and/or peripheral vascular tone is a key mechanistic feature of syncope distinguishing it from other causes of transient LOC. Syncopal episodes are always attended by a loss of postural muscle tone leading to a fall. Patients typically regain consciousness and appropriate orientation within a few seconds or, rarely, minutes.

Syncope is a common clinical condition; some data suggest that up to 20–40% of people report having a fainting spell at least once in their life and about one-third of them will have recurrences within 3 years.

Frequent recurrent syncope is associated with significant morbidity. The risk of physical injury and adverse psychosocial impact of recurrent syncopal episodes may lead to serious lifestyle impairment and professional disability. The mortality risk in patients with syncope is primarily determined by the presence of underlying cardiac condition or other serious comorbidities.

CLASSIFICATION AND TYPES OF SYNCOPE

Syncope is broadly classified based on pathophysiologic mechanisms as reflex (or neurally mediated) syncope, orthostatic hypotension and cardiac syncope (Table 14.1). Although useful for defining prognosis, this classification is limited in providing guidance to specific therapy. Classification of syncope can be further refined based on the underlying rhythm. Arrhythmias are a major mechanism of cardiac syncope while bradycardia is an important component of reflex syncope.

- **Reflex syncope** is the most common type of syncope at any age caused by an inappropriate autonomic-mediated cardiovascular response to certain triggers. The abnormal reflex response results in bradycardia and/or peripheral vasodilatation. Typically, both mechanisms are present. From a practical standpoint, the types of response are grouped into vasodepressor (predominantly vasodilatation), cardioinhibitory (predominantly bradycardia or asystole) or mixed. Reflex syncope is subdivided into several clinical forms based on specific triggers

Table 14.1: Classification of syncope

- Reflex
  - Vasovagal (orthostatic or emotional triggers)
  - Situational (cough, laugh, swallow, defecation, micturition, postprandial, postexercise, etc.)
  - Carotid sinus syncope
- Orthostatic hypotension
  - Drug-induced (e.g. vasodilators and diuretics)
  - Volume depletion (e.g. hemorrhage and dehydration)
  - Primary autonomic failure (e.g. Parkinson's disease and multiple system atrophy)
  - Secondary autonomic failure (e.g. diabetes mellitus and amyloidosis)
- Cardiac
  - Arrhythmias (brady- and tachyarrhythmias)
  - Structural abnormalities (e.g. valvular disease and tumors)
- Other (rare)
  - Acute ischemia, pulmonary embolism, pulmonary hypertension, aortic dissection, cardiac tamponade and subclavian steal syndrome

- **Vasovagal syncope** (VVS), also known as the "common faint", is usually triggered by orthostatic or emotional stress. Classic triggers include prolonged standing or sitting (particularly in a hot crowded environment or hot shower), pain, unpleasant sights or medical procedures. Volume depletion, some medications (e.g. vasodilators and diuretics) or alcohol can facilitate the episodes. Premonitory signs, including feeling hot or cold, diaphoresis, palpitations, nausea, abdominal cramps, blurred vision and others are typically present. Patients usually appear pale and diaphoretic. Severe cardioinhibitory syncope, usually with prolonged asystolic pauses, can be associated with seizure-like activity. Although recovery of consciousness and appropriate orientation are usually rapid, patients characteristically experience fatigue and weakness for many hours following the syncopal event. It is important to emphasize that in some patients, especially in the elderly, characteristic premonitory signs may be absent
- **Situational syncope (faint)** refers to a reflex syncope recurrently caused by specific triggers such as micturition, defecation, swallowing, coughing, laughing, large meals or exercise
- **Carotid sinus (CS) syncope** is a form of reflex syncope thought to be due to CS hypersensitivity, which is an abnormal reflex triggered by stimulation of CS baroreceptors. CSS syncope predominantly occurs in the elderly (often older men) and is rarely diagnosed in patients younger than 50 years of age. In the classical but rare form, clinical events are triggered by mechanical manipulation of the CS, such as neck stretching, neck turning or wearing tight collars. More commonly, a patient presents with unexplained syncope or falls and the diagnosis is made by an abnormal

response to CS massage. An abnormal response to CS massage consistent with CS hypersensitivity is detected in about one-third of elderly patients with unexplained syncope or falls. Of note, CS hypersensitivity is also common in asymptomatic elderly patients; therefore, caution should be exercised in making this diagnosis and other causes of syncope should be excluded.

Reflex syncope is a clinical diagnosis and, in the majority of cases, additional diagnostic tests are not warranted. Tilt testing can be useful in some patients with suspected vasovagal mechanism and atypical presentation. The role of the insertable loop recorder is discussed below.

Although, long-term survival prognosis is favorable, recurrent reflex syncope can result in significant morbidity. Frequency of syncopal events within the past year appears to be the best predictor of future recurrences.

- **Orthostatic hypotension** is an abnormal postural decrease in blood pressure (BP) secondary to inadequate peripheral vasoconstriction in response to orthostatic stress. The "classical" form of orthostatic hypotension is defined as a sustained decline in systolic BP ≥20 mm Hg or in diastolic BP ≥10 mm Hg within 3 minutes of standing or head-up tilt to at least 60° on a tilt table. In the "initial" form, orthostatic hypotension occurs immediately upon standing followed by rapid and spontaneous recovery of BP and symptoms (usually within 30 seconds). The "delayed" form is characterized by a slow (i.e. 20–40 minutes) and progressive BP decline, typically without significant bradycardia. Orthostatic hypotension is an important cause of syncope in the elderly and can cause significant morbidity. It is relatively uncommon in young patients. Orthostatic hypotension is a risk factor for increased cardiovascular and overall mortality, most likely due to its frequent association with other severe comorbidities.

  Causes of orthostatic hypotension include medications, volume depletion or autonomic nervous failure, which can be primary or secondary. Advanced age, diabetes mellitus and Parkinson's disease are frequent contributing factors

- **Postural orthostatic tachycardia syndrome** is a poorly understood form of orthostatic intolerance characterized by a sustained heart rate (HR) increment of ≥30 beats/minute within 10 minutes of standing or head-up tilt in the absence of orthostatic hypotension. The standing HR is usually ≥120 beats/minute. Patients typically complain of posturally induced weakness, fatigue, palpitations and inability to tolerate any physical activities. It occurs mostly in young women and is frequently associated with deconditioning, recent viral infection, chronic fatigue syndrome, limited or restricted autonomic neuropathy and neurally mediated syncope

- **Cardiac syncope** is caused by a sudden drop of CO secondary to either arrhythmias or, rarely, mechanical obstruction to blood flow.
  - **Cardiac arrhythmia** is the leading cause of cardiac syncope. The primary mechanism of cerebral hypoperfusion during arrhythmias

is a sudden fall in CO. A maladaptive cerebral and systemic vascular response to a sudden change in CO also appears to play an important role. Patients frequently regain consciousness despite continuing arrhythmias. Multiple factors can contribute to development of syncope during arrhythmias including underlying heart disease, medications, body position, volume status and others.

Clinical and electrocardiographic (ECG) features consistent with arrhythmic cause of syncope are summarized in Tables 14.2 and 14.3. While palpitations are common in patients with VVS, sudden onset palpitations immediately followed by syncope would strongly suggest an arrhythmia.

- **Causes of bradyarrhythmia** include sinus node dysfunction and atrioventricular (AV) block. Bradyarrhythmia can be due to intrinsic disease of the sinus node or conduction system, medications, metabolic or electrolyte abnormalities, or a reflex response. The latter mechanism should be suspected when both sinus bradycardia/pauses and AV block occur simultaneously. Mobitz type II AV block is highly specific for advanced infranodal conduction system disease. Bradycardia is an important risk factor for QT prolongation. Torsades de pointes

Table 14.2: ECG findings that are diagnostic for arrhythmic syncope

- Alternating bundle branch block
- Mobitz type II second-degree or third-degree AV block
- Sustained VT or fast SVT
- Long QT interval with runs of torsades de pointes VT
- Persistent sinus bradycardia (heart rate <40 bpm) or repetitive sinus pauses (≥3 sec)

AV, atrioventricular; VT, ventricular tachycardia; SVT, supraventricular tachycardia; ECG, electrocardiographic.

Table 14.3: ECG findings suggesting arrhythmic syncope

- Sinus bradycardia (<50 bpm) or a sinus pause (≥3 sec)
- BBB and/or QRS duration >120 ms
- Mobitz type I second-degree AV block
- Brugada pattern
- Long or short QT interval
- Abnormal accentuated J waves in the inferior/lateral leads
- Nonsustained VT
- Pathologic Q waves
- Negative T waves and/or epsilon waves in right precordial leads (ARVC)
- LVH with strain pattern and asymmetric negative T waves (HCM)
- Preexcited QRS

BBB, bundle branch block; AV, atrioventricular; ARVC, arrhythmogenic right ventricular cardiomyopathy; LVH, left ventricular hypertrophy; HCM, hypertrophic cardiomyopathy; VT, ventricular tachycardia; ECG, electrocardiographic.

Table 14.4: Cardiac conditions associated with increased risk of life-threatening ventricular arrhythmias

- Long QT syndrome (congenital or acquired)
- Short QT syndrome
- Brugada syndrome
- Catecholaminergic polymorphic VT
- Prior myocardial infarction
- Arrhythmogenic right ventricular cardiomyopathy
- Hypertrophic cardiomyopathy
- Dilated cardiomyopathies
- Myocarditis
- Cardiac sarcoid*
- Cardiomyopathies secondary to muscular dystrophies*

* Conditions that are also associated with increased risk of atrioventricular block.

polymorphic ventricular tachycardia (VT) is a well-recognized mechanism of syncope in patients with bradycardia
- **Ventricular tachycardia** is more commonly associated with syncope than supraventricular arrhythmia. Self-terminating VT is an important cause of syncope in patients with some cardiomyopathies and inherited arrhythmogenic syndromes (Table 14.4). Recognition of these conditions and early initiation of appropriate therapy are critical for prevention of sudden death. Syncopal idiopathic monomorphic VTs are usually associated with a good survival prognosis
- **Supraventricular arrhythmia** is rarely attended by syncope. Important exceptions are atrial fibrillation/flutter in the setting of a rapidly conducting accessory pathway and atrial flutter with 1:1 AV conduction.
  - **Fixed or dynamic obstruction to blood flow** is a relatively rare mechanism of cardiac syncope. Typical examples are severe aortic stenosis and hypertrophic cardiomyopathy. However, arrhythmias and VVS are also common in these conditions.
- **Unexplained syncope** accounts for up to one-third of all syncope cases seen in the general population and the emergency department setting. The proportion of unexplained syncope seems to be lower among patients evaluated in specialized syncope units.

OTHER CAUSES OF T-LOC

There are a number of conditions associated with true or apparent LOC that can mimic syncope (Table 14.5). In contrast to syncope, their pathophysiological mechanisms do not involve global cerebral hypoperfusion. The differential diagnosis is usually straightforward but, occasionally, may be challenging particularly in some cases of epileptic

Table 14.5: Conditions with transient LOC that can mimic syncope

- Nontraumatic conditions with transient LOC
  - Epilepsy
  - Metabolic disorders (e.g. hypoglycemia, hypoxia, and hypercapnia)
  - Intoxication (e.g. medications, drugs or alcohol)
  - Vertebrobasilar TIA/stroke
- Conditions that mimic transient LOC
  - Psychogenic pseudosyncope
  - Falls
  - Cataplexy
  - Drop attacks

LOC, loss of consciousness; TIA, transient ischemic attack.

seizures and psychogenic pseudosyncope. A thorough history obtained from the patient and eyewitnesses of the event is crucial for establishing the correct diagnosis.

- **Epileptic seizures** are caused by abnormal neuronal cortical activity. Distinguishing syncope from seizures can sometimes be difficult since seizure-like activity is common in syncope. Some important clinical clues that may help distinguish between the two conditions are summarized in Table 14.6. While severe bradycardia and prolonged asystole are noted in up to 2% of patients with complex or simple partial seizures involving the temporal lobes, contrary to syncope, bradycardia typically occurs well after the onset of seizures
- **Psychogenic pseudosyncope** is characterized by apparent rather than true LOC. It is usually diagnosed in young people. There is a female preponderance and a history of psychiatric disorders is common. Notably, many patients also have a history of VVS. Episodes are typically witnessed and prolonged (minutes), have no identifiable triggers and tend to be multiple (frequently several episodes a day). Convulsive activity (i.e. pseudoseizures) may be present but does not exhibit any specific or consistent pattern. Heart rate and BP are within normal range. Eye closure during episodes is characteristic of psychogenic pseudosyncope, while during syncope and epilepsy the eyes are usually open. Tilt testing may be useful for documenting LOC in the absence of significant hypotension or bradycardia. Before making the diagnosis, all other causes need to be carefully excluded. It is important to remember that these episodes are involuntary and patients usually are not willing to accept an explanation about their psychogenic nature. Psychiatric evaluation is essential when psychogenic pseudosyncope is suspected
- **Stroke/transient ischemic attack** is an unlikely cause of transient LOC. Vertebral-basilar transient ischemic attack and subarachnoid hemorrhage are rare exceptions. Typically, other neurological signs are present.

Table 14.6: Clinical features that help differentiate between epilepsy and syncope

	Syncope likely	Epilepsy likely
Posture	Reflex syncope—sitting or standing Orthostatic hypotension—standing Cardiac syncope—any posture	Usually any posture (recurrent episodes of transient LOC consistently occurring only during sitting and/or standing would argue against seizures)
Premonitory symptoms	Premonitory symptoms—nausea, abdominal cramps, lightheadedness, blurred vision, palpitations, etc.	Brief aura (déjà vu, olfactory, gustatory or visual hallucination, etc.) Behavior changes prior to LOC
Convulsive activity	After loss of consciousness and postural tone Usually brief (<15 sec)	Coincide with LOC and can start prior to fall Usually prolonged (minutes) Clonic-tonic movement or hemilateral clonic movement Unusual posturing, head turning, abnormal automatism (chewing or lip-smacking), or tongue biting may be present
Duration of LOC	Brief (typically <30 sec, generally <5 min)	Usually prolonged (>5 min)
Postictal symptoms	Typically brief recovery of orientation and appropriate behavior Prolonged fatigue (typical for vasovagal syncope)	Typically prolonged confusion Arching muscles Occasionally transient neurologic deficit

LOC, loss of consciousness.

- **Metabolic causes** of transient LOC are rare and usually do not represent diagnostic dilemmas.
- **Falls** are an important cause of morbidity in the elderly. It is important to remember that elderly patients commonly have cognitive impairment affecting their memory and are not always able to provide a reliable history of the event (i.e. retrograde amnesia). Eyewitness accounts of the episode should be obtained, whenever possible. Syncope should always be considered as a potential mechanism of falls in elderly patients because of its important therapeutic and prognostic implications.

EVALUATION OF PATIENTS WITH T-LOC AND SYNCOPE

The two major goals in the evaluation of patients with syncope are to (i) establish the mechanism of syncope and (ii) to define prognosis with risk stratification. Effective therapy of syncope is not possible without achieving these goals. A recommended systematic approach to the evaluation of patients with syncope is shown in Figure 14.1. The primary goals of the initial evaluation are to determine the mechanism of transient LOC and identify patients at high short-term risk (days or weeks) for serious clinical events

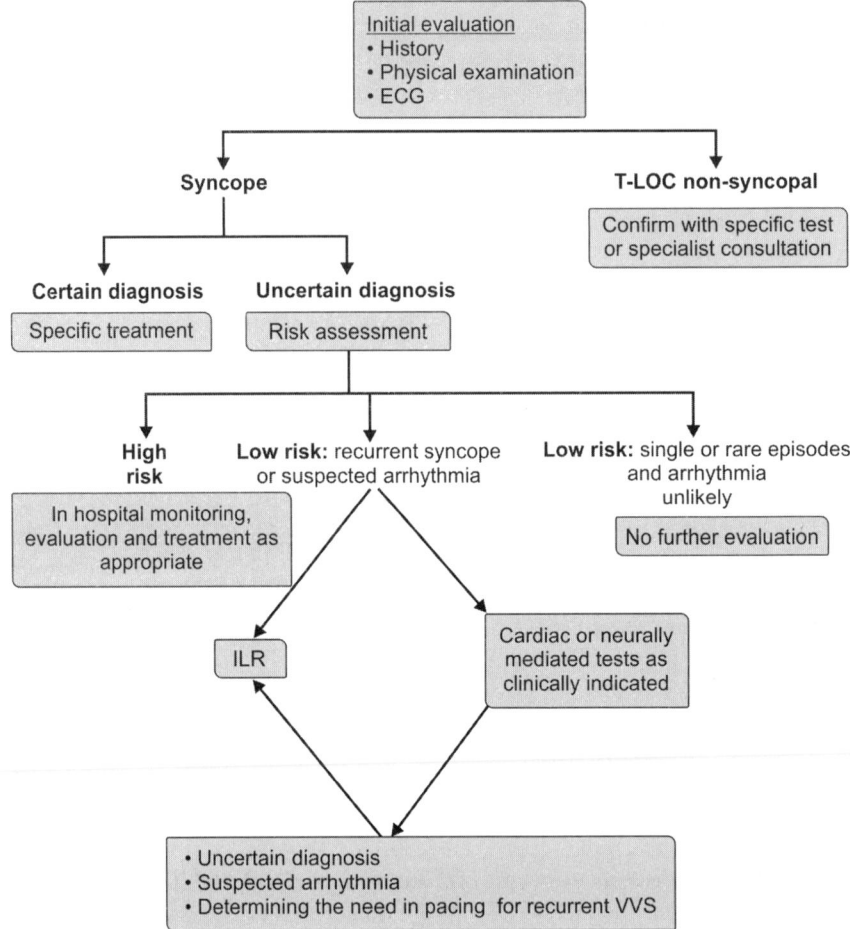

Fig. 14.1: Recommended approach for evaluation of syncope.

T-LOC, transient loss of consciousness; ILR, insertable loop recorder; VVS, vasovagal syncope.

Source: Adapted from the European Society of Cardiology guidelines for the diagnosis and management of syncope (2009).

or mortality who require an intensive in-hospital evaluation. In relatively low-risk patients with uncertain diagnosis, further ambulatory evaluation is guided by likelihood of arrhythmia and frequency of recurrences. Long-term risk assessment should encompass not only the mortality risk but also the risk of recurrent syncope. Patients with a single episode of syncope not resulting in injury and normal initial evaluation can be reassured.

The initial evaluation includes history, physical examination and ECG. Additional diagnostic tests should only be used to confirm suspected clinical diagnosis. Routine use of diagnostic tests not supported by clinical findings should be avoided. In addition to low yield, positive results of some tests may be difficult to interpret if the pretest probability of the disease is low. A thorough initial evaluation can secure diagnosis in up to 50% of patients with

syncope and avoid unnecessary, expensive and, sometimes, unproductive diagnostic testing.
- A **detailed history** is the key element in the evaluation of syncope and should be obtained from both the patient and eyewitnesses of the event. The following clinical features may help to differentiate syncope from other potential causes of transient LOC: (i) transient LOC with rapid onset and short duration (usually <30 seconds but may be a few minutes); (ii) spontaneous and complete recovery; (iii) loss of postural tone. If all these criteria are not met, other causes of transient LOC need to be considered. Important components of history are summarized in Table 14.7
- **Physical examination** may provide additional diagnostic and prognostic information. It should particularly focus on the presence of heart disease (signs of heart failure, valvular disease or arrhythmia), hydration status, including signs of anemia/hemorrhage and neurologic abnormalities suggestive of autonomic abnormalities or focal neurologic deficit.
  - **Orthostatic vital signs** should be obtained in all patients with postural symptoms. Moreover, they should be routinely considered in all elderly patients presenting with syncope or falls. Serial BP and HR measurements should be obtained supine and then each minute for at least 3 minutes while standing. In patients with suspected "delayed" type of orthostatic hypotension, a longer duration of standing period or tilt test may be required to confirm the diagnosis
  - **CS massage** should be performed in patients with clinical events suggestive CS syncope. It may also be considered in adults aged over 40 years with syncope of unknown etiology after initial evaluation and elderly patients with falls. It is contraindicated in patients with a

Table 14.7: Important components of history in patients with syncope
- Circumstances immediately preceding syncope
  - Body position
  - Activity
  - Triggers
- Premonitory signs
- Duration of LOC
- Postictal symptoms
- Frequency and chronicity of syncope
- Eyewitness account:
  - Appearance
  - Presence of seizure-like movements/abnormal automatisms and their temporal relation to the LOC
  - Duration of LOC and seizure-like movements (if present)
  - Postictal confusion and disorientation
- Past cardiac history
- Medications, alcohol and drugs
- Family History of sudden death, arrhythmia, syncope, and neurologic or metabolic conditions

LOC, loss of consciousness.

recent (within 3 months) stroke, prior transient ischemic attacks or carotid bruit (unless significant stenosis has been excluded by carotid Duplex study). The CS is identified either at the anterior border of the sternocleidomastoid muscle at the level of the cricoid cartilage or at the point of maximum carotid pulsation just below the angle of the jaw. Carotid sinus massage is performed for 10–15 seconds sequentially on each side under continuous HR and noninvasive, preferably continuous, BP monitoring. The test is more sensitive when performed in both supine and upright positions using a tilt table. Carotid sinus hypersensitivity is diagnosed if a ventricular pause lasting >3 seconds (either due to sinus pause or AV block) and/or a fall in systolic BP of ≥50 mm Hg are evoked by CS massage. However, these criteria have low specificity for CS syncope if typical patient's symptoms are not reproduced.

Diagnostic Tests

- **Electrocardiography** is part of the initial evaluation recommended for all patients presenting with syncope. Although rarely diagnostic, it is helpful in risk stratification. In patients with a normal ECG, the likelihood of significant cardiac disease is low and survival prognosis is generally excellent, while an abnormal ECG is an independent predictor of cardiac syncope and increased mortality.
- **In-hospital ECG telemetry** is indicated in patients with high-risk features. The duration of the in-hospital monitoring is determined individually and typically does not exceed 48–72 hours.
- **Electrocardiographic ambulatory monitoring** plays a central role in the evaluation of patients with syncope and suspected cardiac arrhythmia. As discussed below, it may also be useful in selected patients with reflex syncope to determine the need for cardiac pacing. Symptom-rhythm correlation during syncope may provide a guide to specific therapy if arrhythmia is documented or direct further evaluation if normal sinus rhythm is found. Electrocardiographic findings may also have important prognostic implications. Monitoring-based strategy has been shown to significantly reduce the recurrence of syncopal episodes and should be considered early in the diagnostic work-up in patients with suspected arrhythmias. Principal characteristics of currently available monitoring options are summarized in Table 14.8.
    - **Holter monitoring** provides continuous ECG recording up to 2 weeks (usually 24–48 hours). The diagnostic data are available only after the completion of the recording period and subsequent analysis.
    - **Event recorders** allow monitoring over longer periods of time, usually up to 1 month. These devices have limited memory capacity (10–20 minutes) and are capable of storing only short intervals of ECG. The information is transmitted trans-telephonically to a centralized monitoring station for interpretation and dispersal to the prescribing physician. There are two principal types of event recorders, loop and postevent.

Table 14.8: Principal characteristics of ambulatory ECG monitors

Features	Duration of monitoring	Continuous ECG Data ("full disclosure")	Remote data transmission
Holter monitor			
Short term	Typically 24-48 h	Yes	No
Long term (patch monitors)	1-2 weeks	Yes	No
Event recorder			
Loop recorder	Up to 1 month	No	Yes
Real-time loop recorder (wireless)	Up to 1 month	Optional	Yes
Postevent (nonlooping)	Up to 1 month	No	Yes
Real-time continuous monitor	Up to 1 month	Yes	Yes
Insertable loop recorder	Up to 3 years	No	Yes

- A *loop recorder* is attached to the chest through electrodes. It continuously records and saves several minutes of the most recent ECG by overwriting earlier data. This allows for storage of ECG recording immediately preceding a triggered event. The device can be activated manually or automatically (auto-trigger) based on specific algorithms for arrhythmia detection.
- A *postevent (nonlooping) recorder* is not worn continuously and records the ECG only prospectively following manual activation by the patient. It has embedded electrodes and is applied directly to the chest during symptoms. This type of monitor is not practical for syncope patients.
- **Real-time monitors** utilize wireless transmission technology. They can be used as an event or a continuous monitor. Continuous type of monitoring affords complete (up to 30 days) ECG data set ("full disclosure"). Some technologies provide real-time streaming of ECG data
- **Insertable loop recorder** requires surgical implantation and allows monitoring for up to 3 years.
- **Patch monitors** are a new generation of miniature leadless ambulatory monitors. They are designed as portable adhesive waterproof patches that can be conveniently applied to the skin for several days. Currently available monitors can be used as a long-term (up to 14 days) Holter-type continuous recorder or a real-time wireless event monitor. Some devices are equipped with an accelerometer for correlation of ECG findings with the patient's activity and documentation of falls.

The yield of the monitoring modalities depends on the frequency of syncopal episodes. As a general rule, the longer the period of monitoring, the higher the diagnostic yield, since syncope recurrences are usually random and unpredictable. A loop monitor with autotrigger capability (preferably with wireless transmission technology) and an insertable loop recorder are the most useful monitoring options in patients with syncope. There is no consensus whether external monitors should be ordered before the placement of an insertable loop recorder. The decision should be made individually based on the type and frequency of syncopal events as well as potential compliance issues with wearing an external monitor.

- **Head-up tilt testing** is indicated in patients with suspected VVS in whom syncopal episodes have apparent orthostatic or emotional stress triggers but clinical presentation is not obvious (no premonitory signs, etc.). It can be used in some patients with classical VVS to provide reassurance that the diagnosis is established. The currently used protocols include an initial supine pretilt stabilization period (5-20 minutes) and a passive phase in the 60-70° tilt position (for 20-40 minutes) frequently followed by the administration of pharmacologic challenge with either intravenous isoproterenol or sublingual nitroglycerin. Pharmacologic challenge increases the sensitivity but decreases the specificity of the test. A positive response is considered when syncope or near syncope attended by hypotension and/or bradycardia are induced. The test has a reported specificity of about 90%. The type of response during the test (i.e. cardioinhibitory, vasodepressor or mixed) poorly correlates with that during clinical events and, therefore, is not useful for defining therapeutic approaches. Also the test is poorly reproducible and is not helpful to monitor the response to therapy.

  Other potentially useful applications include suspected delayed type of orthostatic hypotension and psychogenic pseudosyncope. Patients with orthostatic hypotension show progressive decline in BP usually without significant reflex bradycardia. In patients with psychogenic pseudosyncope, tilt testing may provoke an episode of apparent LOC with no significant change in HR and BP

- **An electrophysiology study** (EPS) should be considered in patients with suspected arrhythmic cause of syncope or structural heart disease. In the latter group, EPS is an important risk stratification tool. Induced ventricular arrhythmia in patients with syncope and structural heart disease is a marker of increased risk of sudden death. Electrophysiology study is not indicated in patients with a normal ECG, no evidence of heart disease and clinical history that is inconsistent with arrhythmia. Even in appropriately selected syncope patients, the diagnostic yield of EPS is usually low. A common limitation is difficulty in determining causal relation of the induced arrhythmia to syncope.

  Electrophysiology study has a limited role in the assessment of the sinus node. Sinus node dysfunction is a clinical diagnosis, which is based on documentation of spontaneous sinus bradycardia or pauses, ideally during symptoms.

  Electrophysiology study is reasonable in patients with syncope and evidence for bundle branch block (BBB) or abnormal AV conduction.

Certain findings strongly suggest a causative role of AV block in patients with syncope. These include documentation of infranodal AV block (spontaneous or pharmacologically provoked) or prolonged HV interval (≥70–100 milliseconds). However, sensitivity of EPS for assessment of AV conduction is low. Normal conduction study in patients with BBB does not generally exclude transient (paroxysmal) AV block as a cause of syncope.

Fast, hemodynamically compromised supraventricular arrhythmias reproducing spontaneous symptoms can be considered potentially causative. This is a rare EPS finding in patients with syncope. Interpretation of the hemodynamic response and symptoms during induced supraventricular tachycardia can be confounded by supine position and sedation.

Ventricular tachycardia is the most common abnormality uncovered during EPS in patients with syncope. Induced sustained monomorphic VT in patients with relatively preserved left ventricular (LV) function or prior myocardial infarction is usually diagnostic. In the latter group, induced monomorphic VT is an indication for an implantable intracardiac defibrillator (ICD). The prognostic significance of induced polymorphic VT or ventricular fibrillation (VF) in these patients is debatable. In patients with severe LV dysfunction, an ICD is indicated and EPS is usually unnecessary unless supraventricular arrhythmia is suspected or ablation of VT is intended to prevent future ICD shocks. Electrophysiology study has a limited role in syncopal patients with nonischemic and hypertrophic cardiomyopathies. The role of EPS in Brugada syndrome is controversial.

- **Echocardiography** is recommended in patients with suspected structural heart disease. While echocardiography is rarely diagnostic for the etiology of syncope, assessment of LV systolic function may have important prognostic implications
- **Exercise stress testing** should be considered in patients with syncope or presyncope that occurs during or immediately after exertion. Syncope occurring during exercise strongly indicates cardiac etiology while syncope that occurs after exercise is usually neurally mediated. Conditions associated with exercise-induced syncope include long QT syndrome, catecholaminergic polymorphic VT, infranodal conduction system disease or hypertrophic cardiomyopathy. Ischemia is usually accompanied by angina
- **Neurologic testing** has a very low yield in patients with syncope and is not routinely indicated. Brain imaging should only be considered if focal neurologic deficit is present or in case of head injury due to syncope. An electroencephalogram should only be obtained if clinical clues suggesting epilepsy are present.

RISK ASSESSMENT

The major goals of risk assessment in patients presenting with syncope are to determine the risks of death and syncope recurrences. As discussed above, syncope is a clinical syndrome, which encompasses a spectrum of

> **Table 14.9:** High-risk clinical features that require in-hospital evaluation
> - Severe structural or coronary artery disease
>   - Heart failure, low ejection fraction, prior myocardial infarction, valvular disease, etc.
> - Clinical or ECG features suggesting arrhythmic syncope
>   - Clinical features: exertional or supine syncope, sudden onset palpitations immediately followed by syncope, brief or no premonitory signs
>   - Family history of sudden death
>   - Abnormal ECG (see Tables 14.2 and 14.3)
> - Suspected life-threatening conditions
>   - Acute ischemia/infarct, pulmonary embolism, aortic dissection, etc.
> - Important comorbidities
>   - Severe electrolyte abnormalities, anemia, etc.

ECG, electrocardiography.

causes, from benign to life threatening. In patients with syncope, survival prognosis is determined by the presence and severity of the underlying, primarily cardiac, disease. However, the presence of structural heart disease, although prognostically important, does not necessarily imply a cardiac cause of syncope. Determining the exact mechanism of syncope is crucial for preventing syncope recurrences and associated morbidity.

Patients with high short-term mortality and morbidity risk (days and weeks) should be admitted to the hospital for further monitoring and evaluation. High-risk features are shown in Table 14.9. A number of risk stratification rules have been developed to simplify risk management of syncopal patients in the ED (Table 14.10). They provide only an approximate assessment of risk and are not intended to replace a comprehensive evaluation by a clinician experienced in the management of syncope patients. Long-term prognosis is mostly determined by the presence and severity of heart disease or other chronic comorbidities. A normal ECG, absence of structural heart disease, and benign family history are usually associated with favorable prognosis.

TREATMENT

Therapeutic goals in patients with syncope are to improve survival and prevent recurrences. To achieve the latter goal, therapeutic approach should ideally target the specific mechanism of syncope. This is not always feasible especially in patients with high-risk cardiac conditions who are frequently undergoing ICD implantation predicated on the assumption that syncope is caused by ventricular arrhythmia. While ICD can improve survival in these patients, it may not necessarily prevent syncope recurrences.

- **Reflex syncope.** There is no truly mechanism-directed or predictably effective therapy for *VVS*. When used in combination, they allow relief of symptoms and improvement in quality of life in the majority of patients with recurrent VVS. Therapy for VVS can be grouped into lifestyle measures, physical maneuvers, medications and cardiac pacing (Table 14.11).

Table 14.10: Examples of risk stratification schemes

Rules/scores	High-risk features	High risk	Outcome
San Francisco syncope rule	• Shortness of breath • Systolic blood pressure <90 mm Hg • Abnormal ECG (arrhythmia or new abnormalities) • Hematocrit <30% • History of congestive heart failure	A single feature	7-day serious events rate
ROSE rule	• Chest pain at time of syncope • Oxygen saturation ≤94% on room air on initial presentation • BNP ≥300 pg/mL • Hemoglobin ≤9 g/dL • Stool positive for occult blood • Bradycardia (heart rate <50 beats/min) • Q-wave on ECG	A single feature	30-day adverse events rate
OESIL (Osservatorio Epidemiologico sulla Sincope nel Lazio)	• Age ≥65-year-old • No prodrome • History of cardiovascular disease • Abnormal ECG (arrhythmia, pathologic Q waves, ST changes, BBB, • LVH)	>1 features	1-year mortality
EGSYS score (Evaluation of Guidelines in Syncope Study)	• Antecedent palpitations (+4) • Abnormal ECG and/or heart disease (+3) • Exertional syncope (+3) • Syncope while supine (+2) • Prodromal symptoms typical for VVS (-1) • Predisposing and/or precipitating factors/environments typical for VVS (-1)	Score ≥3	2-year total mortality

BBB, bundle branch block; BNP, brain natriuretic peptide, LVH, left ventricular hypertrophy; VVS, vasovagal syncope.

- *Lifestyle measures* are the cornerstone in the treatment of VVS. In addition, psychotherapy may need to be considered in patients with psychosocial impairment.
- **Physical maneuvers** can help avert syncopal episodes in patients with premonitory symptoms. However, in about one-third of patients with VVS, premonitory signs may be absent or not sufficiently long to allow for performance of these maneuvers. The role of regular exercise in preventing VVS is not well established. The clinical utility of orthostatic stress training maneuvers ("tilt training" and outpatient standing against the wall one to two times a day for 30 minutes) remains controversial
- **Pharmacological treatment** is recommended only when symptomatic response to lifestyle changes remains unsatisfactory. Although, a

> **Table 14.11:** Treatment of vasovagal syncope
>
> - **Lifestyle measures**
>   - Education: mechanism, precipitating factors and environments, premonitory signs
>   - Reassurance about benign nature and favorable survival prognosis
>   - Adequate hydration and salt intake
>   - Adjustment or discontinuation of potentially contributory medications (diuretics, vasodilators, etc.), if possible
> - **Physical maneuvers**
>   - During premonitory signs: sitting or laying down and isometric counterpressure maneuvers
>   - Orthostatic training: tilt training and standing against the wall
>   - Regular exercise
> - **Pharmacological treatment** (midodrine, fludrocortisone, β-blockers, selective serotonin reuptake inhibitors, etc.)
> - **Cardiac pacing** in patients with prolonged asystolic pauses or severe bradycardia documented during clinical episodes

number of medications have been proposed for treatment of VVS, the data supporting their use are limited. Midodrine and fludrocortisone seem to be the most commonly used medications. They should be avoided in hypertensive patients. Selective serotonin reuptake inhibitors may be useful, in addition to psychotherapy, in patients with psychosocial impairment. Beta blockers may be considered in older, particularly hypertensive, patients

- Cardiac pacing is reserved for patients with refractory recurrent syncope and long asystolic pauses or profound bradycardia documented during spontaneous episodes. Recent studies involving insertable loop recorders suggested beneficial effect of cardiac pacing in preventing VVS in this population of patients. It is important to stress that the type of response during tilt testing correlates poorly with that during spontaneous VVS and should not be used for guiding pacemaker therapy. Another important consideration is that all available data on potentially beneficial effect of pacing in VVS pertain to an adult population aged 40 years and above. The role of pacing in younger patients has not been established. The decision regarding pacing in young patients should take account of long-term risk of potential pacemaker-related complications.

CS Syncope

Treatment of patients with CS syncope is guided by the response to CS massage. The relative contribution of a vasodepressor component to CS syncope is best studied during upright CS massage. Cardiac pacing is an established therapy for patients with predominately cardioinhibitory response. Treatment of patients with vasodepressor physiology is challenging.

Midodrine and fludrocortisone have been advocated, although data on their efficacy are limited.
- **Orthostatic hypotension**. Similar to VVS, treatment of orthostatic hypotension should involve education about the nature of the problem and preventive measures. Iatrogenic cause of orthostatic hypotension is common in older patients. Treatment with vasodilators and diuretics should be adjusted or discontinued, if possible. In patients with autonomic failure, adequate hydration and salt intake are critical. They should be taught standing up slowly and avoid standing motionless for prolonged periods of time. Counterpressure maneuvers such as leg crossing or calf clenching while standing may be helpful. Elevation of the head of the bed (by 15-20 cm) at night can help minimize supine increase in BP and nocturnal diuresis. Waist-high compression stockings have limited efficacy and poorly tolerated, particularly during hot weather.

  Medications are recommended when the response to nonpharmacologic measures is suboptimal. Midodrine and fludrocortisone are the most commonly used medications. Supine hypertension is a common problem in patients with orthostatic hypotension, particularly in the elderly. In these patients, eccentric dosing of short acting medications should be considered. Short acting midodrine is preferred over long-acting fludrocortisone. It should be taken at least 4 hours prior to bedtime. Supine hypertension, in turn, can be treated with bedtime short acting antihypertensives. Mild to moderate permissive systolic supine hypertension is an acceptable strategy for treating this condition.
- **Cardiac syncope**. Treatment of cardiac syncope depends on the etiology and mechanism involved. Detailed discussion of this topic is beyond the scope of this chapter. Patients with arrhythmic cause of syncope should be referred to a cardiac electrophysiologist. Some general principles are outlined below:
  - **Bradyarrhythmias**. Reversible causes of bradyarrhythmia such as medications, electrolyte and metabolic disorder should always be sought. A pacemaker is indicated in patients with intrinsic sinus node or conduction system disease and in selected patients with cardioinhibitory reflex syncope. (Additional details regarding the indications for permanent pacing are discussed in Chapter 16: Bradyarrhythmias.)
  - **Tachyarrhythmias**. Available therapeutic options include antiarrhythmic medications, catheter or surgical ablation and an ICD implantation. In patients with syncopal supraventricular arrhythmias or idiopathic VTs, more definitive ablation approach is preferred over antiarrhythmic medications. An ICD is an important consideration in patients with syncope and structural heart diseases or some inherited arrhythmogenic syndromes associated with high risk of sudden death. Chapter 18: Tachyarrhythmia-provides more detail on the subject.
- **Valvular obstruction or cardiac mass** causing syncope is managed, as a general rule, surgically.

SYNCOPE AND DRIVING

Management of patients with syncope includes the assessment of driving risk and determining the duration of driving restrictions. Factors to consider are etiology of syncope, risk of recurrent syncope, how often and in what capacity the patient drives as well as applicable laws and regulations. Available data suggest that the risk of vehicle accident in patents with a history of syncope is not different from the general population without syncope. However, it is generally recommended that noncommercial driving be restricted for several months unless effective therapy is established.

SUGGESTED READING

1. Brignole M, Hamdan MH. New concepts in the assessment of syncope. J Am Coll Cardiol. 2012;59:1583-91.
2. Freeman R, Wieling W, Axelrod FB, et al. Consensus statement on definition of orthostatic hypotension, neurally mediated syncope and the postural tachycardia syndrome. Clin Auton Res. 2011;21:69-71.
3. Hoefnagles WA, Padberg GW, Overweg J, et al. Transient loss of consciousness: the value of the history for distinguishing seizure from syncope. J Neurol. 1991;238:39-43.
4. Krahn AD, Andrade JG, Deyell MW. Selecting appropriate diagnostic tools for evaluating the patient with syncope/collapse. Prog Cardiovasc Dis. 2013;55:402-9.
5. Moya A, Sutton R, Ammirati F, Blane JJ, Brignola M, Dahm JB, et al. Task force for the diagnosis and management of syncope; European Society of Cardiology (ESC), European Heart Rhythm Association (EHRA), Heart Failure Association (HFA), Heart Rhythm Society (HRS). Guidelines for the diagnosis and management of syncope (version 2009). Eur Heart J. 2009;30:2631-71.
6. Raj SR, Coffin ST. Medical therapy and physical maneuvers in the treatment of vasovagal syncope and orthostatic hypotension. Prog Cardiovasc Dis. 2013;55:425-33.
7. Sakaguchi S, Li H. Syncope and driving, flying and vocational concerns. Prog Cardiovasc Dis. 2013;55:454-63.
8. Seifer C. Carotid sinus syndrome. Cardiol Clin. 2013;31:111-21.
9. Strickberger SA, Benson DW, Biaggioni I, et al. AHA/ACCF Scientific statement on the evaluation of syncope: from the American Heart Association Councils on Clinical Cardiology, Cardiovascular Nursing, Cardiovascular Disease in the Young, and Stroke, and the Quality of Care and Outcomes Research Interdisciplinary Working Group; and the American College of Cardiology Foundation: in collaboration with the Heart Rhythm Society: endorsed by the American Autonomic Society. Circulation. 2006;113:316-27.
10. Van Dijk JG, Weiling W. Pathophysiological basis of syncope and neurological conditions that mimic syncope. Prog Cardiovasc Dis. 2013;55:345-56.

Palpitations

Chapter 15

Uzodinma C Emerenini, Denice Hodgson-Zingman

'Palpitations' is a common term used by patients to describe a sensation of a change from their normal heartbeat. This may be due to an awareness of a more vigorous or forceful heartbeat or of an alteration in the either the rate or cadence of the heartbeat. Other terms, such as fluttering, racing, pounding, skipping, thumping, flip-flopping and extra beats may be used to convey this experience. Some patients notice uncomfortable fullness in the throat, neck or chest. Palpitations are among the most common of symptoms that account for patient disability and healthcare resources utilization.

Generally, thin people are more likely to be aware of the heartbeat. Patients may first be aware of the heartbeat when they lie down or are otherwise in a distraction-free setting. Patients may particularly notice their heartbeat when lying on their left side due to the pressure of the heart against the chest wall in this position. Many patients may be aware of changes in their heartbeat but do not seek medical attention until the frequency of the palpitations increases or they cause symptoms such as dyspnea or lightheadedness.

Palpitations are frequently benign but may be caused by potentially lethal arrhythmias. They may be purely cardiac in etiology or provoked by pathology in other organ systems. A thorough clinical evaluation is necessary (Fig. 15.1), which should begin at a minimum with a detailed history, physical examination and a 12-lead electrocardiogram (ECG).

ETIOLOGY

Palpitations may be caused by sinus rhythm or sinus tachycardia with more forceful contraction, as may occur with adrenergic stimulation, but can also be caused by the following rhythm abnormalities:
- Sinus node: inappropriate sinus tachycardia, sinoatrial node reentry sinoatrial exit block, sinus bradycardia or sinus arrest
- Conduction system: various levels of atrioventricular block, junctional escape, junctional tachycardia, fascicular ectopy or tachycardias, bundle branch reentry, atrioventricular node reentrant tachycardia
- Atrium: premature atrial contractions, atrial tachycardia, atrial flutter, atrial fibrillation
- Ventricle: premature ventricular contractions, ventricular tachycardia, torsades-de-pointes, ventricular fibrillation
- Other: reciprocating tachycardias utilizing an accessory pathway.

The differential for underlying conditions that create the stimulus for palpitations is very broad and includes the following:
- Cardiac: Mitral valve prolapse, Wolff–Parkinson–White, myocardial infarction, myocardial ischemia, congenital abnormalities, channelopathies and other heritable arrhythmia disorders/cardiomyopathies (e.g. Brugada syndrome, long QT syndrome, short QT syndrome, catecholaminergic polymorphic ventricular tachycardia, arrhythmogenic right/left ventricular cardiomyopathy, hypertrophic cardiomyopathy, ventricular noncompaction, muscular/myotonic dystrophies, among others), infiltrative diseases (e.g. amyloidosis, hemochromatosis), tumors (e.g. myxomas, metastases to the myocardium), sarcoidosis, Chagas disease, lupus and pericarditis, among others
- Stress/inflammatory conditions: postoperative state, sepsis, trauma
- Autonomic: postural orthostatic tachycardia syndrome, vasovagal (neurocardiogenic) reflex, dysautonomia
- Pacing devices: antitachycardia pacing, asynchronous pacing, battery depletion, loss of capture, over- and under-sensing, mechanical stimulation from a dislodged lead or a lead with excess slack, irritation from new lead, lead damage, pacemaker mediated tachycardia, upper rate (Wenckebach) behavior, pacing algorithms designed to limit ventricular pacing in dual chamber devices, stimulation of adjacent structures (e.g. pectoral muscle, chest wall, diaphragm or phrenic nerve)
- Respiratory: pulmonary embolus, asthma, chronic obstructive pulmonary disease, pulmonary hypertension, pneumonia, pneumothorax, hypoxia, obstructive sleep apnea
- Medications: vasodilators, sympathomimetic agents, anticholinergic drugs, antiarrhythmic drugs, β-blockers, calcium channel blockers, digoxin, QT prolonging medications, diuretics
- Ingested substances: nicotine, alcohol, caffeine, cocaine, methamphetamine
- Electrolyte abnormalities
- Hormonal: hyper- or hypothyroidism, hypoglycemia, pheochromocytoma, perimenstrual, perimenopausal, pregnancy, peripartum
- Psychiatric: anxiety disorders, depression, somatization.

EVALUATION

The nature of the palpitations may help in identifying the etiology. For example, Are they frequent or infrequent? Are they regular or irregular? Do they last long or are they relatively isolated? Do they occur with exercise or other activities? Is there a positional component? What are the provoking or relieving factors, if any? Is there a relationship between their onset and any other symptoms, medical problems/diagnoses, initiation or discontinuation of any medications? The patients may be asked to tap out the pattern with their fingers on a table top to better illustrate the rate and regularity of their palpitations.

A thorough past medical history, medication list and review of systems are necessary to screen for any of the potential provoking conditions listed in the previous section. Also, taking a careful family history is important to identify any risk for heritable arrhythmia disorders or cardiomyopathies. Patients should be asked not only about any sudden deaths within the family, but also any suspicious deaths, such as due to motor vehicle accidents or drownings that might have been provoked by an arrhythmia. Sudden deaths in family members younger than 50 years should be particularly noted. The social history, including exposures to stimulants or alcohol, should be obtained.

The foremost task in evaluating a patient with palpitations is to determine whether the patient has pre-existing heart disease and the presence of "alarm" symptoms such as diaphoresis, dyspnea, chest pain and syncope. Palpitations with dyspnea can be one of the early signs of heart failure. On the other hand, patients with pre-existing coronary artery disease or heart failure are at increased risk of ventricular arrhythmias as a cause of palpitations, and sudden cardiac death can occur at greatly increased frequency in this population. An ECG should be performed on every patient even in the absence of ongoing symptoms, since a substrate for arrhythmia may be identified. For instance, prior myocardial infarction may be identified by the presence of q waves, hypertrophy may be identified by QRS voltage, a short PR interval may suggest an arrhythmia associated with an accessory pathway, whereas a long QT may suggest polymorphic ventricular tachycardia (torsades-de-pointes) as a cause for symptoms. An echocardiogram should be considered in any patient with palpitations and is essential in any patient at risk for or suspected of having underlying heart disease. Further evaluation may be guided by the algorithm (Fig. 15.1).

PHYSICAL EXAMINATION

The physical examination can be invaluable in the evaluation of patients with palpitations, although the patient may not have ongoing symptoms at the time of the examination. A mid-systolic click as occurs with mitral valve prolapse, murmurs that indicate valvular stenosis or regurgitation, a gallop associated with cardiomyopathy, abnormal jugular venous pulsations and lower extremity edema would all be significant findings. The detection of an irregular rhythm may suggest atrial fibrillation with symptoms occurring during spurts of rapid ventricular conduction. Physical examination findings that suggest underlying provoking conditions can also be helpful such as a goiter or exophthalmos in Graves' disease, or unilateral lower extremity swelling that may indicate a deep venous thrombosis as a source for pulmonary embolism.

TESTING

Testing to identify abnormalities of cardiac rate or rhythm includ: the ECG, rhythm strip recording, treadmill exercise ECG, telemetry, Holter monitoring,

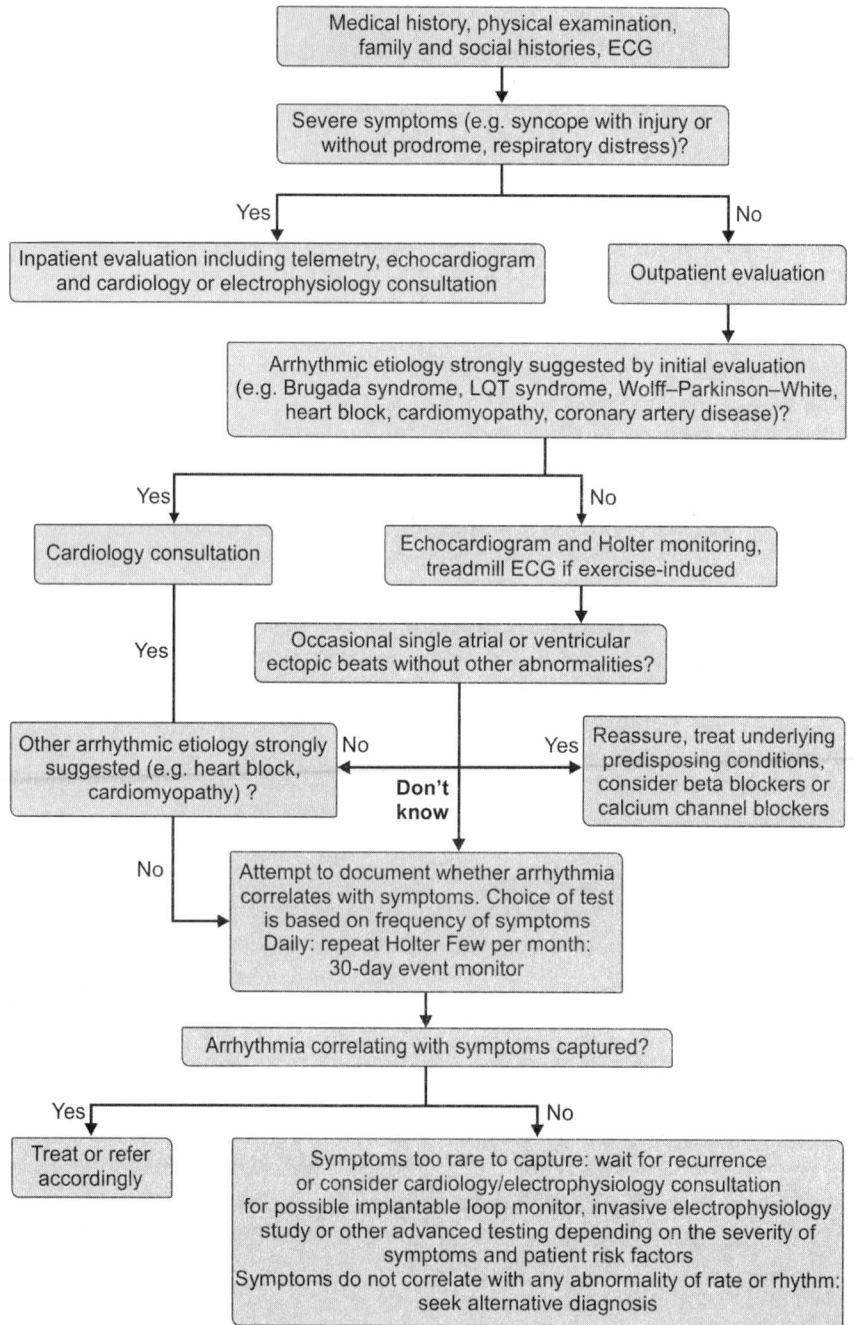

Fig. 15.1: Algorithm for the evaluation and management of palpitation.
ECG, electrocardiogram; LQT, Long-QT.

event monitoring, implantable loop monitoring, signal averaged ECG, cardiac pacing device (pacemaker, implantable cardioverter/defibrillator [ICD, or resynchronization device such as biventricular pacemaker or ICD) interrogation, tilt table testin, and invasive electrophysiology study.

Tests to identify underlying heart disease may includ: echocardiography, stress testing, and other imaging modalities such as cardiac computed tomography or magnetic resonance imaging.

The choice of tests should be based on the risk factors of the patients and appropriate cardiology or electrophysiology consultation in some cases.

PALPITATIONS DURING PREGNANCY

Palpitations are common during pregnancy and may represent a recurrence of previously diagnosed problem or the first manifestation of structural heart disease. In addition, the use of anti-arrhythmic drugs that are safe for both mother and fetus is frequently tha cause of concern for health care providers.

In pregnancy the heart rates increase by 25%; thus, sinus tachycardia is not uncommon. Women with a history of arrhythmias who may have previously been stable on medical therapy may have a recurrence of palpitations due to the increased volume of distribution and increased metabolism associated with pregnancy. Women who may have had repaired congenital heart disease may have an increased incidence of atrial arrhythmias, such as atrial flutter or atrial fibrillation due to the increased plasma volume associated with pregnancy.

An echocardiogram is an essential part of the evaluation of palpitations in pregnancy as this may lead to previously undiagnosed valvular disease such as mitral stenosis that may impact the outcome of the pregnancy. If an arrhythmia is identified, several ant-arrhythmic drugs may be used with caution after organogenesis is complete. A cardiology or electrophysiology consultation is reasonable in any pregnant patient with palpitations.

SUGGESTED READING

1. Adamson DL, Nelson-Piercy C. Managing palpitations and arrhythmias during pregnancy. Heart. 2007;93(12):1630-36.
2. Arrington ME, Mangelsdorff A. The prevalence of symptoms in medical outpatients and the adequacy of therapy. Arch Int Med. 1990;150(8):1685-9.
3. Brugada P, Gürsoy S, Brugada J, Andries E. Investigation of palpitations. Lancet. 1993;341(8855):1254-8.
4. Das MK, Zipes DP. Assessment of the patient with a cardiac arrhythmia. In: DP Zipes, J Jalife (eds). Cardiac Electrophysiology, 5th edition. Philadelphia, PA: Saunders Elsevier; 2009. pp. 831-6.
5. Loscalzo J. Palpitations. In: DL Longo, AS Fauci, DL Kasper, SL Hauser, JL Jameson, J Loscalzo (Eds). Harrison's Principles of Internal Medicine, 18th edition. New York, NY: The McGraw-Hill Companies; 2012; Chapter 37 (online).
6. Raju BS. Palpitation. In: Clinical Methods in Cardiology. Hyderabad: Orient Blackswan; 2003. pp. 149-58.

7. Raviele A, Giada F, Bergfeldt L, Blanc JJ, Blomstrom-Lundquist C, Mont L, et al. Management of patients with palpitations: a position paper from the European Heart Rhythm Associatioc. Europace. 2011;13(7):920-34.
8. Weber BE, Kapoor WN. Evaluation and outcomes of patients with palpitations. Am J Med. 1996;100:138-48.
9. Wexler K, Pleister A, Raman S. Outpatient approach to palpitations. Am Fam Physician. 2011;84(1):63-9.

Bradyarrhythmias

Chapter 16

Hardik Doshi, Prashant Bhave

INTRODUCTION

The lower limit of normal heart rate is generally accepted as a heart rate of <60 beats per minute (bpm). While convenient for the precision and uniformity, such a definition is introduced. This delineation is arbitrary and in isolation conveys little information on the underlying physiologic or pathologic states. Indeed, a large number of intrinsic and extrinsic factors influence the resting heart rate, including age, time of observation, physical condition and activity, autonomic tone, and medications. Broadly, bradyarrhythmias may be classified based on etiology; however, a classification keeping in mind the normal conduction system of the heart is more clinically relevant in diagnosis and management (Fig. 16.1). In general, we can think of bradyarrhythmias as two broad categories involving the sinus node and internodal pathways [i.e. sinoatrial (SA) exit block and sinus node dysfunction (SND)] and the atrioventricular (AV) node and His bundle (i.e. first-, second- or third-degree AV block or AV dissociation).

SINUS PAUSE/SINUS ARREST AND SINOATRIAL EXIT BLOCK

Sinus pause is characterized by simply an interruption in the normal sinus rhythm. There is an apparent increase in the PP cycle length on surface electrocardiogram (ECG) that is not related to the original PP cycle length (i.e. not a multiple of original PP length that would indicate SA exit block) (Fig. 16.2). The presence of significant sinus arrhythmia gives rise to a variable PP interval and can make distinguishing sinus arrest from SA exit block difficult. Sinus pause is felt to be due to slowing of the intrinsic sinus nodal automaticity.

A sinus pause may last from 2 seconds to several seconds and accordingly may range from being completely asymptomatic to causing dizziness, lightheadedness or even frank syncope. A short pause with a structurally normal heart is likely of no hemodynamic consequence and may be well tolerated. In contrast, sinus pauses in patients with structural heart disease may cause a significant drop in cardiac output and give rise to symptoms. The surface ECG may demonstrate escape rhythms from lower-lying pacemakers, depending on the duration of the pause and the general

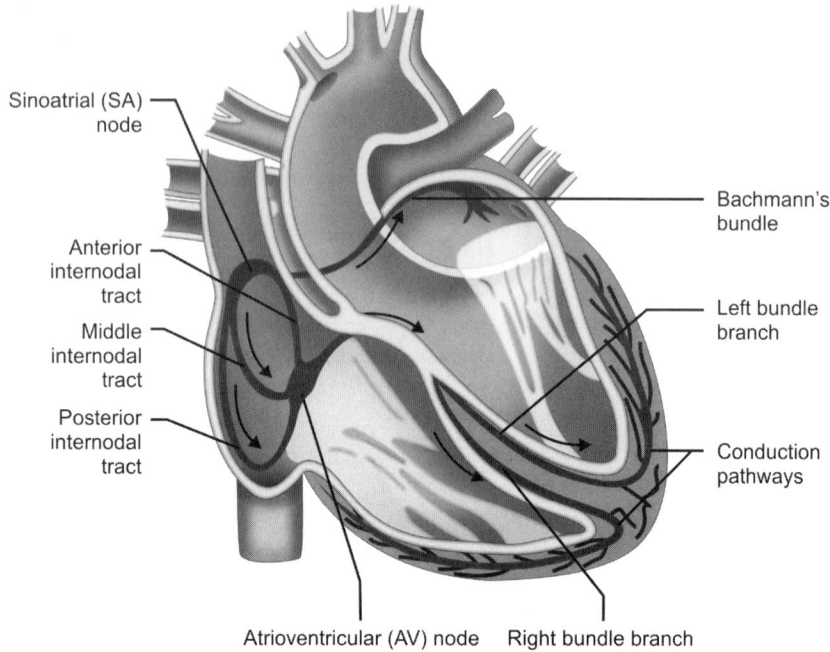

Fig. 16.1: Conduction system of the heart.

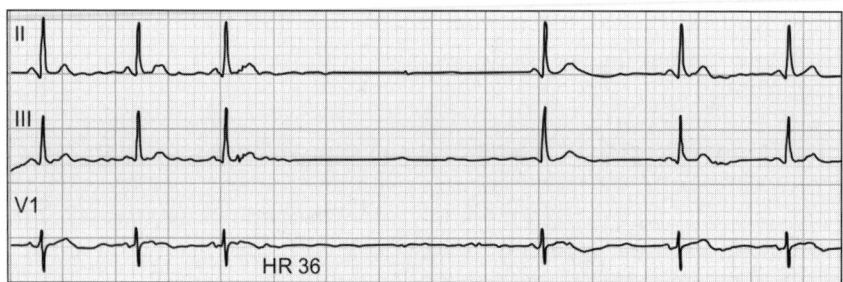

Fig. 16.2: Sinus pause or sinus arrest.

health of the conduction system. Sinoatrial nodal disease secondary to ischemia, inflammation or infiltrative disease, drugs (e.g. digoxin) and even high vagal tone may give rise to sinus pauses or arrest. Sinus pauses are frequently seen with spontaneous termination of atrial tachyarrhythmias (the so-called "tachy–brady syndrome"). This reflects a prolonged sinus nodal recovery time. Medications commonly used for rate control in atrial tachyarrhythmias may prolong sinus nodal recovery time and contribute to a long sinus pause at conversion.

In contrast with sinus pause or arrest, SA exit block is due to failure of propagation (or a delay thereof) of the sinus node impulse to the atrial tissue. The intrinsic automaticity of the sinus node is intact, in contrast with sinus arrest. On the surface ECG, this is manifest as a pause in atrial activity. In keeping with the convention of nodal blocks, SA exit blocks may be thought of as first degree, second degree (types I and II), or third degree. In practice, first-degree SA exit block cannot be recognized on surface ECG while a third-degree SA exit block manifests as a complete absence of sinus P waves on the ECG and cannot be conclusively diagnosed without intracardiac electrograms. Type I (i.e. Wenckebach) second-degree SA exit block features a PP interval that gradually shortens leading to the pause. The duration of the pause is less than two PP cycle lengths. Type II second-degree SA exit block manifests as a sinus pause with a PP cycle length, which is a multiple of the normal PP cycle length (Fig. 16.3).

SINUS NODE DYSFUNCTION

Sinus node dysfunction does not refer to a specific bradyarrhythmia and in fact refers to a spectrum of pathology involving impulse creation and impulse dispersion over the SA tissue. Initially described in the 1960s, SND led to one of the first clinical applications of cardiac pacing. In fact, the pathology in SND is more widespread, beyond the anatomic sinus node and may be referred to as atrial myopathy. Accordingly, a variety of atrial arrhythmias may be seen at different times in people with SND, ranging from inappropriate sinus bradycardia, chronotropic incompetence, sinus pauses and exit blocks to atrial tachyarrhythmias along with tachy–brady syndrome (Fig. 16.4).

SINUS BRADYCARDIA

By definition, sinus bradycardia entails sinus rhythm with the sinus node as the predominant pacemaker discharging at a rate of <60 bpm. This implies a normal P wave morphology (i.e. upright in leads I and II and biphasic in lead V1 on the surface ECG) indicating the sinus node as the predominant pacemaker (Fig. 16.5).

The principal clinical feature is a resting heart rate <60 bpm; however, the symptom spectrum can range from entirely benign and asymptomatic to frank

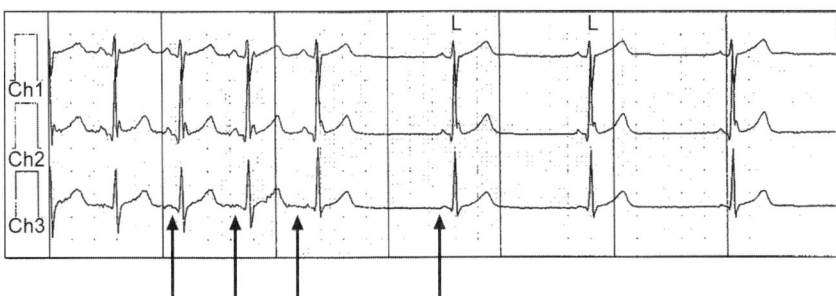

Fig. 16.3: Sinoatrial exit block. Note that the PP interval (arrows) doubles on the right side of the tracing indicating an exit block (see arrows).

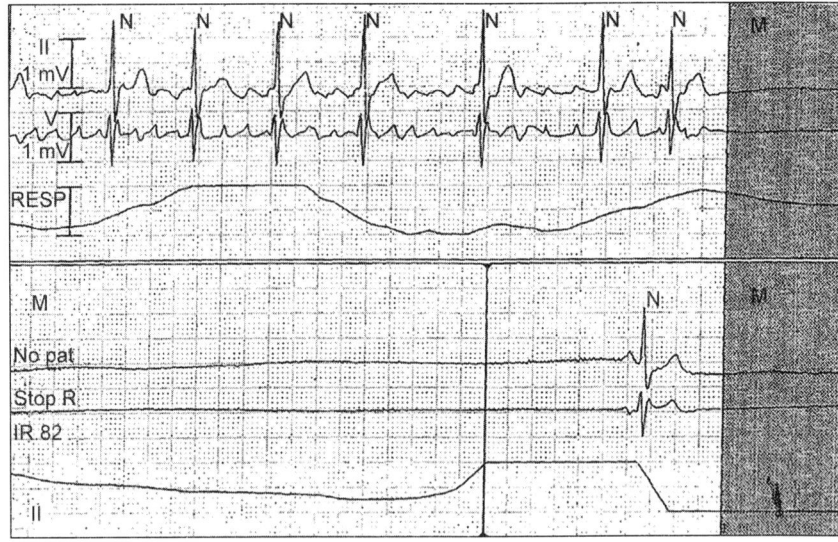

Fig. 16.4: Atrial fibrillation terminating with long sinus pause.

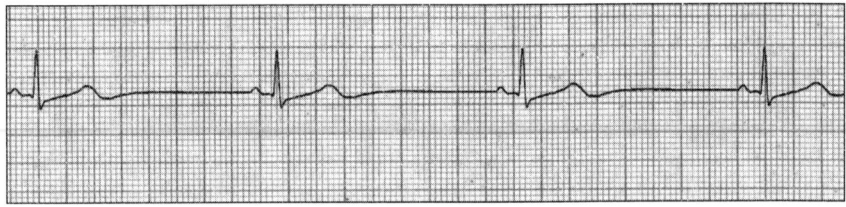

Fig. 16.5: Sinus bradycardia.

syncope, both at different absolute values of heart rates in different patients. Physiologically, daytime resting heart rates have been estimated to be 46–93 bpm for men and 51–95 bpm for women, with nocturnal rates being on an average 24 bpm slower, especially in young adults. Notably, these rates, while meeting the definition of sinus bradycardia, can be entirely asymptomatic.

Cardiac output is a function of both heart rate and stroke volume. Hence, by extension, sinus bradycardia may produce symptoms through its influence on cardiac output. Thus, symptoms of sinus bradycardia are typically due to hypoperfusion: mild reductions causing exertional fatigue and dyspnea while being asymptomatic at rest. Low cardiac output may manifest as chest pain, dizziness and lightheadedness or even syncope and hemodynamic collapse in more severe cases. Evidence of end-organ damage related to ischemia involving cerebrovascular, renal and mesenteric beds may manifest with prolonged periods of low cardiac output.

A wide variety of physiologic and clinical conditions can give rise to sinus bradycardia. Table 16.1 provides a list of etiologies of sinus bradycardia. Importantly, more than one mechanism may be at play in any given clinical situation.

Table 16.1: Causes of sinus bradycardia

1. Physiologic
   a. Physically conditioned athletes
   b. Young adults, especially at rest
   c. Subset of elderly, healthy population
   d. Sleep
2. Associated with pathologic states
   a. Extrinsic:
      i. Hypothyroidism/myxedema
      ii. Hypothermia
      iii. Infections (relative bradycardia, as with Q fever, *Legionella*, diphtheria, Chagas disease, Lyme's disease, etc.)
      iv. Hypoxemia
      v. Metabolic/electrolyte disturbances, e.g. hyperkalemia, hypoglycemia
      vi. Sleep apnea
   b. Intrinsic:
      i. Hypertensive heart disease
      ii. Pericarditis, myocarditis and other cardiomyopathies
      iii. Acute MI
      iv. Post heart transplant
      v. Congenital (familial, with pacemaker HCN4 ion channel mutations)
3. Associated with autonomic tone/autonomic reflexes
   a. Hypervagotonia
      i. Vomiting or coughing
      ii. Valsalva/straining at stool
      iii. Vasovagal or cardioinhibitory syncope
   b. Autonomic reflexes
      i. Hypersensitive carotid sinus syndrome
      ii. Bezold–Jarisch reflex with prolonged standing
      iii. Cushing reflex, with intracranial hypertension
4. Drug-induced
   a. Antiarrhythmic agents
      i. Class IC: Propafenone
      ii. Class II: β-blockers (including topical agents used for glaucoma)
      iii. Class III: Sotalol, amiodarone
      iv. Class IV: Diltiazem, verapamil
   b. Antipsychotic agents
      i. Lithium, amitriptyline
   c. Antihypertensive agents
      i. Clonidine, β-blockers, methyldopa, diltiazem, verapamil
   d. Other (e.g. digoxin, ivabradine)

The natural history of SND can be quite variable, with patients typically seeking medical attention for symptomatic bradycardia. Recurrent syncope is common in this cohort of patients, but the development of concomitant AV nodal and other infranodal conduction abnormalities is relatively rare. The incidence of sudden cardiac death is low in patients with pure SND.

The management of patients with SND is similar regardless of the electrical manifestation of the SND. Asymptomatic rhythms require no specific treatment. Identification and treatment of any underlying etiology are important.

For symptomatic patients, it is important to establish a causal relationship between the underlying rhythm and the reported symptoms so that appropriate treatment can be provided, since symptoms can be vague and nonspecific. Initial evaluation typically includes a 12-lead ECG and often Holter monitoring in the setting of a characteristic history. Exercise testing to evaluate for chronotropic competence and echocardiography to assess for structural heart disease may be useful in the appropriate clinical scenario. For events that occur with a lower frequency, a 30-day event monitor with a symptom diary or rarely, an implantable loop recorder may be useful. Invasive electrophysiology (EP) studies are generally not helpful, as tests of sinus node recovery time are neither sensitive nor specific for the diagnosis of symptomatic SND.

For symptomatic patients, if there is evidence for decreased cardiac output and hypoperfusion, temporizing measures to increase the heart rate and hence cardiac output must be undertaken with ongoing care directed toward any specific etiology. In urgent or emergent clinical situations, vagolytic drugs, such as atropine (at a dose of 0.5 mg IV) can be administered to help increase the heart rate and hence augment cardiac output. Dopamine (dose: 2.5–20 mcg/kg/min) and isoproterenol (dose: 2–20 mcg/min) are sympathomimetic drugs that may be used in the short term to increase heart rate. Glucagon infusion (3–10 mg or 0.05–0.15 mg/kg) bolus followed by an infusion of 3–5 mg/h (or 0.05–0.1 mg/kg/h) may be used for specific drug-induced (e.g. β-blocker or calcium channel blocker) bradycardia. The treatment of symptomatic sinus bradycardia that is due to a reversible cause may require placement of temporary intravenous pacemaker until resolution of the responsible etiology. A permanent pacemaker is indicated for the treatment of symptomatic sinus bradycardia in the absence of a reversible etiology.

Current American Heart Association/Heart Rhythm Society (AHA/HRS) guidelines recommend a permanent pacemaker implantation in symptomatic SND. Pacemakers are not recommended for asymptomatic SND (see guidelines below) and pauses >3 seconds in length do not appear to be predictive of increased mortality. It should be noted that while pacing decreases the morbidity associated with SND, observational studies have failed to show any impact on survival. Often, pacing with drug therapy for tachycardia is necessary in tachy–brady syndrome.

The mode of pacing in SND has been the subject of a number of trials. Modes that preserve AV synchrony (e.g. AAIR or DDDR) seem to be superior to ventricular pacing alone. The DANPACE study found a higher incidence of atrial fibrillation and a twofold increased risk for repeat surgeries (with the majority of them for adding a ventricular lead) for devices programmed to AAIR pacing mode. This lent more support to the routine use of DDDR pacing in patients with SND.

ATRIOVENTRICULAR CONDUCTION BLOCK

Atrioventricular conduction block refers to a condition when impulses from the atria are blocked or delayed on their path to the ventricles. An important caveat is that physiologic AV block can occur with premature atrial beats timed to when the atrial, AV nodal or His-Purkinje tissue is physiologically refractory. It is critically important to distinguish pathologic AV block from physiologic AV block, as the implications for therapy are profound. Based on ECG criteria, AV block is classified as first-, second- or third-degree block, which has important correlations with electrophysiologic recordings, anatomical location of block within the AV node/His–Purkinje system (Fig. 16.6) and clinical findings.

First-degree AV Block

First-degree AV block is something of a misnomer, as it reflects conduction delay and not conduction block. It is defined as a delay in transmission of impulse from the atria to the ventricles, characterized on surface ECG by a PR interval of >200 milliseconds (msec). Each P wave is thus followed by a QRS complex with a fixed, prolonged PR interval (Fig. 16.7).

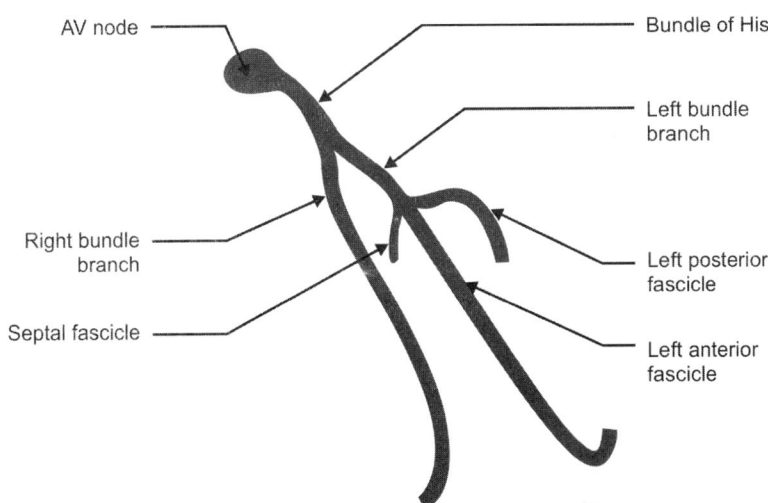

Fig. 16.6: Atrioventricular node and His–Purkinje system.

212 Common Problems in Cardiology

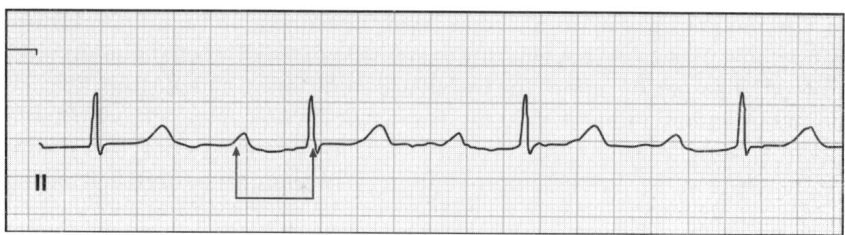

Fig. 16.7: First-degree atrioventricular block. PR interval = 0.38 seconds.

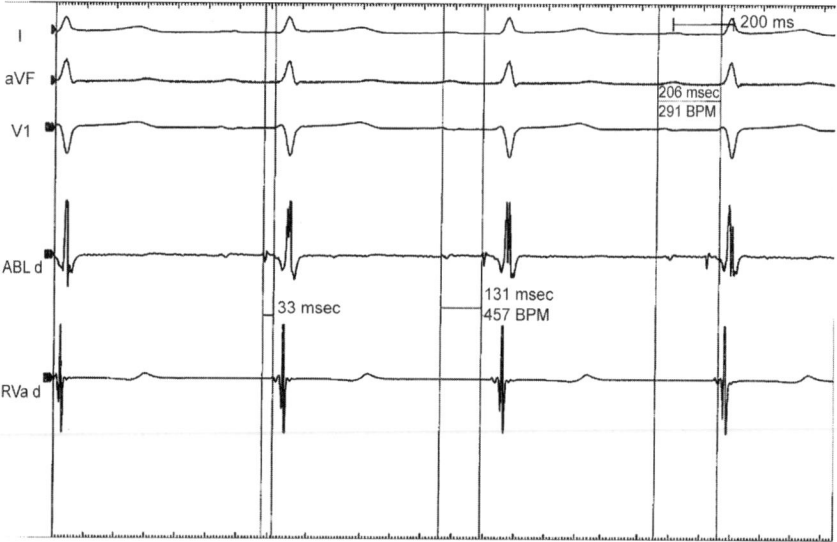

Fig. 16.8: First-degree atrioventricular block with prolonged AH interval. The ablation catheter (ABL) is at the His position.

The PR interval prolongation may be entirely within the AV node or in the His–Purkinje system or both. This can be identified by EP study as prolongation of the AH interval indicating AV nodal delay (Fig. 16.8) or, less commonly, prolongation of the HV interval indicating His–Purkinje delay. Rarely, intra-atrial delay or balanced delay over both the bundle branches can cause a prolonged PR interval, with a normal QRS morphology.

PR interval tends to increase with age. First-degree AV block is usually asymptomatic and no treatment is generally required. Indeed the prevalence of first-degree AV block has been reported to be about 0.5% of healthy young men. In a large cohort of 3,983 men followed over a 30-year period, no significant differences were found in terms of clinical outcomes or development of advanced heart blocks, especially in patients with a "moderate" degree (i.e. PR interval <240 msec) of first-degree AV block. However, a recent study of hypertensive patients with first-degree AV block found a higher incidence of developing atrial fibrillation, advanced AV block and left ventricular dysfunction compared to controls. Also, with acceleration of atrial rate as with exercise, patients with long PR intervals (typically >300 msec) may develop symptoms due to an inability to shorten the PR interval proportionate with shortening of the RR interval, leading to AV dyssynchrony.

Second-degree AV Block

Second-degree AV block is defined as a failure to conduct some atrial impulses to the ventricle when the conduction pathway is not physiologically refractory. On the surface ECG, this is manifest as nonconducted P waves. This type of AV block is often intermittent in nature and may happen at regular intervals or suddenly and unpredictably. Second-degree AV block is divided into Mobitz type I and type II AV block based on surface ECG patterns. The designation of type I versus type II is commonly understood to reflect the anatomical site of the conduction block. The clinical syndrome and the type of escape rhythm, if any, have important clinical implications beyond the mere pattern of block.

Traditionally, type I second-degree AV block has been defined as progressive prolongation of the PR interval on the surface ECG followed by a nonconducted P wave (i.e. Wenckebach phenomenon, Fig. 16.9). The first conducted P wave after the nonconducted P wave has the shortest PR interval of such a cycle. This implies that the pause between the QRS complexes encompassing the nonconducted P wave will be less than twice the PP interval.

However, the PR intervals in type I second-degree AV block can also shorten or show no measurable change anywhere before a single, blocked beat. Long Wenckebach cycles (e.g. 5:4 or 6:5 blocks) are often associated with unusual increases in the atrial rate or AV conduction time. In these long cycles, the last RR interval can actually be longer than prior RR intervals because the PR increment between beats does not have a predictable pattern. Invariably, however, the first beat of the next cycle will have a much shorter PR interval than the last beat of the prior cycle. This is also referred to as atypical type I second-degree AV block. Also, an escape beat (especially junctional escape) can occur during the pause following a nonconducted P wave. This may create the impression of an apparent "shortening" of the PR interval.

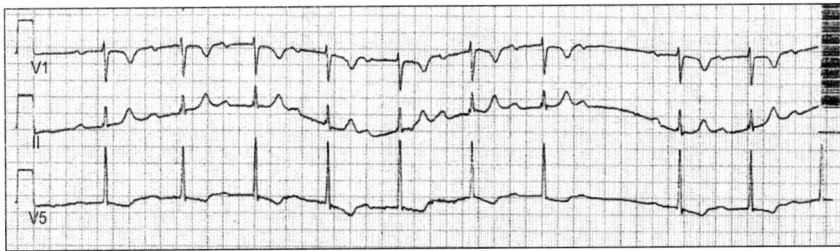

Fig. 16.9: Mobitz type I second-degree atrioventricular block (Wenckebach). Note the gradual prolongation of the PR interval leading into finally a dropped beat with a nonconducted P wave (arrow).

The American College of Cardiology (ACC) defines type I second-degree AV block as the occurrence of a single nonconducted P wave associated with inconstant PR intervals before and after the blocked impulse as long as there are at least two consecutive conducted P waves (e.g. 3:2 AV block) to determine the behavior of the PR intervals. Note that it is not possible to accurately classify a 2:1 AV block as type I or type II based on surface ECG alone. Associated features like the length of the PR interval and presence of an accompanying bundle branch block may be valuable clues in determining the location and hence the clinical significance of the block (see below).

Type I second-degree AV block with a narrow QRS complex (i.e. <0.12 seconds) almost always involves the AV node as the site of conduction delay. Often the block is physiologic, especially during sleep and in young individuals with high vagal tone. No treatment is generally required for such asymptomatic type I block. Infra-nodal type I blocks are rare, but can be seen in patients with baseline bundle branch block (Fig. 16.10).

A modified Wenckebach ladder diagram (Fig. 16.11) may be helpful in understanding the physiology of second-degree AV blocks. Atrial, AV junction and ventricular activation are represented in three different levels. AV conduction in any cycle is represented by slanted lines of varying inclination (representing AV delays) in the AV bar. The first AV delay of the Wenckebach periodicity is represented by AV with the increments being represented as Δ1, Δ2 and Δ3 accompanying AV2, AV3 and AV4 (the lag in numbering is due to the fact that AV1 has no increment) respectively. Hence, AV3 = AV2+ Δ2 etc. where AV2 is the duration of the previous AV delay in the first ventricular interval (RR1). A ladder diagram demonstrates the progressive increase in

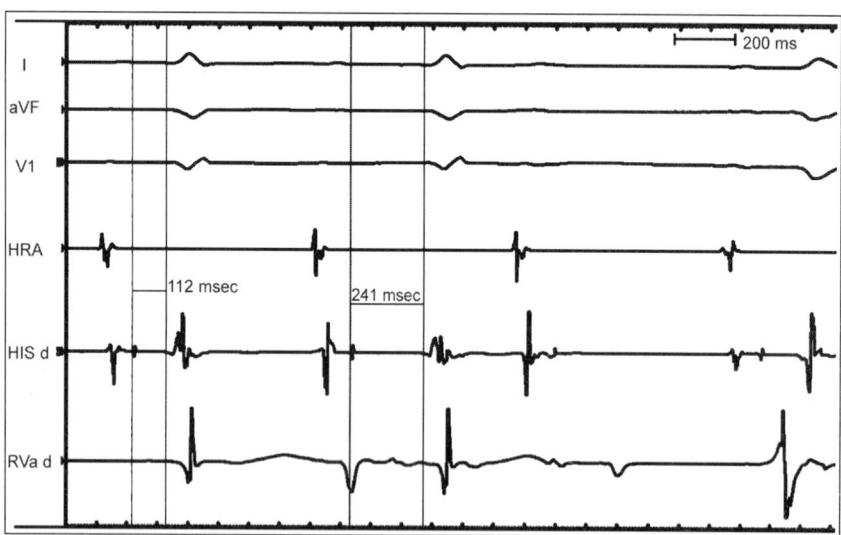

Fig. 16.10: Infra-His Wenckebach on intracardiac electrogram. Note the gradual prolongation of the HV interval from 112 to 241 msec followed by subsequently nonconducted beat. The top 3 are the surface electrodes. HRA, high right atrium.

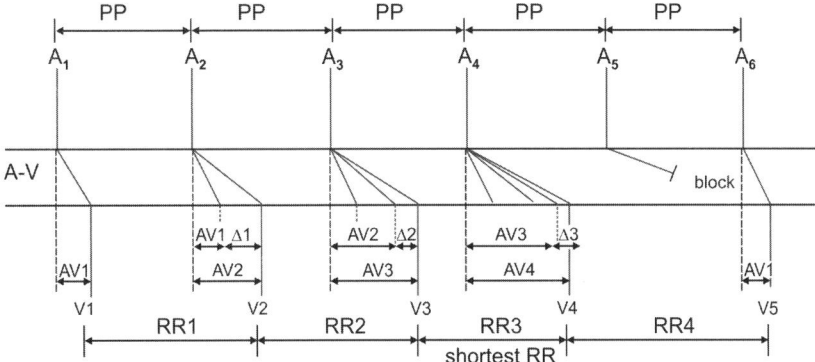

Fig. 16.11: Modified ladder diagram for second-degree atrioventricular block.

Source: Reprinted from Barold SS, Stroobandt RX, Sinnaeve AF, Andries E, Herweg B. Reappraisal of the traditional Wenckebach phenomenon with a modified ladder diagram. Ann Noninvasive Electrocardiol. 2012;17:3-7 *with permission* from John Wiley and Sons.

PR intervals with progressive decline in RR intervals and the inverse relation between PR and RP intervals.

Mobitz Type II Second-degree AV Block

Mobitz type II second-degree AV block is defined as the occurrence of a single nonconducted P wave associated with constant PR intervals before and after the blocked impulse, provided the sinus rate or the PP interval is constant (i.e. no slowing) and there are at least two consecutive conducted P waves to reveal the behavior of the PR interval (Fig. 16.12).

While a stable sinus rate is considered to be important to the diagnosis by many entities, this is not specifically incorporated in the ACC/AHA/HRS guidelines. The diagnosis of type II AV block cannot be made if the P wave after a blocked impulse is not conducted with the same PR interval as all the other conducted P waves, since a shorter PR interval after the blocked P wave may either be caused by improved conduction (i.e. type I block) or AV dissociation from an escape AV junctional beat bearing no relationship to the preceding P wave. However, this is difficult to discern form a surface ECG alone. Type II second-degree AV block always occurs in the His–Purkinje system and may be associated with bundle branch block in up to 70% of cases.

The differentiation between type I and type II second-degree AV block is very important clinically. Even in asymptomatic patients, type II AV block is associated with a high risk of progressing to advanced heart block and is a reasonable recommendation for pacemaker implantation. On the other hand, type I AV block with a narrow QRS is generally felt to be benign. Also, type I AV blocks associated with an inferior myocardial infarction rarely herald advanced AV blocks and seldom require permanent pacing. Conversely, type II AV blocks in the setting of ischemia are often associated with anterior myocardial infarction and indicate extensive septal infarction.

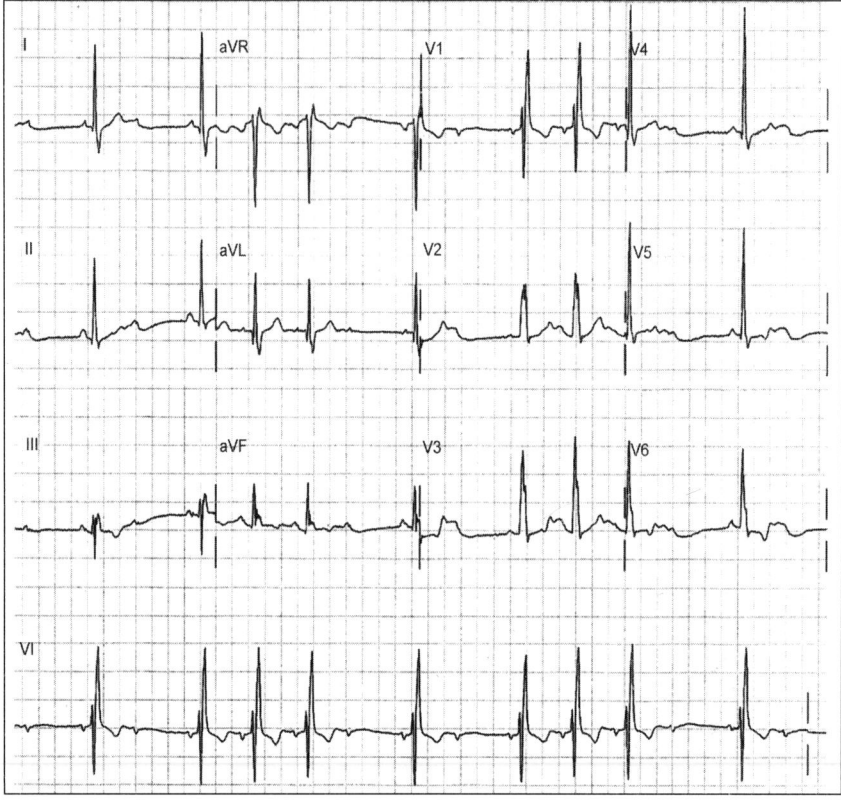

Fig. 16.12: Mobitz type II second-degree atrioventricular block.

Type II AV block with a bundle branch block is an indication for a permanent pacemaker even in the absence of symptoms.

High-grade AV Block/2:1 AV Block

It is not possible to reliably attribute a 2:1 second-degree AV block as type I or type II AV block since the relationship between the P wave and the following QRS complex is difficult to establish (Fig. 16.13). However, such a distinction is important since the prognosis and management for type I and type II AV blocks clearly differ. EP studies can help identify the anatomic site of block in these situations. Alternatively, carotid sinus massage can help unmask this rhythm by slowing the sinus rate and allowing the AV node more time to recover. In case of a type I AV block, slowing the sinus rate may change the AV block to 3:2 or longer while demonstrating gradually prolonging PR intervals, while a type II AV block may not change significantly (or may "improve" with slower sinus rate) since the enhanced vagal tone has little influence on the His–Purkinje system. Alternatively, administration of atropine or exercise testing may enhance AV nodal conduction and unmask type I AV block by improving the conduction through the AV node (via vagolytic and

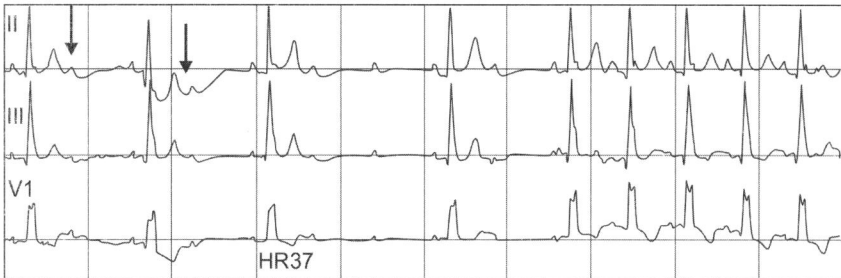

Fig. 16.13: 2:1 atrioventricular block. Note that it is not possible to differentiate the nature of the AV relationship in the first 2 blocked beats (arrows) from surface ECG alone. However, the relatively short conducted PR interval and the wide QRS complex suggest infra-Hisian block.

sympathomimetic actions, respectively); however, these maneuvers will typically not influence a true 2:1 infra-Hisian block given the relatively poor influence that autonomic tone exerts to this part of the conduction tissue. In fact, they may make infra-Hisian block worse because a greater frequency of impulses will stress the His-Purkinje system. A wide QRS complex and a relatively short PR interval may also be clues suggesting a type II AV block.

Miscellaneous Clinical Conditions Associated with AV Blocks

Several clinical conditions may be associated with transient AV block. Generally, in these situations, intermittent AV blocks are provoked by an increase or decrease in the sinus rate, sometimes in the face of pre-existing bundle branch blocks. This suggests a rate-dependent site of block within the AV node/His-Purkinje system. Enhanced vagotonia (e.g. athletes, deep sleep) or maneuvers (e.g. tracheal suctioning in intubated patients, bronchoscopy) that increase vagal tone may give rise to intermittent AV blocks that can be symptomatic, but are generally self-limited to the inciting maneuver. No specific therapy may be necessary in such a situation. Clues suggesting underlying sleep apnea must be sought for and evaluated in the appropriate clinical scenario.

Contrasting from this scenario is the situation with paroxysmal AV block (PAVB), which is defined as a sudden and unexpected repetitive block in the conduction of the atrial impulse, often with delayed escape rhythm leading to syncope. PAVB may arise with an increase in the rate of impulses to the AV node (i.e. tachycardia-dependent PAVB or phase 3 block) or may arise due to a supraventricular pause, as may be induced by a premature ventricular contraction (i.e. bradycardia-dependent PAVB). In the latter scenario, they may be described as phase 4 blocks or pause-dependent PAVB (Fig. 16.14). Pacemaker placement is generally necessary for PAVB.

Third-degree AV Block/Complete Heart Block

Third-degree AV block is manifest by the lack of any conduction of atrial impulses to the ventricles (Fig. 16.15); hence, the atria and ventricles are

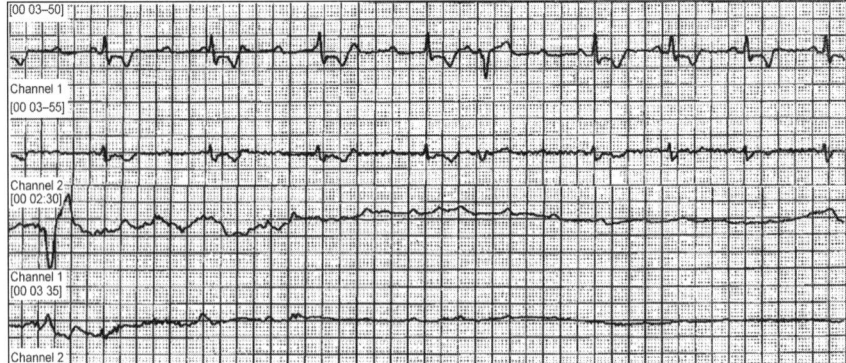

Fig. 16.14: Paroxysmal atrioventricular (AV) block or phase 4 AV block. Note the premature ventricular contraction preceding the AV block. This patient had received a diagnosis of seizures for his multiple syncopal episodes and had been treated for the same prior to the diagnosis of paroxysmal AV block and subsequent pacemaker placement.

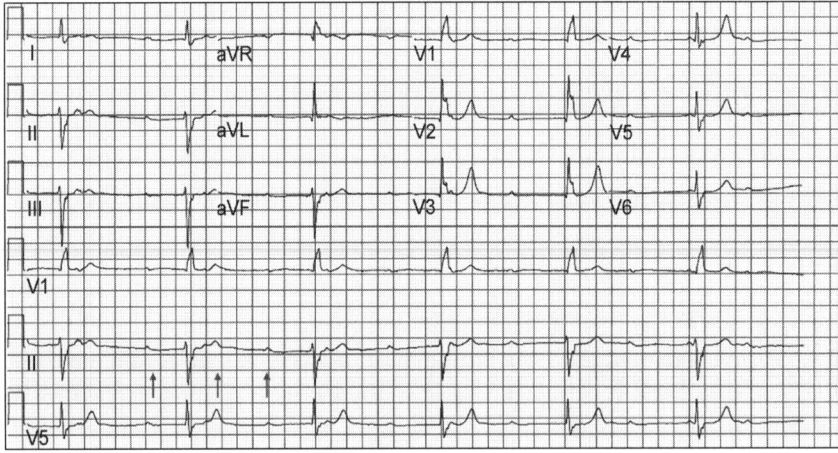

Fig. 16.15: Complete heart block. Arrows indicate the P waves.

under the control of different pacemakers. The atrial pacemakers may be sinus or ectopic or even retrograde from AV nodal junction; the ventricular pacemaker may lie in the AV node, His bundle, Purkinje fibers, or ventricular myocardium. Escape rhythms proximal to the His bundle may have narrow QRS complexes on surface ECG with a ventricular rate of 45–60 bpm. Infra-Hisian and more distal escape rhythms generally give rise to a wide QRS complex (at a slower rate). Intracardiac tracings can reveal the site of block by the presence or absence of a His-deflection preceding each ventricular impulse. Generally, higher ventricular pacemakers are more reliable and may exhibit some degree of clinical stability.

Complete heart block (CHB) may be congenital with an incidence estimated between 1 in 15,000 and 20,000 live births. Congenital CHB by definition is diagnosed *in utero*, at birth or in the neonatal period (i.e. at 0–27 days of life); however, sometimes the manifestation of CHB may be delayed. The pathophysiology of congenital CHB is generally attributed to an autoimmune phenomenon with transplacental passage of maternal anti-SSA/Ro-SSB/La antibodies, but overt rheumatologic disease may not be manifested in many mothers. Other conditions like congenitally corrected transposition of great arteries are also associated with congenital CHB. Sometimes, this may manifest later in life as well. Congenital CHB is generally at the level of the AV node, while intra- or infra-Hisian block is generally acquired in nature. An exception is that heart block in transposition of great arteries generally occurs at the level of the His bundle. Blunt chest wall trauma, cardiac surgery, electrolyte abnormalities, some infectious diseases (e.g. Lyme's disease and Chagas disease), amyloidosis, and sarcoidosis can also be associated with CHB. Progressive AV block can occur with Lyme's disease (Fig. 16.16).

Clinical Features of AV Blocks

First-degree AV blocks generally tend to be clinically asymptomatic unless the PR interval is very significantly prolonged (i.e. typically >0.3 seconds). Patients may report palpitations or "skipped beats". The jugular venous pressure may demonstrate prolonged a-c wave duration, occasionally with a soft first heart sound. Second- and third-degree AV blocks can cause the entire spectrum of symptoms associated with low cardiac output, including

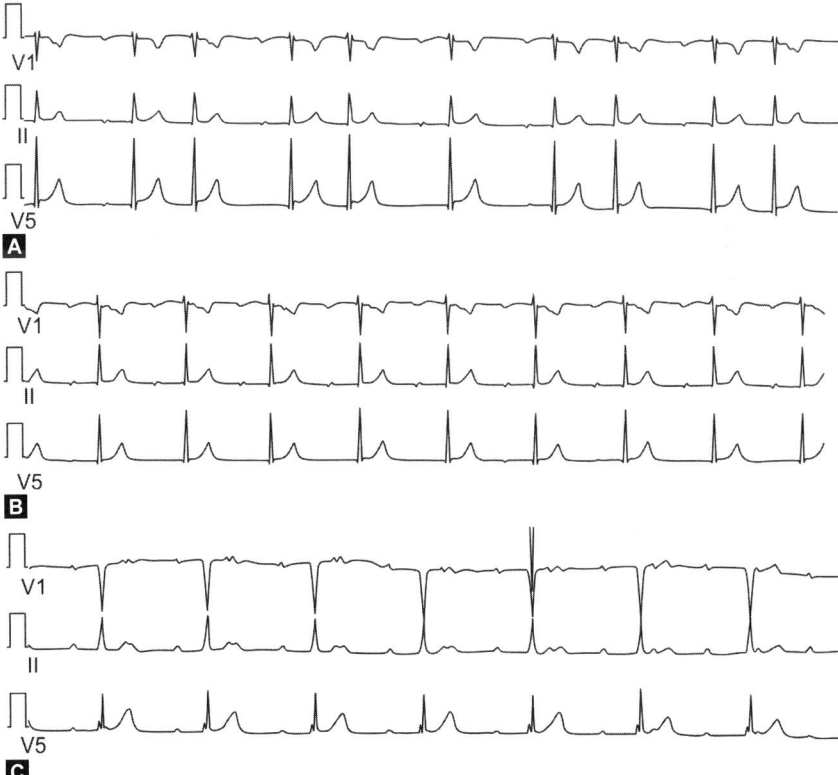

Fig. 16.16: Progressive atrioventricular (AV) block in Lyme's disease; (A) Sinus rhythm with Mobitz type I second-degree AV block. Note the 3:2 AV block pattern; (B) Sinus rhythm with second-degree AV block. Note the 2:1 AV block pattern; (C) Sinus rhythm with AV dissociation and complete heart block.

Table 16.2: Indications for permanent pacing

Recommended indications

- SND with documented symptomatic bradycardia
- Symptomatic chronotropic incompetence
- Symptomatic sinus bradycardia from required drug therapy for medical conditions
- Third-degree and advanced second-degree AV block at any anatomic level associated with bradycardia with symptoms or ventricular arrhythmias presumed to be due to AV block
- Third-degree and advanced second-degree AV block at any level associated with arrhythmias or other medical conditions that require drug therapy resulting in symptomatic bradycardia
- Third-degree and advanced second-degree AV block at any level in awake, asymptomatic patients in sinus rhythm with document asystole ≥3 seconds or any escape < 40 bpm or with an escape from below AV node
- Third-degree and advanced second-degree AV block at any level in awake, asymptomatic patients with AF and bradycardia with 1 or more pauses ≥5 seconds
- Third-degree and advanced second-degree AV block at any level after AV junction ablation
- Third-degree and advanced second-degree AV block at any level associated with cardiac postoperative state that is not expected to resolve
- Third-degree and advanced second-degree AV block at any level with neuromuscular diseases with AV block, with or without symptoms
- Second-degree AV block with symptoms, regardless of type or site of block
- Asymptomatic, persistent third degree with average awake ventricular rates ≥40 bpm if cardiomegaly or LV dysfunction is present or if block is below AV node
- Second- or third-degree AV block during exercise in the absence of myocardial ischemia

Reasonable indications

- SND with HR <40 bpm when a clear association between symptoms and actual bradycardia has not been documented
- Unexplained syncope when clinically significant sinus node abnormalities are discovered or provoked during EP study
- Third-degree AV block with escape rate >40 bpm in asymptomatic patients without cardiomegaly
- Asymptomatic second-degree AV block at intra- or infra-His level on EP study
- First- or second-degree AV block with symptoms of pacemaker syndrome or hemodynamic compromise
- Asymptomatic type II second-degree AV block with narrow QRS (note that type II second-degree AV block with wide QRS or with isolated RBBB earns a class I indication)

Permanent pacing not indicated

- Asymptomatic patients with SND
- SND with symptoms clearly documented as occurring in the absence of bradycardia
- SND with symptomatic bradycardia occurring with nonessential medical therapy
- Asymptomatic first-degree AV block
- Asymptomatic type I second-degree AV block at supra-His level, not known to be intra- or infra-Hisian
- AV block expected to resolve and unlikely to recur (e.g. drug toxicity and Lyme's disease)

SND, sinus node dysfunction; LV, left ventricular; AV, atrioventricular; AF, atrial fibrillation; EP, electrophysiology; RBBB, right bundle branch block.

Source: Adapted from Epstein AE, DiMarco JP, Ellenbogen KA, Estes III NA, Freedman RA, Gettes LS, et al. ACC/AHA/HRS 2008 guidelines for device-based therapy of cardiac rhythm abnormalities. J Am Coll Cardiol. 2008;51:e1-62.

dizziness, angina, presyncope and syncope, although type I second-degree AV blocks tend to be asymptomatic. Physical findings associated with CHB include cannon a-waves and a variable first heart sound.

Management

Management of symptomatic high grade and complete AV block is identical to the management of symptomatic bradycardia in that the immediate measures are directed toward maintenance of cardiac output. Vagolytic drugs like atropine and chronotropic agents like dopamine or isoproterenol may be used acutely for short durations of time; however, these are best avoided when AV block is associated with acute myocardial infarction. Temporary RV pacing with a transvenous pacing wire is preferable in this situation. Ultimately, for any symptomatic AV block that is not due to reversible causes, permanent pacing is the treatment of choice (Table 16.2).

SUGGESTED READING

1. Barold SS, Hayes DL. Second-degree atrioventricular block: a reappraisal. Mayo Clin Proc. 2001;76:44-57.
2. Barold SS, Stroobandt RX, Sinnaeve AF, Andries E, Herweg B. Reappraisal of the traditional Wenckebach phenomenon with a modified ladder diagram. Ann Noninvasive Electrocardiol. 2012;17:3-7.
3. Bergman G, Skog A, Tingstrom J, Ottosson V, Hoxha A, Ambrosi A, et al. Late development of complete atrioventricular block may be immune mediated and congenital in origin. Acta Pædiatrica. 2014;103:275-81.
4. Connolly SJ, Kerr CR, Gent M, Roberts RS, Yusuf S, Gillis AM, et al. Effects of physiologic pacing versus ventricular pacing on the risk of stroke and death due to cardiovascular causes. N Engl J Med. 2000;342:1385-91.
5. Epstein AE, DiMarco JP, Ellenbogen KA, Estes III NA, Freedman RA, Gettes LS, et al. ACC/AHA/HRS 2008 guidelines for device-based therapy of cardiac rhythm abnormalities. J Am Coll Cardiol. 2008;51:e1-62.
6. Lamas GA, Orav EJ, Stambler BS, Ellenbogen KA, Sgarbossa EB, Huang SK, et al. Quality of life and clinical outcomes in elderly patients treated with ventricular pacing as compared with dual-chamber pacing. N Engl J Med. 1998;338:1097-104.
7. Lamas GA, Lee KL, Sweeney MO, Silverman R, Leon A, Yee R, et al. Mode selection trial in sinus-node dysfunction. Ventricular pacing or dual-chamber pacing for sinus-node dysfunction. N Engl J Med. 2002;346:1854-62.
8. Menozzi C, Brignole M, Alboni P, Boni L, Paparella N, Gaggioli G, et al. The natural course of untreated sick sinus syndrome and identification of the variables predictive of unfavorable outcome. Am J Cardiol. 1998;82:1205-9.
9. Mymin D, Mathewson FA, Tate RB, Manfreda J. The natural history of primary first-degree atrioventricular heart block. N Engl J Med. 1986;315:1183-7.
10. Nielsen JC, Kristensen L, Andersen HR, Mortensen PT, Pedersen OL, Pedersen AK. A randomized comparison of atrial and dual-chamber pacing in 177 consecutive patients with sick sinus syndrome: echocardiographic and clinical outcome. J Am Coll Cardiol. 2003;42:614-23.
11. Nielsen JC, Thomsen PE, Hojberg S, Moller M, Vesterlund T, Dalsgaard D, et al. DANPACE Investigators. A comparison of single-lead atrial pacing with dual chamber pacing in sick sinus syndrome. Eur Heart J. 2011;32:686-96.

12. Saba MM, Donahue TP, Panotopoulos PT, Ibrahim SS, Abi-Samra FM. Long-term mortality in patients with pauses in ventricular electrical activity. Pacing Clin Electrophysiol. 2005;28:1203-7.
13. Sanders P, Morton JB, Kistler PM, Spence SJ, Davidson NC, Hussin A, et al. Electrophysiological and electroanatomic characterization of the atria in sinus node disease: evidence of diffuse atrial remodeling. Circulation. 2004;109(12):1514-22.
14. Spodick DH, Raju P, Bishop RL, et al. Operational definition of normal sinus heart rate. Am J Cardiol. 1992;69:1245-6.
15. Surawicz B, Uhley H, Borun R, Laks M, Crevasse L, Rosen K, et al. The quest for optimal electrocardiography. Task Force I: standardization of terminology and interpretation. Am J Cardiol. 1978;41:130-45.
16. Tracy CM, Epstein AE, Darbar D, DiMarco JP, Dunbar SB, Estes NA III, et al. 2012 ACCF/AHA/HRS focused update incorporated into the ACCF/AHA/HRS 2008 guidelines for device-based therapy of cardiac rhythm abnormalities. J Am Coll Cardiol. 2013;61(3):e6-75.
17. Uhm JS, Hwang IU, Oh YS, Choi MS, Jang SW, Shin WS, et al. Prevalence of electrocardiographic findings suggestive of sudden cardiac death risk in 10867 apparently healthy young Korean men. Pacing Clini Electrophysiol. 2011;34:717-23.
18. Wang NC. Immediate pacing for traumatic complete atrioventricular block and ventricular asystole. Am J Med. 2010;123(1):e3-4.

17

Atrial Fibrillation

Chapter

Michael C Giudici, Basil Abu-El-Haija

INCIDENCE

Atrial fibrillation (AF) is the most common arrhythmia in adults. An earlier report in 2001 estimated that 2.3 million individuals in the United States alone had AF at that time.[1] A recent study in 2013 estimated that around 5.2 million individuals in the United States had AF.[2] This increase in prevalence is due to the increase in the incidence of AF (total number of new cases per year), which was estimated at 1.2 million cases in 2010. The incidence is estimated to double by 2030 with an estimated total AF population of 12.1 million cases.[2] Atrial fibrillation is more common in men than in women (1.1% vs. 0.8%; P < 0.001), and is a disease of aging (the prevalence of AF has been estimated to be around 0.1% among adults younger than 55 years and as high as 9.0% in persons aged 80 years or older).[1]

PRESENTATION

Patient presentation with AF is widely variable and runs the gamut from urgent emergency department visits for severe symptoms of palpitations, chest pain, dizziness, lightheadedness, dyspnea or presyncope to completely asymptomatic with AF found on a routine examination.

When clinicians see a patient with AF, they should have three main concerns: symptoms, stroke and long-term injury to the heart.
- The *symptoms* listed above may be subtle or dramatic and it is important to take a probing history as many seemingly asymptomatic patients will admit that their exercise tolerance has declined or that they are napping more frequently, etc. There are also many patients who truly think they are asymptomatic and function fully, but after being put back in sinus rhythm notice a significant improvement and are more aware of a decline in function the second time they go into AF
- Concern for *stroke* is a major issue. Studies vary in the duration of an AF episode considered at risk for thrombus formation and embolization. In general, if a patient's episodes of AF are <24 hours, they should be at low risk and anticoagulation should not be necessary. If they have other major risks, such as a previous history of stroke, pulmonary embolism or hypercoagulable state, then the benefit of anticoagulation may exceed the risk. Discussion of risk scoring and the agents available for anticoagulation will be later in the chapter

- *Long-term damage* to the heart can be due to a tachycardia-mediated cardiomyopathy[3] or simply due to a cardiomyopathy brought on by the irregular rhythm. A nonischemic cardiomyopathy in a patient without a bundle branch block whose only other presenting abnormality is AF has an AF-induced cardiomyopathy until proven otherwise.

PATHOPHYSIOLOGY

Atrial fibrillation was initially felt to be due to reentry based on the work of Lewis in the 1920s.[4] The studies of Scherf[5] in the 1940s suggested automaticity was the initiator and reentry the propagator. Gordon Moe's[6] "multiple wavelet" hypothesis again established reentry as the presumed mechanism until the observations of Haïssaguerre et al. in 1996,[7] which clearly demonstrated rapid automatic firing from pulmonary veins as the inciting event.

The complexities of initiation and propagation of AF are too great for a full discussion in this text, but current thought is that AF originates with a rapidly firing atrial focus. These foci are usually found in muscular sleeves extending out from the atrium around the pulmonary veins and are referred to as pulmonary vein potentials. They have also been seen in the coronary sinus,[8] the vein of Marshall,[9] the superior vena cava[10] and the base of the left atrial appendage (LAA). Areas of fibrosis in the atrium can serve as "rotors" and propagate the arrhythmia,[11] which may explain why patients with less atrial fibrosis tend to have paroxysmal AF (PAF) and those with more fibrosis have persistent AF. That is probably a useful oversimplification. There are also autonomic ganglionic plexi that play a role in the initiation and propagation of AF. Exactly how they alter atrial physiology is still under investigation as is the potential role of "low-voltage bridges" within the tissue.

EPIDEMIOLOGY

Established risk factors for AF include increasing age, male gender, obesity, hypertension, diabetes, left ventricular hypertrophy and mitral valve disease. A recent epidemiologic study looking at a biracial cohort also showed that Caucasian race, being tall in stature, left atrial enlargement, cigarette smoking, coronary artery disease (CAD) and heart failure are risk factors for AF.[12]

MANAGEMENT

Acute Atrial Fibrillation

If the episode of AF is <24 hours in duration and the person has no significant structural heart disease, the options for conversion include (i) "pill-in-the-pocket" amiodarone (800–1,200 mg as a single dose), flecainide (200–400 mg as a single dose) or propafenone (450–600 mg as a single dose);[13] (ii) intravenous (IV) therapy with ibutilide (1 mg over 10–15 minutes followed by a 15-minute waiting period, and a single repeat dose of 1 mg IV over 10–15 minutes, if needed.[14] Maximum dose is 2 mg); or (iii) sedate and cardiovert.

We recommend always using the maximum output of the defibrillator for the synchronized shock. Lower outputs result in lower efficacy and the need for repeat shocks. If there is concern that the 24-hour window is ending, a 1.5 mg/kg subcutaneous dose of enoxaparin or an oral dose of one of the new anticoagulants will quickly achieve therapeutic anticoagulation and obviate the need for longer-term anticoagulation and a transesophageal echocardiogram (TEE) prior to cardioversion.

If the episode has been >24 hours at the time of diagnosis, then there are two paths. If a controlled rate (<100 beats/minute) is either present or can be achieved with a β-blocker, verapamil or diltiazem, and the patient is minimally symptomatic, one can begin either warfarin or a newer anticoagulant and consider a chemical or electrical cardioversion after 3–4 weeks of therapeutic anticoagulation. Again, using the newer anticoagulant agents, the patient is immediately therapeutic and a cardioversion can be planned in 3–4 weeks. With warfarin, there is a concern as to whether bridging with enoxaparin or heparin is indicated (higher-risk patients) and then a therapeutic range [international normalized ratio [(INR)] ≥ 2.0] must be maintained until cardioversion. If the symptoms are too great to wait 3–4 weeks or the rate is unable to be controlled, once therapeutic anticoagulation is achieved a TEE can be performed to rule out left atrial thrombus and, if negative, one can proceed with cardioversion.

Recurrent Paroxysmal Atrial Fibrillation

If you are seeing a patient with recurrent PAF, your choice of treatment options will depend on the duration of the individual episodes, level of symptoms and desires of the patient. For example, an asymptomatic patient with a low CHA_2DS_2-VASc score and episodes lasting seconds to minutes may do well with aspirin or no anticoagulation and observation or a β-blocker or calcium channel blocker if their episodes are >100 beats/minute. Patients with episodes lasting over 24 hours and a CHA_2DS_2-VASc score >1 may need chronic anticoagulation.

The treatment options available for AF include rate control and appropriate anticoagulation, rhythm control medications and cardioversions (if needed), AF ablation, pacemaker placement (with or without AV nodal ablation) and surgical options.

Rate Control and Appropriate Anticoagulation

Rate control agents include the various β-blockers, diltiazem and verapamil. We try to avoid digoxin due to its poor rate control with exercise and narrow therapeutic window. It is also important to note that carvedilol is predominantly an α-blocker and provides minimal AV nodal blockade. The criteria used to determine good rate control are an average heart rate ≤ 80 beats/minute on a 24-hour Holter monitor and no single hour averaging >110 beats/minute unless during exercise.[15] There are recent data, however, suggesting those criteria can be relaxed with good long-term results.[16,17] The goal with this therapy in an asymptomatic person is to avoid a cardiomyopathy due to either the high rate or irregular rhythm. We usually perform follow-up Holter monitors and echocardiograms every 2–3 years and intervene if there is a change in status. There will be some patients who require either an up or down titration of their AV nodal blocking agents.

Rhythm Control Medications and Cardioversions

Tailoring the appropriate rhythm control agent to the patient is critical. For PAF, if the patient has a structurally normal heart, your choices include disopyramide, flecainide, propafenone, sotalol, dronedarone and dofetilide.[17] We will briefly discuss each agent.

- Disopyramide is a vagolytic class Ia antiarrhythmic. Its best use is in women who tend toward bradycardia when in sinus rhythm. It is the only currently used agent that will speed up the sinus node. The usual starting dose is 100–150 mg bid or tid. We usually start low and check an ECG for QT prolongation in a week, then titrate the drug as needed. Serum drug levels can be measured. Side effects are usually dryness of mucus membranes and occasional mild constipation. There is a risk of a lupus-like syndrome in the long term. It can also be used in younger men but it can exacerbate prostatic hypertrophy and cause urinary retention in older men. Other common uses for disopyramide in the past years were AF associated with hypertrophic cardiomyopathy and also treatment of neurogenic syncope
- Flecainide is a class Ic drug that is quite potent at suppressing AF. It is best used in patients with structurally normal hearts and no evidence of ischemia. Side effects are minimal—patients occasionally report a mild headache or slightly blurred vision for the first few days—and there are no known long-term toxicities. The usual starting dose is 50–100 mg bid with a maximum of 200 bid[18]
- Propafenone is a class Ic and somewhat similar to flecainide with the addition of weak β-blocking effect that can be an issue in patients with reactive airway disease. It tends to be more efficacious and better tolerated in women. Side effects can be mild constipation and a metallic taste. The usual starting dose is 150–225 mg bid or tid. Most people do well on the bid dosing. There are no known long-term toxicities. Propafenone may interact with warfarin to produce a modest rise in the INR[18]
- Sotalol is a class III agent that is also a β-blocker. This is convenient for patients who are already on a β-blocker for either hypertension or rate control. Switching from 50 mg bid of metoprolol to 60 or 80 mg of sotalol may obviate the need for taking two different drugs. We will often, in men, start this low-dose of sotalol as an outpatient and check an ECG in 4–7 days to check for QT prolongation. This is very rarely an issue as ≤80 mg of sotalol is predominantly β-blocker with little class III effect. We then can titrate up to 120–160 bid, if needed, and follow serial ECGs. Sotalol use in women is a bit more hazardous. Metabolism is variable and late torsade de pointes can occur even if the QTc was normal after achieving steady state. Use extra care when prescribing sotalol in women. We would recommend inpatient initiation of sotalol in women and any patient being given over

80 mg bid to start. Sotalol can be used in the presence of ischemia, left ventricular hypertrophy and hypertrophic cardiomyopathy. Side effects are mainly asthenic symptoms related to the β-blocker. Occasional patients will report diarrhea and some report weight gain
- Dronedarone is a class III drug that is similar to amiodarone but lacks the iodine moiety. It does not have the potential long-term toxicities of amiodarone, but also lacks its efficacy. It is presently used, and is reasonably effective, for PAF in patients without congestive heart failure. The dosing is 400 mg bid. Side effects are usually GI, such as abdominal bloating and discomfort or diarrhea
- Dofetilide is a class III agent that must be started as an inpatient, which greatly limits its use. It is metabolized by the kidneys and is strictly dosed based on renal function. The QTc must be closely monitored and the patient must be observant of any changes in his or her medical regimen including over-the-counter medications as a multitude of other medications interact with dofetilide and can result in dangerous spikes in blood levels and risk of torsades de pointes. The usual starting dose is 125–250 mg bid.

Atrial Fibrillation Ablation

Atrial fibrillation ablation is an excellent option in patients with PAF who either fail medical therapy or opt for a potential curative therapy rather than long-term medical treatment. Atrial fibrillation ablation has made slow progress over the last 10 years, but recent improvements in both catheter technology and the understanding of the pathophysiology of PAF have improved the efficacy of the procedures.

Atrial fibrillation ablation is still most commonly done with a double transseptal puncture and both a "lasso" catheter for recording pulmonary vein (PV) potentials and a radiofrequency (RF) ablation catheter to perform circumferential antral PV ablation (Fig. 17.1). A more recent advance for PAF is the Arctic Front cryoballoon system, which produces a wider antral PV ablation with a single transseptal puncture (Fig. 17.2). The balloon is advanced to occlude the PV and the distal half of the balloon is cooled with liquid nitrogen achieving temperatures as low as –60° C. This achieves similar results to RF ablation and may spare tissue endothelium around the PVs.[19] The risks of cryoablation are injury to the esophagus and phrenic nerve palsy. A third catheter technology currently available in Europe and Canada, and under study in the United States, is the Ablation Frontiers pulmonary vein ablation catheter (PVAC)[20] (Fig. 17.3). This is a duty-cycled RF catheter that can perform a circumferential antral PV isolation using both bipolar and unipolar ablation simultaneously. Success rate for all these ablation modalities is up to 90% for PAF.

Pacemaker Placement—with or without AV Nodal Ablation

For patients who fail medical therapy and are not candidates for AF ablation, an AV nodal ablation and pacemaker placement is an excellent option for restoring a reliable regular rhythm and peace of mind to the patient.

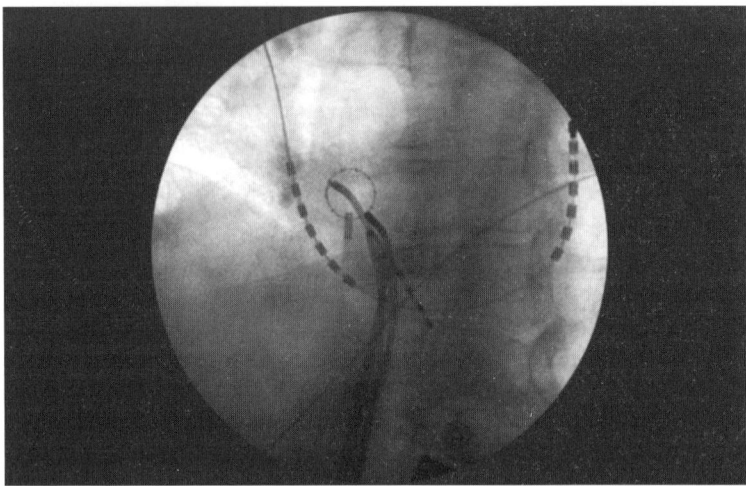

Fig. 17.1: Left anterior oblique view of radiofrequency ablation of the right inferior pulmonary vein using a multipolar circular catheter (Map) to record pulmonary vein potentials and a deflectable tip ablation catheter (RF) to isolate the pulmonary vein.

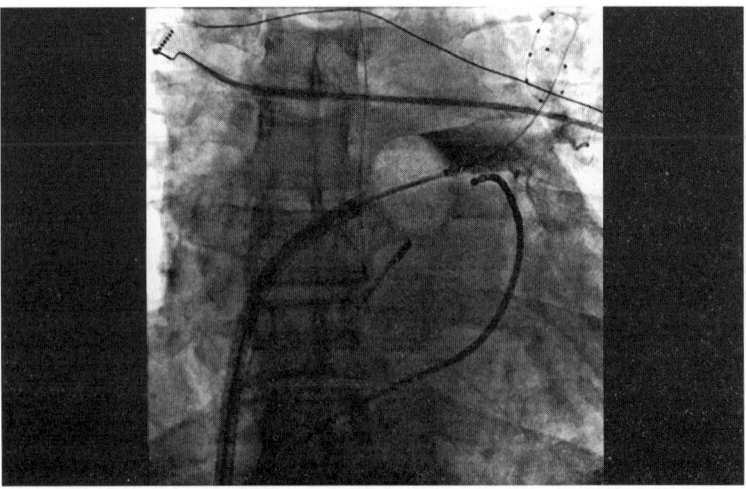

Fig. 17.2: Left anterior oblique view of cryoballoon ablation of the left superior pulmonary vein.

Studies have shown that quality of life (QOL) in patients with PAF is as low as patients with heart failure. The Ablate and Pace Trial demonstrated that patients who undergo AV nodal ablation and pacemaker placement have a dramatic improvement in QOL scores across the entire spectrum—physical, emotional, social—and improvement in ejection fraction and cardiac output.[21] Patients who undergo this therapy will need to remain on anticoagulation, if appropriate, but are able to discontinue both rate and rhythm control medications.

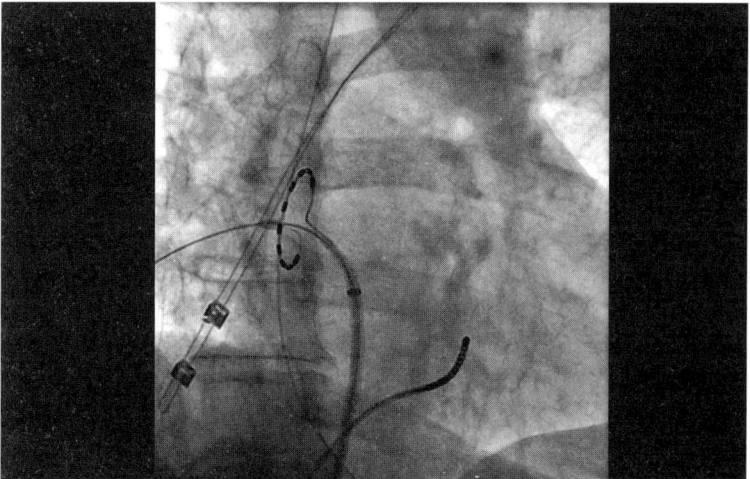

Fig. 17.3: Right anterior oblique view of duty-cycled radiofrequency ablation using the pulmonary vein ablation catheter (Ablation Frontiers, Carlsbad, CA) in the right inferior pulmonary vein.

Pacemaker selection is important in this group, as mode-switching varies among manufacturers. Some company devices will have a sudden increase in rate before the mode-switch and others have rate-smoothing properties to render the mode-switch asymptomatic.[22]

Surgical Options

A discussion of the many open and thoracoscopic surgical procedures is beyond the scope of this text. Surgery for PAF is usually an open procedure done as an adjunct to valve surgery or bypass grafting. Like AF ablation, there are RF and cryoprocedures, and also true surgical procedures like the MAZE, which usually includes a left atrial appendectomy.[23]

Persistent Atrial Fibrillation

Persistent AF has essentially the same therapeutic options as PAF. The approach, however, is different as these patients tend to be older and have more structural heart disease. There is more rate control compared to rhythm control and more AV nodal ablation and pacing compared with AF ablation. The medications are also different—dronedarone is out and amiodarone is in.

The approach to a patient who presents with persistent AF should be a big-picture view. How old is this patient? How symptomatic are they? What do we have to work with in terms of ejection fraction, left ventricular wall thickness, left atrial dimensions and valve function? Are there other issues such as sleep apnea, diabetes or hypertension that will make us lean toward one therapy over another?

Patients aged 70 years or above should be approached with caution for AF ablation. Their procedural stroke rate is higher and their success rate is lower. Having said that, we have done many AF ablations, both RF and cryoablation, in patients well over 70 years if their heart is structurally healthy and they have few comorbidities, with good results. The cryoballoon procedure is especially well-tolerated in older patients.

The issue of symptoms is an important one. Many patients who report fewer or no symptoms have simply adjusted to their "new normal" and feel much better back in sinus rhythm. We try to get nearly every patient back into sinus rhythm for at least 2 weeks to give the patient an opportunity to compare how he or she feels in sinus rhythm versus AF. If they can tell a significant difference, then we are much more aggressive about trying to maintain either sinus rhythm with drugs or ablation, or consider an AV nodal ablation and pacemaker, if needed. For those truly asymptomatic in AF, the rate control strategy is employed.

Medications for persistent AF include all the above with the exception of dronedarone. Amiodarone is the most effective drug therapy for persistent AF. It is a unique agent that has effects across all Vaughan–Williams classes. The usual loading dose is 800 mg daily in divided doses for 7–14 days followed by 200–400 mg daily with the dose tapered over time to 100–200 mg daily. Amiodarone is safe to start as an outpatient. We will usually try to load amiodarone for 4–6 weeks in patients with longer-term AF prior to cardioversion. Amiodarone has little in the way of side effects, such as headache and nausea. It can cause constipation and photosensitivity. It has significant toxicities to the lungs, liver, thyroid and possibly the eyes that should be monitored with quarterly liver enzymes and thyroid studies, and annual spirometry with diffusing capacity and a chest X-ray. A drop in the diffusing capacity may be the first sign of toxicity and the drug should be discontinued.

Atrial fibrillation ablation is a reasonable option for selected patients with persistent AF. Radio frequency has been the mainstay of therapy and the new Ablation Frontiers system of catheters for the pulmonary veins (i.e. PVAC), the septum [i.e. the multiarray septal catheter (MASC)] and the remainder of the left atrium [i.e. the multiarray ablation catheter (MAAC)] may offer better long-term success.[20]

Surgical options for persistent AF are, again, usually performed in conjunction with other cardiac surgeries, but there has been interest in hybrid procedures where the electrophysiologist performs endocardial ablation and a surgeon performs epicardial ablation through a thoracoscopic approach.[24]

Upstream Therapies for Atrial Fibrillation

As mentioned earlier, atrial inflammation and fibrosis are the key mechanisms for the development of AF. Atrial fibrillation can be the result of continuous remodeling (electrical and structural) of the atria, as well as autonomic changes secondary to aging. Therapies that target the formation and evolution of the substrate for AF have been an active area of research and investigations in the recent years. Upstream therapy refers to the use of nonantiarrhythmic medications that modify the atrial substrate and target specific mechanisms of AF to prevent the occurrence of this arrhythmia in a high-risk population (primary prevention), or prevent the recurrence of AF in patients with prior episodes. Angiotensin converting enzyme inhibitors (ACEIs), angiotensin receptor blockers (ARBs), statins and omega-3 polyunsaturated fatty acids are among the most commonly used agents for this purpose. The key targets for these medications are electrical remodeling of the atria, structural changes, oxidative stress, inflammation and fibrosis.[25] A sustained reduction of new onset AF was noticed with the use of these agents with the most promising results seen with the use of ACEIs or ARBs in patients with congestive heart failure (CHF) and the use of statins after cardiac surgery.[25]

The renin–angiotensin–aldosterone-system (RAAS) promotes stimulation of atrial remodeling, fibrosis and hypertrophy; therefore, it is not surprising that RAAS inhibition would decrease AF occurrence. The occurrence of AF post cardiac surgery, which is known to be due to a strong inflammatory response, can be decreased significantly with the use of statins because of their anti-inflammatory and antioxidant effects. Omega-3 polyunsaturated fatty acids decreased AF recurrence but their effect is less pronounced than RAAS inhibitors and statins. We recommend considering these agents for high-risk patients, especially if they have another indication (CHF, CAD, hypertension etc.). Accordingly, if a patient with a history of AF or strong risk factors for AF develops hypertension, an ACEI or ARB would be the preferred antihypertensive agent since there is potential that these agents may also help prevent AF in addition to controlling blood pressure.

Anticoagulation in Atrial Fibrillation

A major sociomedical consequence of AF is its association with embolic stroke.[26] Strong evidence suggests that the LAA is the primary site of thrombus formation[27,28] and subsequent embolization of thrombi can occur in any form of AF (paroxysmal, persistent or permanent) at any time, if adequate anticoagulation is not achieved.

The CHADS2 and CHA2DS2-VASc Scores

Chronic anticoagulation is indicated for most patients with AF to prevent thrombus formation and subsequent embolization leading to ischemic stroke. Since the risk of thromboembolism is variable among patients and depends on the presence of various comorbidities, multiple studies have investigated the pathogenesis and risk factors for thrombus formation and embolization in AF. Multivariate risk models have been constructed to help guide the clinician in identifying the patients who would benefit most from anticoagulation. The risk score most commonly used is the $CHADS_2$ score, where 1 point is assigned for the presence of congestive heart failure, hypertension, age over 75 years, and diabetes mellitus, and assigning 2 points for history of stroke or transient ischemic attack. The $CHADS_2$ score has been validated in large studies.[29] The more detailed CHA_2DS_2-VASc model was introduced with the intent to improve risk stratification.[30] The CHA_2DS_2-VASc score emphasizes the importance of age over 74 years and includes vascular disease, aged 65–74 years and female sex as risk factors.[30] Because of its proven reliability and better prediction of stroke risk, the ACC/AHA/HRS guidelines recommend using the CHA_2DS_2-VASc score for evaluating the risk of stroke and arterial embolization in patients with AF.

Oral anticoagulants are strongly recommended for most patients with AF and CHA_2DS_2-VASc score of 2 or higher according to ACC/AHA and ESC guidelines.[17,31,32] The rationale for this approach is that patients with CHA_2DS_2-VASc score of 2 or higher are at a relatively higher risk of stroke (around 2.2% per year). Patients with CHA_2DS_2-VASc score of 0 are at low risk (rate of 0.5% per year) and oral anticoagulation is not recommended.[17] Patients with a CHA_2DS_2-VASc score of 1 are at intermediate risk of stroke (2% per year), and one can consider treating with oral anticoagulation especially in patients who have low bleeding risk. Many physicians, however, decide not to treat AF patients with CHA_2DS_2-VASc score of 1 with anticoagulation, and choose aspirin as the preventive measure for stroke. The choice between anticoagulation and aspirin will depend upon the physician's assessment of the risk of bleeding and stroke and patient preference.

Antithrombotic Regimens (Oral Anticoagulants)

Many antithrombotic regimens to prevent stroke in AF have been studied. There are numerous randomized trials that have demonstrated the efficacy of warfarin and compared it with aspirin and placebo. The newer oral anticoagulants—dabigatran, rivaroxaban and apixaban—were studied and compared to warfarin in randomized trials.

Warfarin as an Anticoagulant

Warfarin is presently the most widely used anticoagulant. The SPAF-I, SPAF-II and SPAF-III trials and AFASAK, BAATAF, SPINAF and CAFA trials are among the many studies that have demonstrated the efficacy of warfarin.[33-38] In these trials, patients were randomly assigned to warfarin, aspirin or placebo. The main finding of these studies was that anticoagulation with adjusted-dose warfarin (equivalent to INR 2–3) significantly reduced clinical stroke risk in patients with AF when compared with aspirin (relative risk reduction 50%) or placebo (warfarin reduces the risk of stroke by two-thirds).[39] The target INR when warfarin is used should be between 2.0 and 3.0 per the current guidelines.[17,31,32] A major disadvantage of warfarin is the need of continuous INR monitoring and dose adjustments since warfarin interacts with many food products and other medications. International normalized ratio monitoring is very important during therapy because sub- and supratherapeutic INR levels are frequently encountered and are responsible for increased incidence of stroke, and intracranial hemorrhage, respectively.[26]

Newer (Novel) Oral Anticoagulants

Because of the challenges associated with warfarin use, mainly food and drug interactions, and the need for frequent INR monitoring and dose adjustments, newer oral anticoagulants were introduced with the hope of eliminating those issues.

The direct thrombin inhibitor dabigatran, and factor Xa inhibitors rivaroxaban and apixaban are the newer oral anticoagulants that have been studied and compared to warfarin in clinical trials. The three largest trials that assessed these novel agents are the RE-LY (dabigatran), ARISTOTLE (apixaban) and ROCKET AF (rivaroxaban) trials.[40-42] Each of these trials showed that the newer oral anticoagulants dabigatran, apixaban and rivaroxaban have comparable or superior efficacy and safety to warfarin, do not require serial laboratory test monitoring and have fewer food and medication interactions.

More than one meta-analyses have been done of the three clinical trials above and reached the conclusion that the newer oral agents are not only a reasonable alternative to warfarin but actually decreased the risk of stroke [odds ratio (OR) 0.85, 95% CI 0.74-0.99; absolute risk reduction, 0.7%] and major bleeding (OR 0.86, 95% CI 0.75-0.99; absolute risk reduction 0.8%) when compared to warfarin.[43,44] Does this mean that the newer agents are superior to warfarin? Probably, however, they do have limitations and challenges as well. First, the use of dabigatran and rivaroxaban is limited in patients with chronic kidney disease and are contraindicated if the creatinine clearance is <30 mL/min. Second, there is no antidote to reverse their action that can be problematic in patients with life-threatening bleeding. Dabigatran is associated with more severe gastrointestinal (GI) bleeding when compared to warfarin, and should be avoided in patients with prior history of significant GI bleed. Other disadvantages of the newer agents that might limit their use include twice-daily dosing (dabigatran, apixaban) and higher cost. They are also contraindicated in patients with mechanical prosthetic heart valves.

As mentioned previously, patients with AF duration longer than 24 hours or of unknown duration undergoing cardioversion should be anticoagulated prior to the procedure due to the increased risk of thromboembolic events associated with conversion from AF to sinus rhythm. Adequate anticoagulation for 4 weeks prior and 4 weeks after cardioversion decreases the risk of thromboembolism significantly (<1%).[45]

Finally, no significant difference in the rate of stroke within 30 days of cardioversion was noted between patients who received dabigatran or warfarin,[46] which makes dabigatran a reasonable alternative to warfarin for patients undergoing cardioversion. However, unlike dabigatran, the oral factor Xa inhibitors, rivaroxaban and apixaban, have not been studied and evaluated in the pericardioversion period, which limits their use for the prevention of thromboembolic events prior to or immediately after cardioversion until more studies are conducted.

Bleeding Risk

A thorough assessment of the bleeding risk for each individual patient should be carried out prior to initiation of antithrombotic therapy. Initiation of anticoagulation is indicated when the benefits outweigh the bleeding risk. An important fact to keep in mind is that dual antiplatelet therapy and oral anticoagulation have similar bleeding risks, as shown in the ACTIVE W trial[47]; therefore, dual antiplatelet therapy should not be chosen as a substitute for anticoagulation if bleeding is a concern. Elevated INR levels >3.0 are associated with increased bleeding tendency; the most dangerous of all is intracranial hemorrhage. Unlike the newer anticoagulants, patients on warfarin can be treated with vitamin K, which can reverse the INR assuming a normal synthetic function of the liver. Fresh frozen plasma can be given if fast reversal of INR is needed or in cases of liver failure and decreased synthetic function.

CONCLUSION

Atrial fibrillation is the most common arrhythmia affecting the US population. The incidence of AF increases with age. The presentation of AF is widely variable it has and multiple long-term consequences. Proper management of AF patients requires an understanding of the pathophysiological mechanisms responsible for this arrhythmia and the therapies available. Hypertension, valvular or structural heart disease and metabolic causes are among the most common causes of AF. Chronic inflammation, fibrosis and structural remodeling (dilatation) result in electrical changes to the atria that make AF more likely to occur and more difficult to manage. The choice between rate control and antiarrhythmic drugs should be based on thorough evaluation of each individual patient as well as the side effect profile of each medication. Prevention of tachycardia-induced cardiomyopathy and stroke, as well as symptom control, is the main goals of long-term management. Upstream therapies for AF show some promise for the prevention of AF and decreasing the recurrence rate, but more definitive studies are needed. The newer anticoagulants are gaining popularity due to ease of administration, elimination of frequent testing and better efficacy in terms of prevention of embolic stroke and intracranial hemorrhage.

REFERENCES

1. Go AS, Hylek EM, Phillips KA, Chang Y, Henault LE, Selby JV, et al. Prevalence of diagnosed atrial fibrillation in adults: national implications for rhythm management and stroke prevention: the AnTicoagulation and Risk Factors in Atrial Fibrillation (ATRIA) Study. JAMA. 2001;285:237-5.
2. Colilla S, Crow A, Petkun W, Singer DE, Simon T, Liu X. Estimates of current and future incidence and prevalence of atrial fibrillation in the U.S. adult population. Am J Cardiol. 2013;112(8):1142-7.
3. Gupta S, Fiqueredo VM. Tachycardia mediated cardiomyopathy pathophysiology, mechanisms, clinical features and management. Int J Cardiol. 2014;172(1):40-6.

4. Lewis T. Report CXIX. Auricular fibrillation: a common clinical condition. Br Med J. 1909;2(2552):1528.
5. Scherf D, Romano FJ, Terranova R. Experimental studies on auricular flutter and auricular fibrillation. Am Heart J. 1948;36(2):241-51.
6. Moe GK, Abildskov JA. Atrial fibrillation as a self-sustaining arrhythmia independent of focal discharge. Am Heart J. 1959;58(1):59-70.
7. Haïssaguerre M, Jais P, Shah DC, Takahashi A, Hocini M, Quiniou G, et al. Spontaneous initiation of atrial fibrillation by ectopic beats originating in the pulmonary veins. N Engl J Med. 1998;339(10):659-66.
8. Morita H, Zipes DP, Morita ST, Wu J. The role of coronary sinus musculature in the induction of atrial fibrillation. Heart Rhythm. 2012;9(4):581-9.
9. Okuyama Y, Miyauchi Y, Park AM, Hamabe A, Zhou S, Hayashi H, et al. High resolution mapping of the pulmonary vein and the vein of Marshall during induced atrial fibrillation and atrial tachycardia in a canine model of pacing-induced congestive heart failure. J Am Coll Cardiol. 2003;42(2):348-60.
10. Fukumoto K, Takatsuki S, Kimura T, Nishiyama N, Tanimoto K, Aizawa Y, et al. Electrophysiological properties of the superior vena cava and venoatrial junction in patients with atrial fibrillation: relevance to catheter ablation. J Cardiovasc Electrophysiol. 2014;25(1):16-22.
11. Pandit SV, Jalife J. Rotors and the dynamics of cardiac fibrillation. Circ Res. 2013;112(5):849-62.
12. Chamberlain AM, Agarwal SK, Folsom AR, Soliman EZ, Chambless LE, Crow R, et al. A clinical risk score for atrial fibrillation in a biracial prospective cohort (from the Atherosclerosis Risk in Communities [ARIC] study). Am J Cardiol. 2011;107(1):85-91.
13. Alboni P, Botto GL, Baldi N, Luzi M, Russo V, Gianfranchi L, et al. Outpatient treatment of recent-onset atrial fibrillation with the "pill-in-the-pocket" approach. N Engl J Med. 2004;351(23):2384-91.
14. Giudici MFischer WJ 3rdIII, Cervantes DG, Schrumpf PE, Paul DL, Sentman KE, et al. Ibutilide therapy for atrial fibrillation: 5-year experience in a community hospital. J Cardiovasc Nus. 2008;23(6):484-8.
15. Reiffel JA, Kowey PR, Myerburg R, Naccarelli GV, Packer DL, Pratt CM, et al. AFFECTS Scientific Advisory Committee and Investigators. Practice patterns among United States cardiologists for managing adults with atrial fibrillation (from the AFFECTS Registry). Am J Cardiol. 2010;105(8):1122-9.
16. Van Gelder IC, Wyse DG, Chandler ML, Cooper HA, Olshansky B, Hagens VE, et al. RACE and AFFIRM Investigators. Does intensity of rate-control influence outcome in atrial fibrillation? An analysis of pooled data from the RACE and AFFIRM studies. Europace. 2006;8(11):935-42.
17. January CT, Wann LS, Alpert JS, Calkins H, Cleveland Jr JC, Cigarroa JE, et al. 2014 AHA/ACC/HRS Guideline for the Management of Patients With Atrial Fibrillation: Executive Summary. J Am Coll Cardiol. 2014; doi: 10.1016/j.jacc.2014.03.021.
18. Wann LS, Curtis AB, January CT, Ellenbogen KA, Lowe Estes NA III[3rd], et al. 2011 ACCF/AHA/HRS focused update on the management of patients with atrial fibrillation (Updating the 2006 Guideline): a report of the American College of Cardiology Foundation/American Heart Association Task Force on Practice Guidelines. J Am Coll Cardiol. 2011;57:223-42.
19. Andrade JG, Khairy P, Macle L, Packer DL, Lehmann JW, Holcomb RG, et al. Incidence and significance of early recurrences of atrial fibrillation after cryoballoon ablation: insights from the multicenter sustained treatment of paroxysmal atrial fibrillation (STOP AF) Trial. Circ Arrhythm Electrophysiol. 2014;7(1):69-75.

20. Hummel J, Michaud G, Hoyt R, DeLurgio D, Rasekh A, Kusumoto F, et al. TTOP-AF investigators. Phased RF ablation in persistent atrial fibrillation. Heart Rhythm. 2014;11(2):202-9.
21. Kay GN, Ellenbogen KA, Giudici M, Redfield MM, Jenkins LS, Mianulli M, et al. The Ablate and Pace Trial: a prospective study of catheter ablation of the AV conduction system and permanent pacemaker implantation for treatment of atrial fibrillation. APT Investigators. J Interv Card Electrophysiol. 1998;2(2):121-35.
22. Giudici MC, Orias DW. Mode switching anomalies: a patient who remained symptomatic during paroxysmal atrial tachyarrhythmias despite a mode switching pacemaker. Pacing Clin Electrophysiol. 1997;20(7):1883-4.
23. La Meir M. Surgical options for treatment of atrial fibrillation. Ann Cardiothorac Surg. 2014;3(1):30-7.
24. Pison L, Gelsomino S, Lucà F, Parise O, Maessen JG, Crijns HJ, et al. Effectiveness and safety of simultaneous hybrid thoracoscopic and endocardial catheter ablation of lone atrial fibrillation. Ann Cardiothorac Surg. 2014;3(1):38-44.
25. Savelieva I, Kakouros N, Kourliouros A, Camm AJ. Upstream therapies for management of atrial fibrillation: review of clinical evidence and implications for European Society of Cardiology guidelines. Part II: secondary prevention. Europace. 2011;13(5):610-25.
26. Walker AM, Bennett D. Epidemiology and outcomes in patients with atrial fibrillation in the United States. Heart Rhythm. 2008;5(10):1365-72.
27. Sievert H, Lesh MD, Trepels T, Omran H, Bartorelli A, Della Bella P, et al. Percutaneous left atrial appendage transcatheter occlusion to prevent stroke in high-risk patients with atrial fibrillation: early clinical experience. Circulation. 2002;105(16):1887-9.
28. Sick PB, Schuler G, Hauptmann KE, Grube E, Yakubov S, Turi ZG, et al. Initial worldwide experience with the WATCHMAN left atrial appendage system for stroke prevention in atrial fibrillation. J Am Coll Cardiol. 2007;49(13):1490-5.
29. Gage BF, Waterman AD, Shannon W, Boechler M, Rich MW, Radford MJ. Validation of clinical classification schemes for predicting stroke: results from the National Registry of Atrial Fibrillation. JAMA. 2001;285(22):2864-70.
30. Friberg L, Rosenqvist M, Lip GY. Evaluation of risk stratification schemes for ischaemic stroke and bleeding in 182 678 patients with atrial fibrillation: the Swedish Atrial Fibrillation cohort study. Eur Heart J. 2012;33(12):1500-10.
31. Fuster V, Ryden LE, Cannom DS, Crijin HJ, Curtis AB, Ellenbogen KA, et al. ACC/AHA/ESC 2006 Guidelines for the Management of Patients w Atrial Fibrillation---executive summary: a Report of the American College of Cardiology/American Heart Association Task Force on Practice Guidelines and the European Society of Cardiology Committee for Practice Guidelines (Writing Committee to Revise the 2001 Guidelines for the Management of Patients With Atrial Fibrillation). J Am Coll Cardiol. 2006; 48(4):854-906.
32. Camm AJ, Lip GY, De Caterina R, Savelieva I, Atar D, Hohnloser SH, et al. 2012 focused update of the ESC Guidelines for the management of atrial fibrillation: an update of the 2010 ESC Guidelines for the management of atrial fibrillation. Developed with the special contribution of the European Heart Rhythm Association.Eur Heart J. 2012;33 (21):2719-47.
33. The effect of low-dose warfarin on the risk of stroke in patients with nonrheumatic atrial fibrillation. The Boston Area Anticoagulation Trial for Atrial Fibrillation Investigators. N Engl J Med. 1990;323(22):1505-11.
34. Stroke Prevention in Atrial Fibrillation Study. Final results. Circulation. 1991;84(2):527-39.
35. Warfarin versus aspirin for prevention of thromboembolism in atrial fibrillation: Stroke Prevention in Atrial Fibrillation II Study. Lancet. 1994;343(8899):687-91.

36. Petersen P, Boysen G, Godtfredsen J, Andersen ED, Andersen B. Placebo-controlled, randomised trial of warfarin and aspirin for prevention of thromboembolic complications in chronic atrial fibrillation. The Copenhagen AFASAK study. Lancet. 1989;1(8631):175-9.
37. Ezekowitz MD, Bridgers SL, James KE, Carliner NH, Colling CL, Gornick CC, et al. Warfarin in the prevention of stroke associated with nonrheumatic atrial fibrillation. Veterans Affairs Stroke Prevention in Nonrheumatic Atrial Fibrillation Investigators. N Engl J Med. 1992;327(20):1406-12.
38. Connolly SJ, Laupacis A, Gent M, Robert RS, Cairns JA, Joyner C. Canadian Atrial Fibrillation Anticoagulation (CAFA) Study. J Am Coll Cardiol. 1991;18(2):349-55.
39. Risk factors for stroke and efficacy of antithrombotic therapy in atrial fibrillation. Analysis of pooled data from five randomized controlled trials. Arch Intern Med. 1994;154(13):1449-57.
40. Connolly SJ, Ezekowitz MD, Yusuf S, Eikelboom J, Oldgren J, Parekh A, et al. RE-LY Steering Committee and Investigators. Dabigatran versus warfarin in patients with atrial fibrillation. N Engl J Med. 2009;361(12):1139-51.
41. Patel MR, Mahaffey KW, Garg J, Pan G, Singer DE, Hacke W, et al. ROCKET AF Investigators. Rivaroxaban versus warfarin in nonvalvular atrial fibrillation. N Engl J Med. 2011;365(10):883-91.
42. Granger CB, Alexander JH, McMurray JJ, Lopes RD, Hylek EM, Hanna M, et al. ARISTOTLE Committees and Investigators. Apixaban versus warfarin in patients with atrial fibrillation. N Engl J Med. 2011;365(11):981-92.
43. Adam SS, McDuffie JR, Ortel TL, Williams JW Jr. Comparative effectiveness of warfarin and new oral anticoagulants for the management of atrial fibrillation and venous thromboembolism: a systematic review. Ann Intern Med. 2012;157(11):796-807.
44. Ntaios G, Papavasileiou V, Diener HC, Makaritsis K, Michel P. Nonvitamin-K-antagonist oral anticoagulants in patients with atrial fibrillation and previous stroke or transient ischemic attack: a systematic review and meta-analysis of randomized controlled trials. Stroke. 2012;43(12):3298-304.
45. Gentile F, Elhendy A, Khandheria BK, Seward JB, Lohse CM, Shen WK, et al. Safety of electrical cardioversion in patients with atrial fibrillation. Mayo Clin Proc. 2002;77(9):897-904.
46. Nagarakanti R, Ezekowitz MD, Oldgren J, Yang S, Chernick M, Aikens TH, et al. Dabigatran versus warfarin in patients with atrial fibrillation: an analysis of patients undergoing cardioversion. Circulation. 2011;123(2):131-6.
47. ACTIVE Writing Group of the ACTIVE Investigators, Conolly S, Pogue J, Hart R, Pfeffer M, Hohnloser S, et al. Clopidogrel plus aspirin versus oral anticoagulation for atrial fibrillation in the Atrial fibrillation Clopidogrel Trial with Irbesartan for prevention of Vascular Events (ACTIVE W): a randomised controlled trial. Lancet. 2006;367(9526):1903-12.

Tachyarrhythmia

18
Chapter

Min Luo, Dwayne Campbell

DIVISION

Tachyarrhythmias can be divided into two major categories: narrow QRS complex (<120 milliseconds) tachycardia and widened QRS complex (≥120 milliseconds) tachycardia (Fig. 18.1).

NARROW COMPLEX TACHYCARDIAS

Division

Narrow complex tachycardias can be divided into those that require only atrial tissue for initiation and maintenance, and those that are AV node

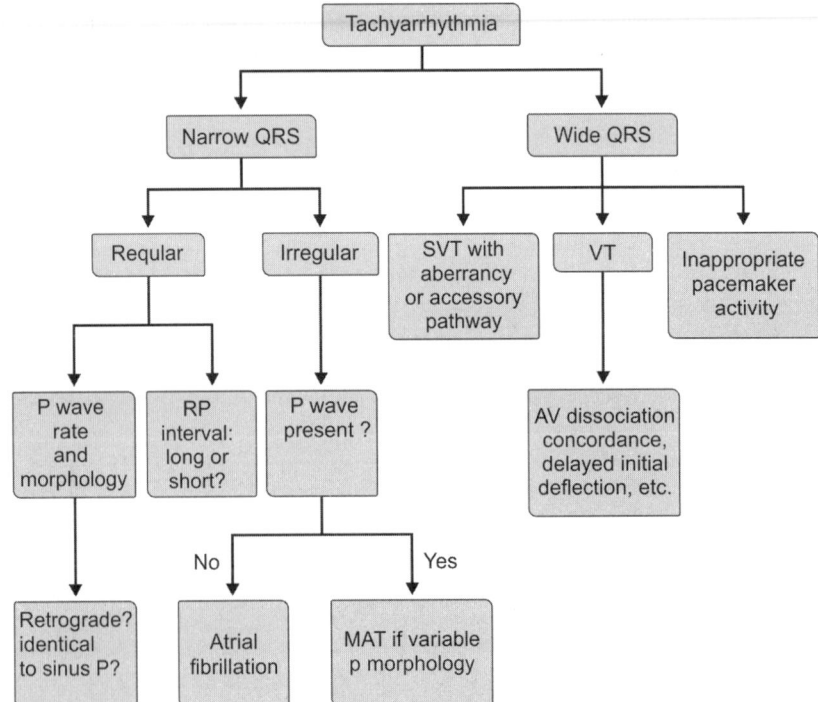

Fig. 18.1: Tachyarrhythmia—diagnostic approach.

dependent. It can also be divided into regular and irregular narrow complex tachycardia. Common types include the following.

Regular Narrow Complex Tachycardias

- **Atrioventricular nodal reentrant tachycardia** (AVNRT) is the most common cause for paroxysmal supraventricular tachycardia (PSVT) and accounts for approximately 60% of cases. Atrioventricular nodal reentrant tachycardia is due to reentry involving two pathways within the AV node or perinodal atrial tissue. There is typical AVNRT (i.e. antegrade conduction down the slow pathway and retrograde conduction up the fast pathway) and atypical AVNRT (i.e. antegrade conduction down a fast pathway and retrograde conduction through a slow pathway)
- **Atrioventricular reentrant tachycardia** (AVRT, Fig. 18.2) accounts for approximately 30% of cases. It is caused by reentry involving both AV node

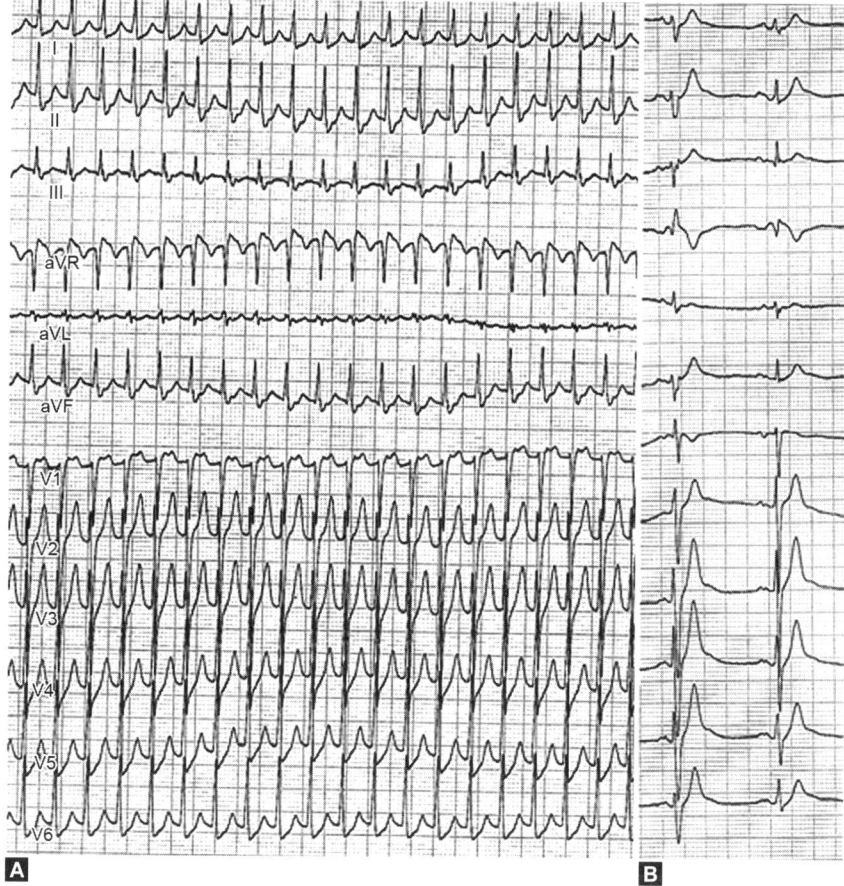

Fig. 18.2: Atrioventricular nodal reentrant tachycardia (A) before and (B) after (right panel) termination with adenosine; note negative retrograde P waves in inferior leads and short RP interval and R' in V1.

and an extranodal accessory pathway connecting the atrium and ventricle with two potential forms of conduction: antidromic versus orthodromic. Orthodromic AVRT occurs via antegrade conduction through the AV node and retrograde conduction through an accessory pathway. Antidromic AVRT conducts antegrade through an accessory pathway and retrograde through the AV node with a morphology resembling a wide complex tachycardia (WCT)

- **Atrial flutter** is a rapid atrial arrhythmia due to microreentrant mechanisms or unclassified mechanisms. Typical atrial flutter is cavo-isthmus-dependent and has distinct electrocardiographic (ECG) features (Figs 18.3 and 18.4)
- **Atrial tachycardia** occurs usually as a result of enhanced automaticity of ectopic atrial focus secondary to conditions, such as catecholamine surges or lung disease.
- **Junctional ectopic tachycardia (JET)** is also called nonparoxysmal junctional tachycardia (NPJT) and is rare in adults. It is commonly misdiagnosed as AVNRT or AVRT. It is an arrhythmia typically arising from a focus within the AV node or His bundle, as a result of enhanced automaticity, digitalis toxicity, excessive exogenous catecholamines or theophylline. It is more common in children, where it is known as JET and usually associated with significant underlying heart disease
- **Sinus tachycardia** is caused by underlying conditions, such as coronary ischemia, heart failure or systemic illness. *Inappropriate sinus tachycardia (IST)* occurs in patients without apparent heart diseases or underlying illness. It is presumed to be due to abnormal autonomic tone

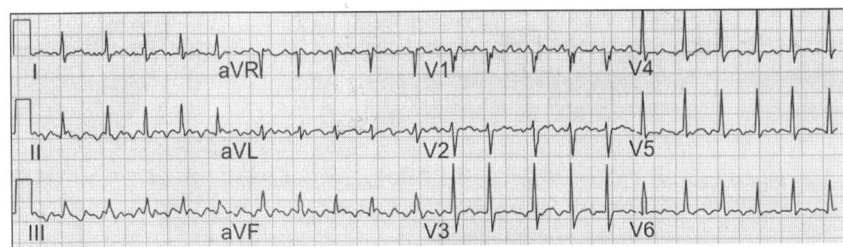

Fig. 18.3: Typical clockwise isthmus dependent atrial flutter positive p ("F" waves in V1) and negative flutter ("F") waves in inferior leads.

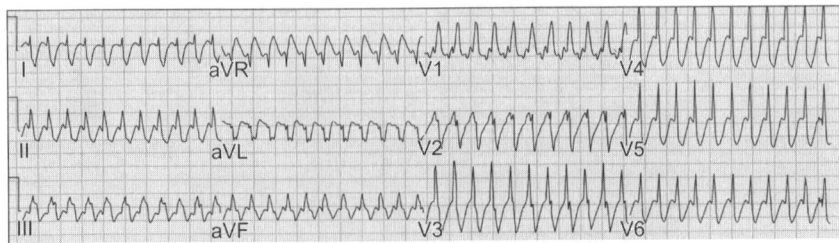

Fig. 18.4: Same patient as in Figure 18.3 now with 1:1 atrioventricular conduction rate-related right bundle branch block (note typical bundle branch block morphology).

- **Sinoatrial nodal reentrant tachycardia (SANRT) and intraatrial reentrant tachycardia (IART)** are microreentrant arrhythmias that do not involve the AV node or accessory pathways. Sinoatrial nodal reentrant tachycardia has P waves identical to sinus P waves whereas IART has a different P wave morphology from normal sinus rhythm.

Irregular Narrow Complex Tachycardia

Irregular SVT includes atrial fibrillation, atrial flutter/tachycardia with variable block or multifocal atrial tachycardia. Atrial fibrillation with digoxin toxicity can manifest as regular SVT. Additional detail on atrial fibrillation is provided in the chapter on atrial fibrillation.

Diagnosis

Initial clinical evaluation should focus on the assessment of hemodynamic stability. Signs and symptoms include palpitations, dyspnea, hypotension, chest pain, altered mental status, shock, and/or presyncope or syncope. Other assessments should target to determine the etiology, duration of the arrhythmia (> or <48 hours), left ventricular function, presence of the Wolff-Parkinson-White syndrome. Electrocardiographic features of atrial activity are essential to the diagnosis of SVT as below:

- *Atrial rate:* Very fast atrial rates [i.e. >250 beats per minute (bpm)] are generally associated with atrial flutter or atrial tachycardia. In atrial flutter, the atrial rate is typically close to 300 bpm with 2:1 AV conduction, resulting in a ventricular rate of 150 bpm. The P waves typically exhibit a classic "sawtooth" pattern ("F" waves); vagal stimulation and intravenous adenosine can slow down the ventricular rate and make the "F" waves more evident. Both SANRT and atrial tachycardia have an abrupt onset and offset whereas in sinus tachycardia and IST (the rate typically ranges from 100 to 180 bpm) the changes in rate are typically smooth and gradual
- *P wave morphology:* The P wave indicates the origin of atrial activity and if a sinus P wave is present, SVT could be sinus tachycardia, IST or SANRT. Abnormal P waves that are not retrograde most likely represent atrial tachycardia. Retrograde P waves can be associated with AVNRT, AVRT or junctional tachycardia. Retrograde P waves are negative in the inferior leads and positive in lead V1 due to the direction of activation from inferior to superior and posterior to anterior. Retrograde P waves can blend in with the terminal portion of the QRS, producing an S wave in the inferior leads or an R' in V1 that is not present during sinus rhythm. Junctional tachycardia can have variable atrial activity, including retrograde atrial activation or independent atrial activity with complete AV dissociation
- *RP relationship:* If the RP interval is short (less than one-half of the RR interval) and the P waves appear to be retrograde, it is likely caused by the typical AVNRT or orthodromic AVRT. If the RP interval is long (more than one-half of the RR interval) with an abnormal P wave morphology, it usually indicates atrial tachycardia. If the RP interval is long with retrograde P waves, it is usually caused by atypical AVNRT or AVRT with a

slowly conducting accessory pathway [permanent junctional reciprocating tachycardia (PJRT)].

Management

Urgent direct current cardioversion (DCCV) is indicated for those patients who are hemodynamically unstable. Following appropriate conscious sedation, an initial synchronized shock of 200–360 joules (monophasic) is administered. Cardioversion is often ineffective in multifocal atrial tachycardia, junctional tachycardia and atrial tachycardia.

In a stable patient, vagotonic maneuvers, such as carotid sinus pressure, Valsalva maneuver or intravenous (IV) adenosine can be attempted to terminate AVNRT or AVRT. Patient should have ECG and blood pressure monitoring when receiving IV adenosine (in a dose of 6 or 12 mg administered rapidly). Termination of SVT by adenosine with a P wave after the last QRS complex suggests AVRT or AVNRT. If SVT continues despite successful AV nodal blockade, it suggests that SVT is independent of AV node and indicates atrial arrhythmia. Hemodynamically stable patients can also be treated with AV nodal blocking, including calcium channel blocker or β-blockers. Caution should be exercised when using AV nodal blocking agents in patients with heart failure as these medications can potentially exacerbate heart failure. Consider digoxin and amiodarone in these patients.

For sinus tachycardia, management should be focused on investigating and treating underlying causes (such as coronary ischemia, heart failure, respiratory distress, hypovolemia, anemia, infection or uncontrolled pain).

For atrial fibrillation, first, the optimal strategy (i.e. rate vs. rhythm control) should be determined. If a rhythm control strategy is chosen and the duration is <48 hours, DCCV is the preferred treatment in the absence of contraindications (e.g. valvular heart disease, heart failure or prior history of thromboembolism). Pharmacologic therapy may be considered if electrical cardioversion is not feasible using antiarrhythmics, including amiodarone, ibutilide, flecainide, propafenone, sotalol and procainamide. Class Ic agents (e.g. flecainide and propafenone) should only be used when there are no significant structural heart diseases, conduction abnormality or coronary artery disease. If the duration is >48 hours or unknown, DCCV should be delayed until there has been at least 3 weeks of adequate anticoagulation [i.e. target international normalized ratio (INR) of 2.0–3.0] or exclusion of LA thrombus using a transesophageal echocardiogram or cardiac computed tomography (CT). Anticoagulation should be continued for 4 weeks after DCCV due to an increased risk of thromboembolism from atrial stunning. In patients with atrial fibrillation and an accessory pathway (Fig. 18.5), atrial fibrillation can degenerate into ventricular fibrillation. In this case, adenosine should be avoided. In addition to DCCV, antiarrhythmic drugs, such as IV procainamide are often very effective for pharmacologic conversion.

For junctional tachycardia and atrial tachycardia, the recommended therapy in the absence of LV dysfunction is an AV nodal blocking agent; in the presence of LV dysfunction, the recommended therapy is amiodarone.

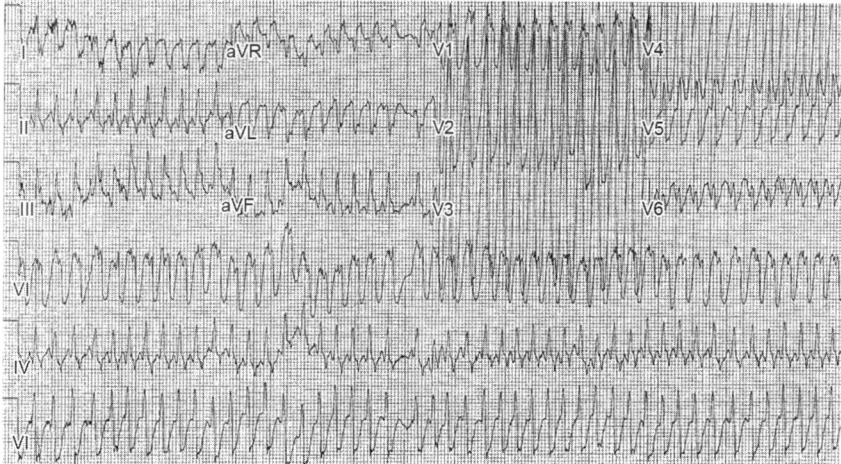

Fig. 18.5: Atrial fibrillation with rapid conduction over accessory pathway note irregularity in RR intervals and variable QRS morphology.

One may consider antiarrhythmics such as flecainide and propafenone if AV nodal blocker fails.

WIDE COMPLEX TACHYCARDIA

Division

Wide complex tachycardia can be due to ventricular tachycardia (VT), SVT with aberrant conduction, SVT with accessory pathway or inappropriate pacemaker activity.

VT

Ventricular tachycardia (Fig. 18.6) is the most common cause of WCT and accounts for up to 80% of cases of WCT, among which >90% of patients have history of prior myocardial infarction (MI). Ventricular activation originates within the ventricular myocardium, is slower, and proceeds in a different sequence compared to the normal conduction system, thus making the QRS complex wide and abnormal. *Ventricular tachycardia* may be monomorphic or polymorphic. Torsades de pointes (TdP) is a polymorphic VT associated with a prolonged QT. It is often triggered by a premature ventricular contraction (PVC) that occurs during the prolonged repolarization period. QT prolongation could be due to congenital long QT syndrome or acquired from drug therapy, hypomagnesemia or hypokalemia.

SVT

It can cause widened QRS by a number of mechanisms, including the following:
- Aberrant conduction (e.g. delayed or blocked conduction in the bundle branches or distal Purkinje system). Conduction may be rate-related

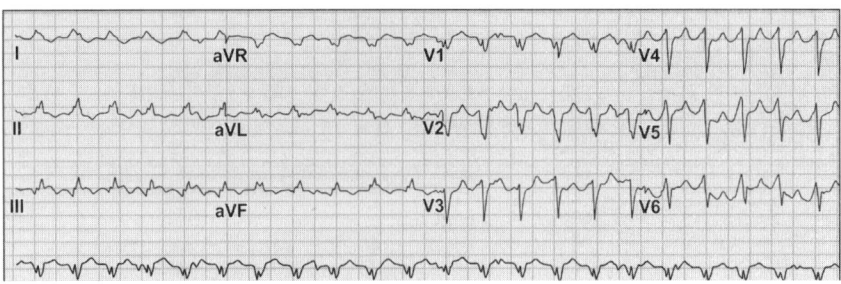

Fig. 18.6: Relatively slow ventricular tachycardia with atrioventricular dissociation and atypical left bundle branch block pattern.

aberrant (i.e. functional bundle branch block) as rapidly generated impulses reach the conducting fibers before fully recovered from the previous impulse, hyperkalemia or antiarrhythmic drugs (e.g. class IC agents such as flecainide and propafenone)
- Baseline conduction abnormality due to left bundle branch block (LBBB), right bundle branch block (RBBB) or a nonspecific intraventricular conduction delay (IVCD). The more similar the QRS during the WCT is to the QRS during sinus rhythm, the more likely it is that the WCT is an SVT with aberrancy
- Antidromic AVRT. Supraventricular tachycardia with antidromic conduction (i.e. antegrade conduction through an accessory pathway and retrograde through the AV node) will produce a wide QRS and is difficult to differentiate from VT.

Inappropriate Pacemaker Activity

Paced QRS complexes can often be identified by a pacing "spike" or stimulus artifact. Dual chamber pacemaker often produces QRS complexes of LBBB morphology (e.g. a broad R wave in lead I) as most ventricular pacemakers pace the right ventricle, causing delayed activation of the LV. Biventricular (BiV) pacemakers produce a different QRS morphology with Q wave in lead I as a result of initial activation from left to right. In the presence of SVT, the device may "track" the atrial impulse and pace the ventricle at the rapid rate, resulting in WCT. However, this is uncommon as this device is programmed with upper tracking rate and function of mode switches when atrial rates increase up to the preset limit. Pacemaker-mediated tachycardia can occur when ventricular paced beats are conducted retrograde through the AV node, resulting in an atrial signal that the pacemaker senses and tracks with another ventricular stimulus, causing pacemaker-mediated tachycardia or endless loop tachycardia. This can also be avoided by increasing "postventricular atrial refractory period."

The presence of narrow-complex beats that "march" through the supposed WCT at a fixed rate strongly supports the diagnosis of artifact.

Diagnosis

Management of WCT often relies on the differentiation of VT from SVT, which requires an adequate ECG analysis using both 12-lead ECG and a rhythm strip and comparing with prior baseline ECG as described below:

- *Rate:* The rate of WCT is of limited use in distinguishing VT from SVT
- *Regularity:* Monomorphic VT is generally regular with a slight irregularity, which is more notable during the onset of the arrhythmia (i.e. the "warm-up phenomenon"). Polymorphic VT and atrial fibrillation with aberrant conduction are typically irregular
- *Axis:* The axis of VT is often indeterminate or "northwest" (i.e. an axis from –90° to –180°). An axis shift during the WCT of >40° compared to sinus rhythm suggests VT. The QRS axis to the left of –30° in RBBB-like WCT suggests VT. QRS axis to the right of +90° in LBBB-like WCT suggests VT
- *QRS duration:* In general, a wider QRS favors VT over SVT. However, it does not preclude SVT. Supraventricular tachycardia with aberrant conduction or accessory pathway, use of class I antiarrhythmic drugs and hyperkalemia can also produce wide QRS. A relatively narrow QRS does not exclude VT, since VT originating from the septum or within the His-Purkinje system (as opposed to the myocardium) may be associated with a relatively narrow QRS complex
- *Concordance:* Concordance is present when the QRS complexes in all precordial leads are monophasic with the same polarity. While the presence of concordance strongly suggests VT, its absence does not exclude VT
- *AV dissociation:* AV dissociation is characterized by atrial activity that is independent of ventricular activity [e.g. dissociated P waves (as evidenced by different PP and RR intervals), variable PR intervals, no association between P and QRS complexes]. In a WCT with AV dissociation, an atrial rate slower than the ventricular rate strongly suggests VT. While the presence of AV dissociation largely establishes VT as the diagnosis, its absence is not as helpful in the case of AV dissociation with retrograde atrial activation
- *Fusion beats and capture beats:* Fusion occurs when the impulses originating from the ventricle and from supraventricular source simultaneously activate the ventricular myocardium. The resulting QRS complex has a morphology intermediate between that of a sinus beat and a purely ventricular complex. Intermittent fusion beats during a WCT are diagnostic of AV dissociation and therefore of VT. Capture beats are QRS complexes that are identical to the sinus QRS complexes as a result of the capturing of ventricular activation by the normal conduction system
- *Brugada criteria:* This is a widely used algorithm for diagnosis of VT. It uses a stepwise approach in which four criteria are sequentially assessed. If any of the criterion is satisfied, the diagnosis of VT is made. The first criterion is

the absence of an RS complex in leads V1–V6, which suggests the presence of concordance. The second criterion is that the RS interval (the interval between the onset of the R wave and the nadir of the S wave) is >100 milliseconds and the R wave is wider than the S wave. This is due to the slower ventricular activation in VT compared to SVT. The third criterion is the presence of AV dissociation as discussed above. The fourth criterion is based on QRS morphology: for RBBB pattern, a monophasic R or biphasic qR complex in lead V1 favors VT; for LBBB pattern, a broad initial R wave (40 milliseconds duration or longer) in lead V1 or V2 favors VT. A slurred or notched downstroke of the S wave in lead V1 or V2 and a duration from the onset of QRS to the nadir of the S wave of ≥60 milliseconds in lead V1 or V2 also favor the diagnosis of VT. The presence of any Q or QS wave in lead V6 favors VT
- Alternative criteria that are diagnostic of VT include an initial R wave in aVR, and the ratio of Vi:Vt (i.e. magnitude of voltage change in the initial and terminal 40 milliseconds of a QRS, respectively) ≤1.

An electrophysiologic study can provide a definitive diagnosis, but is not necessary unless it will influence therapy and can potentially be curative.

Management

General Approach

Wide complex tachycardia should be managed as VT if diagnostic certainty is in question. Presumption of VT will prevent potentially dangerous therapies targeted to treat SVT, such as AV nodal blockers (e.g. β-blockers, adenosine and calcium channel blocker) that can precipitate cardiac arrest in patients with VT or cause deterioration of WCT due to SVT with accessary pathway to ventricular fibrillation. In contrary, treatment of SVT as if it were VT is often safe and effective.

The first priority when evaluating a patient with a WCT is the assessment of hemodynamic stability. Symptoms and signs of unstable hemodynamics include angina, altered mental stats, hypotension or shock. Emergent cardioversion should be performed using synchronized shocks. If the QRS complex and T wave cannot be distinguished accurately, immediate defibrillation with unsynchronized shocks should be performed. After hemodynamic stability is established, further evaluation includes the determination of the WCT etiology (e.g. heart failure, myocardial ischemia, drug reaction or electrolyte abnormalities) as described below:
- *History:* A history of structural heart diseases, such as coronary artery disease, implantation of pacemaker or implantable cardioverter-defibrillator (ICD), strongly suggests VT as an etiology
- *Age:* Supraventricular tachycardia is more likely in younger patients and VT is more likely in older patients. However, VT must be considered in younger patients particularly if there is a family history of ventricular arrhythmias or premature sudden cardiac death

- *Medications:* Many medications have proarrhythmic effects and the most common drug-induced WCT is orsades de pointes. Drugs that can cause TdP include the class III antiarrhythmic agents, quinidine and certain antimicrobials such as erythromycin and the quinolones. The class I antiarrhythmics, especially class Ic agents, can cause aberrancy during an SVT and also VT. These drugs can cause rate-related aberration and a wide QRS complex during SVT via a mechanism of "use-dependency" (i.e. a progressive decrease in impulse conduction velocity at faster heart rates). It can also cause incessant VT with a very wide QRS. Digoxin can cause cardiac arrhythmia including VT, especially at plasma concentrations above 2.0 ng/mL or at any given plasma concentration if hypokalemia is also present. Diuretics can cause hypokalemia and hypomagnesemia, which may predispose to ventricular tachyarrhythmias, particularly TdP
- *Physical examination:* Physical findings suggestive of heart failure and AV dissociation (e.g. fluctuations in blood pressure and heart sounds, cannon "A" waves due to simultaneous atrial and ventricular activation). Vagal maneuvers such as carotid massage can terminate AVNRT or AVRT. Sinus tachycardia will gradually slow with carotid message and accelerate upon release. Atrial arrhythmia is usually unaffected but the ventricular response may slow due to increased AV nodal blockade. Ventricular tachycardia is unaffected by vagal maneuver except retrograde conduction
- *Labs:* Electrolyte abnormalities such as hypokalemia, hyperkalemia and hypomagnesemia should be evaluated. Plasma levels of medications such as digoxin, quinidine and procainamide should be measured to rule out toxicities
- *Other:* A chest X-ray can provide information, such as cardiomegaly, previous cardiothoracic surgery and the presence of a pacemaker or ICD. Electrophysiologic testing allows definitive diagnosis of a WCT, but is rarely feasible and used in the acute setting.

Targeted Approach

Idiopathic VT can be treated with calcium channel blockers or β-blockers. Class I and III antiarrhythmics are generally reserved for refractory or recurrent arrhythmias such as amiodarone (bolus of 150 mg IV over 10 minutes followed by an infusion of 1 mg/min for 6 hours, then 0.5 mg/min for 18 hours). Procainamide (15-18 mg/kg administered as slow infusion followed by 1-4 mg/min by continuous infusion) can effectively treat both SVT (antidromic AVRT) and VT. Intravenous lidocaine (1-1.5 mg/kg over 2-3 minutes) is preferred if cardiac ischemia is present. In patients with VT and impaired LV function, amiodarone and lidocaine are recommended. For recurrent or refractory VT, evaluation should also focus on potential arrhythmia triggers (e.g. ischemia, electrolyte abnormalities and drug toxicity).

Torsades de pointes associated with congenital QT prolongation can be triggered by increased heart rate or tachycardia and hence the recommended therapy is to slow down the heart rate. In contrast, TdP associated with acquired QT prolongation is triggered by bradycardia or pause and therefore therapies are targeted to treat bradycardia using pacing or isoproterenol. Other management includes withdrawal of offending drugs, correction of electrolyte abnormalities and IV Magnesium sulfate infusion. For patients with TdP due to long QT syndrome type 3, lidocaine, mexiletine or flecainide can be used.

If WCT is caused by inappropriate pacemaker activity, the pacemaker can be reprogrammed or a magnet can be placed to terminate inappropriate tracking of atrial impulses. In patients with an ICD and recurrent WCT, the ICD should be interrogated to potentially provide a diagnosis based on intracardiac recordings of the arrhythmia, history of device therapies or adjust therapy parameters to avoid inappropriate device discharges. For WCT terminated effectively by ICD, evaluation should focus on potential arrhythmic triggers such as ischemia, decompensated heart failure, electrolyte abnormalities or medication changes. For WCT not terminated by ICD, tachytherapy parameters or defibrillation threshold should be evaluated and adjusted accordingly. Defibrillation thresholds can increase as a result of the addition of a new medication or clinical deterioration. Wide complex tachycardia due to SVT usually does not convert with the device shocks.

SUGGESTED READING

1. Akhtar M, Jazayeri MR, Sra J, Blanck Z, Deshpande S, Dhala A. Atrioventricular nodal reentry. Clinical, electrophysiological, and therapeutic considerations. Circulation. 1993;88(1):282-95.
2. Akhtar M, Shenasa M, Jazayeri M, Caceres J, Tchou PJ. Wide QRS complex tachycardia. Reappraisal of a common clinical problem. Ann Int Med. 1988;109(11):905-12.
3. Bash SE, Shah JJ, Albers WH, Geiss DM. Hypothermia for the treatment of postsurgical greatly accelerated junctional ectopic tachycardia. J Am Coll Cardiol. 1987;10(5): 1095-9.
4. Blomstrom-Lundqvist C, Scheinman MM, Aliot EM, Alpert JS, Calkins H, Camm AJ, et al. ACC/AHA/ESC guidelines for the management of patients with supraventricular arrhythmias—executive summary: a report of the American College of Cardiology/American Heart Association Task Force on Practice Guidelines and the European Society of Cardiology Committee for Practice Guidelines. Circulation. 2003;108(15):1871-909.
5. Brugada P, Brugada J, Mont L, Smeets J, Andries EW. A new approach to the differential diagnosis of a regular tachycardia with a wide QRS complex. Circulation. 1991;83(5):1649-59.
6. Buxton AE, Marchlinski FE, Doherty JU, Flores B, Josephson ME. Hazards of intravenous verapamil for sustained ventricular tachycardia. Am J Cardiol. 1987;59(12):1107-10.
7. Chauhan VS, Krahn AD, Klein GJ, Skanes AC, Yee R. Supraventricular tachycardia. The Med Clin North Am. 2001;85(2):193-223.
8. Collins KK, Van Hare GF, Kertesz NJ, Law IH, Bar-Cohen Y, Dubin AM, et al. Pediatric nonpost-operative junctional ectopic tachycardia medical management and interventional therapies. J Am Coll Cardiol. 2009;53(8):690-7.

9. Ganz LI, Friedman PL. Supraventricular tachycardia. New Engl J Med. 1995;332(3):162-73.
10. Gupta AK, Thakur RK. Wide QRS complex tachycardias. Med Clin North Am. 2001;85(2):245-66.
11. Haines DE, DiMarco JP. Sustained intraatrial reentrant tachycardia: clinical, electrocardiographic and electrophysiologic characteristics and long-term follow-up. J Am Coll Cardiol. 1990;15(6):1345-54.
12. Kalbfleisch SJ, Williamson B, Man KC, Vorperian V, Hummel JD, Hasse C, et al. Prospective, randomized comparison of conventional and high dose loading regimens of amiodarone in the treatment of ventricular tachycardia. J Am Coll Cardiol. 1993;22(6):1723-9.
13. Krikler DM. Torsades de pointes. J Am Coll Cardiol. 1993;22(2):632-3.
14. Olshansky B, Sullivan RM. Inappropriate sinus tachycardia. J Am Coll Cardiol. 2013;61(8):793-801.Or magniet ea poruntis dolupta volorum que dus rectatiunt dellant ecuptatibus si utempostrum qui re libus, ut fugition eos debita quibeatusti ant poratio rrovide reperrum explaboris delenihicae. Nam quidebis aut elictemque consequatem quam, officiu sanissi tem ut lati dolest eaquam exerrunt ea nossusc iatem. Et fuga. Ut aut ernatur?
15. Nus modi sitas a dolo evelles am dolore dolo ipsandus eossitasped ut dolupta ssitat.

Claudication and Peripheral Artery Disease

Chapter 19

Lee Joseph

EPIDEMIOLOGY AND RISK FACTORS

Lower extremity peripheral artery disease (PAD) is a common atherosclerotic syndrome associated with significant morbidity and mortality. The prevalence of PAD in primary care practices is as high as 29% among individuals aged 70 years or older or aged 50-69 years with history of cigarette smoking or diabetes. Peripheral artery disease affects >5 million adults in the United States based on the 1999-2000 nationally representative PAD prevalence estimates of 4.3% among adults aged 40 years and over.

Peripheral artery disease, a coronary artery disease (CAD) risk equivalent, increases the risk for cardiovascular (CV) mortality by three- to sixfold. Tobacco use and diabetes mellitus are the strongest risk factors for PAD. There is a 2.3-fold greater prevalence of symptomatic PAD in current smokers compared with nonsmokers. Hypertension, hyperlipidemia, older age, black race, hyperhomocysteinemia, chronic kidney disease and inflammatory markers are associated with higher risk for PAD.

CLINICAL PRESENTATION AND NATURAL HISTORY

Patients with PAD can initially present with a wide clinical spectrum and 20-50% of patients with PAD may have no symptoms. While only up to a third of these patients develop intermittent claudication, 30-40% patients with PAD have atypical leg pain. Critical limb ischemia (CLI) is defined as the presence of ischemic rest pain or tissue loss (e.g. nonhealing ulceration or gangrene). It occurs in 1-2% of patients initially presenting with PAD and has 25% mortality rate and 30% amputation rate at 1 year.

Within 5 years after initial presentation of PAD, there is 15% risk for a fatal event, three out of four times from CV causes, and a 20% risk for nonfatal CV event. Even though claudication symptoms remain stable in the majority of patients (i.e. 70-80%), it worsens in 10-20% of claudicants, and even leads to CLI in 5-10% patients. Of note, PAD patients who smoke or have diabetes are at a higher risk for developing CLI requiring amputation.

DIAGNOSTIC METHODS

Individuals with or at risk for PAD should be identified with a thorough vascular assessment, including history, examination and measurement of

Table 19.1: Interpretation of ABI values	
ABI values	**Interpretation**
≤0.90	PAD
0.91–0.99	Borderline
1.00–1.40	Normal
>1.40	Noncompressible vessel

ABI, ankle-brachial index; PAD, peripheral artery disease.

the ankle-brachial index (ABI). The interpretation for ABI values is shown in Table 19.1. An exercise ABI measurement in individuals who have a normal ABI (i.e. 1.0–1.30) and a toe–brachial index or pulse volume recording (PVR) measurement in individuals who have an ABI >1.30 are useful diagnostic tools for PAD. If the individual has normal postexercise ABI, no further PAD evaluation is required unless there is clinical suspicion for other vascular etiologies such as entrapment syndromes or isolated internal iliac artery occlusive disease. Anatomic localization of lower extremity PAD can be achieved by means of PVR with leg segmental pressure measurements.

In the absence of contraindication, noninvasive imaging modalities, including color flow duplex imaging, magnetic resonance angiography with gadolinium enhancement and computed tomographic angiography, are useful to diagnose lower extremity PAD location and severity and to select candidates for endovascular intervention and for postrevascularization surveillance. Contrast angiography utilizing digital subtraction technique is indicated in patients in whom revascularization is contemplated.

MANAGEMENT

The goals of PAD management are secondary prevention of CV events, relief of lower extremity symptoms, protection of limb and improvement of functional status.

Risk Factors
- **Hypertension**: The goal BP should be <140/90 mm Hg (<150/90 mm Hg for persons aged 60 years or older). Angiotensin converting enzyme (ACE) inhibitors, angiotensin receptor blockers (ARB), calcium-channel blockers or thiazide-type diuretics are the recommended first-line drugs to achieve this BP goal. Ramipril, an ACE inhibitor, showed a 22% significant relative risk reduction in the rates of death, myocardial infarction and stroke independent of BP-lowering effect in the Heart Outcomes Prevention Evaluation (HOPE) trial of 9,297 high-risk patients, including PAD. The ACE inhibitor therapy is preferred in PAD patients with and without hypertension. Use of β-blocker in PAD is not associated with worsening of claudication, and thus β-blocker is not contraindicated in PAD patients.

- **Diabetes mellitus**: For adults with type 2 diabetes, the target hemoglobin A1C is <7%
- **Lipids**: High-intensity statin therapy in adults aged 75 years or younger with known CV disease, and statin therapy after risk benefit assessment for persons aged 75 years or older is the recommended lipid control strategy. In addition to reducing the risk for CV events in patients with PAD, statin therapy can also improve intermittent claudication and mean pain-free walking time
- **Smoking cessation**: It can reduce severity of limb symptoms, the risk for CV events and progression of PAD. Pharmacological and behavioral treatment strategies must be utilized for achieving smoking cessation. Varenicline (nicotine receptor partial agonist), bupropion (antidepressant) and nicotine replacement therapy (NRT) are the commonly available pharmacological agents for smoking cessation
- **Antiplatelets therapy**: Patients with symptomatic PAD must be treated with aspirin 75–325 mg per day. Aspirin therapy must be considered for secondary prevention in patients with asymptomatic PAD. Current evidence does not support the combination of oral anticoagulation therapy and antiplatelet therapy for atherosclerotic risk reduction among patients with PAD. Patients with allergy, intolerance or nonresponsiveness to aspirin should be treated with clopidogrel 75 mg per day. Peripheral artery disease patients with lower extremity claudication, CLI, prior limb revascularization or amputation and no increase in bleeding risk may be candidates for aspirin and clopidogrel. Newer antiplatelet agents may prove to have a role in PAD management, particularly for nonresponders to aspirin and clopidogrel. However, robust evidence is lacking to support their clinical use.

Claudication

Pharmacotherapy, exercise rehabilitation programs and revascularization are the principal strategies for managing claudication.
- **Pharmacological therapy for claudication**

    There are limited drugs with proven efficacy in improving claudication. Currently, cilostazol and pentoxifylline are the only two FDA-approved drugs for treatment of claudication.

    Cilostazol, a phosphodiesterase type III inhibitor, has antiplatelet and weak vasodilator effects. In the absence of heart failure, PAD patients with claudication should be treated with cilostazol, for at least a trial period of 3 months. Headache, diarrhea, palpitations and dizziness are the side effects commonly associated with cilostazol. The administered dose of cilostazol is 100 mg orally two times a day.

    A second-line alternate option to cilostazol for claudication therapy is pentoxifylline. Pentoxifylline is a methylxanthine derivative with potent hemorheologic and antithrombotic properties. It has marginal benefit in treating claudication. The oral pentoxifylline dose for managing claudication is 400 mg three times a day.

Naftidrofuryl, a vasoactive drug, is a cost-effective agent for claudication treatment compared with cilostazol and pentoxifylline. However, it is not available in the United States.

The efficacy of ACE inhibitors and oral sodium nitrite for improving claudication is not yet clear. Ramipril (at a dose of 10 mg/day) significantly improved mean pain-free walking time, maximum walking time and quality of life (QoL) measures compared with placebo in a randomized controlled trial.

There is no role for ginkgo biloba, vitamin E, buflomedil (a vasoactive agent), L-arginine supplementation (precursor of endothelium-derived nitric oxide), oral vasodilator prostaglandins, such as beraprost and iloprost, chelation therapy and propionyl-L-carnitine for the treatment of claudication

- **Exercise therapy**
  Supervised exercise training program is indicated for management of intermittent claudication in PAD patients. Patient should participate in such a program for a minimum of 3 months, in sessions of at least 30–45 minutes performed at least three times per week under one-to-one supervision by an exercise physiologist, physical therapist or nurse. The session initially has 35 minutes of intermittent walking, which is gradually increased by 5 minutes for a goal of 50 minutes of intermittent walking. A motorized treadmill or a track can be utilized. The claudication threshold and CV status are monitored.

  Several studies concluded that supervised exercise improved pain-free walking distance, maximal walking distance and QoL of PAD participants with and without intermittent claudication. Such a favorable response to exercise therapy can be explained by measurable improvements in endothelial function, muscle metabolism, blood viscosity and inflammatory responses, and possibly, promotion of vascular angiogenesis. Although supervised exercise therapy is more cost-effective than catheter-based revascularization, its widespread use is limited due to poor availability of reimbursement. There is not enough evidence yet to support unsupervised exercise therapy as an equivalent alternative to supervised programs for claudication

- **Revascularization therapy**
  Lifestyle limiting intermittent claudication (in the absence of other comorbidities) resulting in a significant functional impairment and favorable anatomy is an indication for an evaluation for revascularization by endovascular or surgical means. However, in the absence of a significant translesional gradient or symptoms, surgical or endovascular intervention is not indicated.

  Since aortoiliac/inflow disease results in greater disability than infrainguinal/outflow disease, revascularization of inflow lesion is more common. Among patients with inflow and outflow disease, inflow lesions should be revascularized initially. If symptoms persist despite treatment of inflow disease, infrainguinal revascularization should be considered.

For aortoiliac, femoral and popliteal artery disease, the Trans-Atlantic Inter-Society Consensus (TASC) classification is utilized to choose between surgery and endovascular intervention as an initial approach for managing lifestyle limiting claudication (Tables 19.2 and 19.3). The TASC type A and B lesions benefit from endovascular therapy as initial approach. Primary stent placement is indicated for treatment of lesions in the iliac arteries.

For the treatment of femoral, popliteal and infrapopliteal arterial lesions, stents, atherectomy, cutting balloons, thermal devices and lasers can be used to salvage a suboptimal or failed result from balloon dilation, such as persistent translesional gradient, residual diameter stenosis >50% or flow-limiting dissection.

Surgical approach is the preferred initial revascularization strategy for TASC type C and D lesions. Autogenous vein bypass graft from ipsilateral or contralateral leg or arms if available is preferred to a prosthetic material graft.

The TASC classification is not applicable to the treatment of tibial vessel disease or multilevel disease.

Table 19.2: TASC II classification scheme: aortoiliac lesions

Type A	Type B
• Unilateral or bilateral stenosis of the common iliac artery • Unilateral or bilateral single short (≤3 cm) stenosis of the external iliac artery	• Short (≤3 cm) stenosis of the infrarenal aorta • Unilateral common iliac artery occlusion • Single or multiple stenoses totaling 3–10 cm of the external iliac artery not extending into the common femoral artery • Unilateral external iliac artery occlusion not involving the origins of the internal iliac artery or common femoral artery
Type C	**Type D**
• Bilateral common iliac artery occlusions • Bilateral external iliac artery stenosis 3–10 cm not extending into the common femoral artery • Unilateral external iliac artery stenosis extending into the common femoral artery • Unilateral external iliac artery occlusion of the origins of the internal iliac and/or common femoral artery • Heavily calcified unilateral external iliac artery occlusion with or without involvement of the origins of the internal iliac and/or common femoral artery	• Infrarenal aortoiliac occlusion • Diffuse disease of the aorta and both iliac arteries requiring treatment • Diffuse multiple stenoses of the unilateral common and iliac artery, and common femoral artery • Unilateral occlusions of the common iliac and external iliac arteries • Bilateral occlusions of external iliac arteries • Iliac stenoses in patients with abdominal aortic aneurysm (that require treatment and are not amenable to endograft placement) or other lesions requiring open aortic or iliac surgery

TASC, Trans-Atlantic Inter-Society Consensus.

Source: Norgren L, Hiatt WR, Dormandy JA, Nehler MR, Harris KA, Fowkes FG, et al. Inter-Society Consensus for the Management of Peripheral Arterial Disease (TASC II). Eur J Vasc Endovasc Surg. 2007;33 (Suppl 1):S1-75.

Table 19.3: TASC II classification scheme: femoral popliteal lesions

Type A	Type B
• Single stenosis ≤10 cm in length • Single occlusion ≤5 cm in length	• Multiple lesions (stenoses or occlusions), each ≤5 cm • Stenosis or occlusion ≤15 cm not involving the infrageniculate popliteal artery • Single or multiple lesions in the absence of continuous tibial vessels to improve inflow for a distal bypass • Heavily calcified occlusion ≤5 cm in length • Single popliteal stenosis
Type C	**Type D**
• Multiple stenoses or occlusion totaling >15 cm with or without heavy calcification • Recurrent stenoses or occlusion that needs treatment after two endovascular interventions	• Chronic total occlusion of the common femoral artery or superficial femoral artery (>20 cm, involving the popliteal artery) • Chronic total occlusion of the popliteal artery and proximal trifurcation vessels

TASC, Trans-Atlantic Inter-Society Consensus.

Source: Norgren L, Hiatt WR, Dormandy JA, Nehler MR, Harris KA, Fowkes FG, et al. Inter-Society Consensus for the Management of Peripheral Arterial Disease (TASC II). Eur J Vasc Endovasc Surg. 2007;33(Suppl 1):S1-75.

Following revascularization, periodic clinic follow-up and imaging studies are important to identify progressive or new stenotic lesions involving the graft or native vessel, and address appropriately.

In patients with significant aortoiliac disease unsuitable or unresponsive to endovascular therapy, aortobifemoral bypass needs to be considered. Surgical options for patients with unilateral iliac artery disease with acceptable aortic inflow include iliac endarterectomy, patch angioplasty, or aortoiliac or iliofemoral bypass. If aortobifemoral bypass is not feasible for bilateral iliac artery disease, one of the above unilateral procedures in conjunction with femoral–femoral bypass can be performed. Axillofemoral–femoral bypass is reserved for limited instances, such as chronically occluded infrarenal aorta.

- **Optimal management strategy**

  Medical therapy including exercise regimens has been compared with endovascular or surgical revascularization in a limited number of studies thus far. The CLEVER trial performed a head to head comparison of optimal medical care (OMC) with CV risk reduction plus cilostazol, OMC plus supervised exercise rehabilitation (three times a week for 26 weeks) and OMC plus stenting revascularization in 111 patients with aortoiliac PAD. At 6 months, supervised exercise group achieved significantly higher peak walking time, and stenting showed significant improvement in QoL measures compared with the other two arms. Given the disagreement between the treadmill performance and QoL measures, the optimal strategy for claudication management and the optimal outcome measure remains unclear.

Critical Limb Ischemia

Restoration of adequate perfusion by surgical or endovascular means and wound care form the cornerstones of CLI management to prevent limb loss.

Assessment of CV risk must be performed in individuals who are planned for open surgical repair. Surgical revascularization is the recommended initial approach for improving distal blood flow in a patient with CLI whose estimated life expectancy is >2 years and who has an autogenous vein conduit available. If the estimated life expectancy is 2 years or less, or an autogenous vein conduit is unavailable, balloon angioplasty is a reasonable initial approach. The ACC/AHA guidelines suggest primary amputation of a symptomatic leg if there is marked necrosis of the weightbearing portions of the foot (in ambulatory patients), an uncorrectable flexion contracture, paresis of the extremity, refractory ischemic rest pain, sepsis or a very limited life expectancy.

- **Wound care principles**

Wound care management requires a multidisciplinary approach with a focus on appropriate assessment and optimization of local, regional and systemic factors that play a crucial role in wound healing. The local components include etiologic basis, wound bed debridement, maintenance of adequate moisture balance in the wound and control of infection. Restoring perfusion, pressure offloading and management of edema play critical roles in promoting wound healing. Optimization of systemic disease states, such as diabetes, malnutrition, obesity, anemia and vitamin deficiencies, and smoking cessation have significant impact on wound healing prospects.

Acute Limb Ischemia

Emergent endovascular or surgical revascularization is indicated for patients with acute limb ischemia and a salvageable limb. In the absence of a salvageable extremity, such measures are futile. Catheter-based thrombolysis is indicated for patients with acute limb ischemia of <14 days' duration. In conjunction with catheter-based thrombolysis, mechanical thrombectomy can be used for patients with acute limb ischemia.

SUGGESTED READING

1. Ahimastos AA, Walker PJ, Askew C, Leicht A, Pappas E, Blombery P, et al. Effect of ramipril on walking times and quality of life among patients with peripheral artery disease and intermittent claudication: a randomized controlled trial. JAMA. 2013;309(5):453-60.
2. Anand S, Yusuf S, Xie C, Pogue J, Eikelboom J, Budaj A, et al. Oral anticoagulant and antiplatelet therapy and peripheral arterial disease. N Engl J Med. 2007;357(3):217-27.
3. Anderson JL, Halperin JL, Albert NM, Bozkurt B, Brindis RG, Curtis LH, et al. Management of patients with peripheral artery disease (compilation of 2005 and 2011 ACCF/AHA guideline recommendations): a report of the American College of Cardiology Foundation/American Heart Association Task Force on Practice Guidelines. Circulation. 2013;127(13):1425-43.

4. Bonaca MP, Scirica BM, Creager MA, Olin J, Bounameaux H, Dellborg M, et al. Vorapaxar in patients with peripheral artery disease: results from TRA2{degrees} P-TIMI 50. Circulation. 2013;127(14):1522-9, 9e1-6.
5. Bumpus K, Maier MA. The ABC's of wound care. Curr Cardiol Rep. 2013;15(4):346.
6. Criqui MH, Langer RD, Fronek A, Feigelson HS, Klauber MR, McCann TJ, et al. Mortality over a period of 10 years in patients with peripheral arterial disease. N Engl J Med. 1992;326(6):381-6.
7. Gardner AW, Poehlman ET. Exercise rehabilitation programs for the treatment of claudication pain. a meta-analysis. JAMA. 1995;274(12):975-80.
8. Hirsch AT, Criqui MH, Treat-Jacobson D, Regensteiner JG, Creager MA, Olin JW, et al. Peripheral arterial disease detection, awareness, and treatment in primary care. JAMA. 2001;286(11):1317-24.
9. Hood SC, Moher D, Barber GG. Management of intermittent claudication with pentoxifylline: meta-analysis of randomized controlled trials. CMAJ. 1996;155(8):1053-9.
10. Howell MA, Colgan MP, Seeger RW, Ramsey DE, Sumner DS. Relationship of severity of lower limb peripheral vascular disease to mortality and morbidity: a six-year follow-up study. J Vasc Surg. 1989;9(5):691-7.
11. James PA, Oparil S, Carter BL, Cushman WC, Dennison-Himmelfarb C, Handler J, et al. 2014 evidence-based guideline for the management of high blood pressure in adults: report from the panel members appointed to the Eighth Joint National Committee (JNC 8). JAMA. 2014;311(5):507-20.
12. Kavalukas SL, Barbul A. Nutrition and wound healing: an update. Plast Reconstr Surg. 2011;127(Suppl 1):38S-43S.
13. McDermott MM, Ades P, Guralnik JM, Dyer A, Ferrucci L, Liu K, et al. Treadmill exercise and resistance training in patients with peripheral arterial disease with and without intermittent claudication: a randomized controlled trial. JAMA. 2009;301(2):165-74.
14. McKenna M, Wolfson S, Kuller L. The ratio of ankle and arm arterial pressure as an independent predictor of mortality. Atherosclerosis. 1991;87(2-3):119-28.
15. Meng Y, Squires H, Stevens JW, Simpson E, Harnan S, Thomas S, et al. Cost-effectiveness of cilostazol, naftidrofuryl oxalate, and pentoxifylline for the treatment of intermittent claudication in people with peripheral arterial disease. Angiology. 2014;65(3):190-7.
16. Mohler ER III, Hiatt WR, Gornik HL, Kevil CG, Quyyumi A, Haynes WG, et al. Sodium nitrite in patients with peripheral artery disease and diabetes mellitus: safety, walking distance and endothelial function. Vasc Med. 2014;19(1):9-17.
17. Murphy TP, Cutlip DE, Regensteiner JG, Mohler ER, Cohen DJ, Reynolds MR, et al. Supervised exercise versus primary stenting for claudication resulting from aortoiliac peripheral artery disease: six-month outcomes from the claudication: exercise versus endoluminal revascularization (CLEVER) study. Circulation. 2012;125(1):130-9.
18. Nathan DM, Buse JB, Davidson MB, Ferrannini E, Holman RR, Sherwin R, et al. Medical management of hyperglycemia in type 2 diabetes: a consensus algorithm for the initiation and adjustment of therapy: a consensus statement of the American Diabetes Association and the European Association for the Study of Diabetes. Diabetes Care. 2009;32(1):193-203.
19. Norgren L, Hiatt WR, Dormandy JA, Nehler MR, Harris KA, Fowkes FG, et al. Inter-Society Consensus for the Management of Peripheral Arterial Disease (TASC II). Eur J Vasc Endovasc Surg. 2007;33(Suppl 1):S1-75.
20. Pedersen TR, Kjekshus J, Pyorala K, Olsson AG, Cook TJ, Musliner TA, et al. Effect of simvastatin on ischemic signs and symptoms in the Scandinavian simvastatin survival study (4S). Am J Cardiol. 1998;81(3):333-5.

21. Porter JM, Cutler BS, Lee BY, Reich T, Reichle FA, Scogin JT, et al. Pentoxifylline efficacy in the treatment of intermittent claudication: multicenter controlled double-blind trial with objective assessment of chronic occlusive arterial disease patients. Am Heart J. 1982;104(1):66-72.
22. Radack K, Deck C. Beta-adrenergic blocker therapy does not worsen intermittent claudication in subjects with peripheral arterial disease. A meta-analysis of randomized controlled trials. Arch Intern Med. 1991;151(9):1769-76.
23. Salhiyyah K, Senanayake E, Abdel-Hadi M, Booth A, Michaels JA. Pentoxifylline for intermittent claudication. Cochrane Database Syst Rev. 2012;1:CD005262.
24. Samlaska CP, Winfield EA. Pentoxifylline. J Am Acad Dermatol. 1994;30(4):603-21.
25. Selvin E, Erlinger TP. Prevalence of and risk factors for peripheral arterial disease in the United States: results from the National Health and Nutrition Examination Survey, 1999-2000. Circulation. 2004;110(6):738-43.
26. Stewart KJ, Hiatt WR, Regensteiner JG, Hirsch AT. Exercise training for claudication. N Engl J Med. 2002;347(24):1941-51.
27. Stone NJ, Robinson J, Lichtenstein AH, Merz CN, Blum CB, Eckel RH, et al. 2013 ACC/AHA Guideline on the treatment of blood cholesterol to reduce atherosclerotic cardiovascular risk in adults: a report of the American college of cardiology/American Heart Association Task Force on Practice Guidelines. Circulation. 2014;129:S1-S45.
28. Torngren K, Ohman J, Salmi H, Larsson J, Erlinge D. Ticagrelor improves peripheral arterial function in patients with a previous acute coronary syndrome. Cardiology. 2013;124(4):252-8.
29. Treesak C, Kasemsup V, Treat-Jacobson D, Nyman JA, Hirsch AT. Cost-effectiveness of exercise training to improve claudication symptoms in patients with peripheral arterial disease. Vasc Med. 2004;9(4):279-85.
30. Weitz JI, Byrne J, Clagett GP, Farkouh ME, Porter JM, Sackett DL, et al. Diagnosis and treatment of chronic arterial insufficiency of the lower extremities: a critical review. Circulation. 1996;94(11):3026-49.
31. Willigendael EM, Teijink JA, Bartelink ML, Kuiken BW, Boiten J, Moll FL, et al. Influence of smoking on incidence and prevalence of peripheral arterial disease. J Vasc Surg. 2004;40(6):1158-65.
32. Wiviott SD, Braunwald E, McCabe CH, Montalescot G, Ruzyllo W, Gottlieb S, et al. Prasugrel versus clopidogrel in patients with acute coronary syndromes. N Engl J Med. 2007;357(20):2001-15.
33. Yusuf S, Sleight P, Pogue J, Bosch J, Davies R, Dagenais G. Effects of an angiotensin-converting-enzyme inhibitor, ramipril, on cardiovascular events in high-risk patients. The heart outcomes prevention evaluation study investigators. N Engl J Med. 2000;342(3):145-53.

20
Acute Aortic Syndromes

Chapter

Belal Al Khiami

INTRODUCTION

Acute aortic syndromes (AAS) consist of three related conditions with similar clinical presentation and include acute aortic dissection (AD), intramural hematoma (IMH) and penetrating aortic ulcer (PAU). This syndrome is rapidly fatal; thus, having high clinical index of suspicion is essential to provide an expedited diagnosis and definitive treatment.

DEFINITIONS

- **Aortic dissection** is defined as a disruption of the media layer of the aorta with bleeding within and along the wall of the aorta resulting in separation of aortic wall layers to create double lumen: a true and a false lumen, separated by an intimal flap. Intimal tear is present in approximately 90% of these patients
- **Intramural hematoma** is defined as a collection of static blood or hematoma within the aortic wall. A small tear in the aortic intima or a hemorrhage of the vasa vasorum located within the medial layer of the aorta have been suggested as possible mechanisms for development of IMH. Progression to frank dissection occurs in many cases
- **Penetrating aortic ulcer** refers to an atherosclerotic lesion with ulceration that penetrates the internal elastic lamina and allows hematoma formation within the media of the aortic wall. This can lead to IMH, AD or frank aortic rupture.

EPIDEMIOLOGY

The true incidence of acute AD is difficult to define as many deaths resulting from this syndrome are mistakenly classified as nondissection-related deaths, which include both cases that die from AD before presentation to healthcare facilities and cases where the diagnosis of AD was not made at the initial presentation.

Epidemiological studies showed that the incidence of AD ranges from 2 to 3.5 cases per 100,000 person-years, which corresponds with approximately 6,000–10,000 cases annually in the United States. Thus, it is estimated that a single case of AAS would be expected in only 1 in 100,000 emergency department visits, which can be easily missed given the significant overlap of symptoms at presentations with other diseases. The mean age of patients at presentation with AD is 63 years, with men accounting for 63% of cases according to the International Registry of Aortic Dissection (IRAD).

AORTIC DISSECTION CLASSIFICATION

The DeBakey and Stanford classification systems are the most common systems used for AD classification (Fig. 20.1).
- The DeBakey system classifies AD based on the origin of the intimal tear and the extent of the dissection as follows:
    - Type I: Dissection originates in the ascending aorta and propagates distally to include at least the aortic arch and typically the descending aorta
    - Type II: Dissection originates in and is confined to the ascending aorta
    - Type III: Dissection originates in the descending aorta and propagates most often distally
    - Type IIIa: Limited to the descending thoracic aorta
    - Type IIIb: Extending below the diaphragm
- The Stanford system classifies AD based on the involvement of the ascending aorta as follows:
    - Type A: Dissection involves the ascending aorta regardless of the site of origin.
    - Type B: Dissection does not involve the ascending aorta.

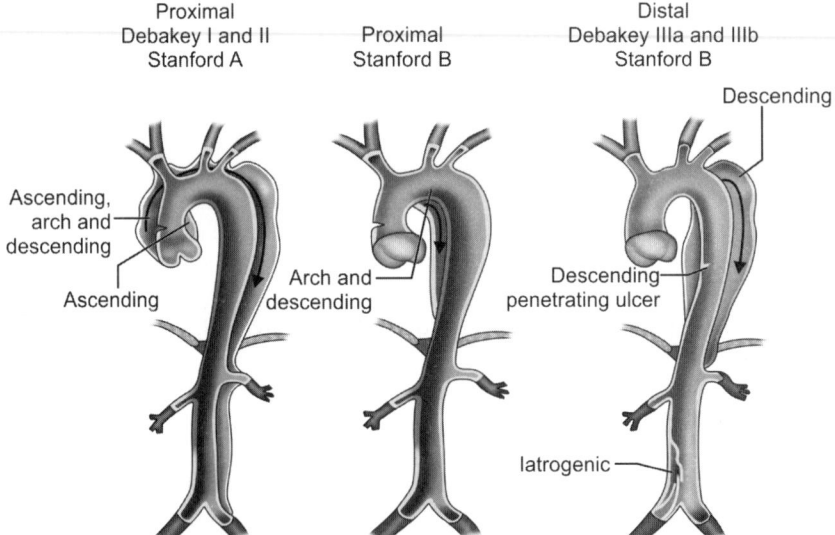

Fig. 20.1: The DeBakey and Stanford classifications of aortic dissection.

Source: Reproduced from Hiratzka LF, Bakris GL, Beckman JA, Bersin RM, Carr VF, Casey DE Jr, et al. 2010 ACCF/AHA/AATS/ACR/ASA/SCA/SCAI/SIR/STS/SVM. Guidelines for the diagnosis and management of patients with thoracic aortic disease. A Report of the American College of Cardiology Foundation/American Heart Association Task Force on Practice Guidelines, American Association for Thoracic Surgery, American College of Radiology, American Stroke Association, Society of Cardiovascular Anesthesiologists, Society for Cardiovascular Angiography and Interventions, Society of Interventional Radiology, Society of Thoracic Surgeons, and Society for Vascular Medicine. J Am Coll Cardiol. 2010; 55(14):e27-e129, *with permission.*

The terms "communicating" and "noncommunicating" refer to the presence or absence, respectively, of blood flow between the true and false lumens of the aorta.

An aortic syndrome considered to be acute if presentation occurs within 2 weeks of the onset of symptoms and subacute/chronic if beyond that.

RISK FACTORS AND PATHOGENESIS

Acquired or inherited conditions that result in aortic medial layer weakness (e.g. cystic degeneration) or conditions that place significant stress on the aortic wall (e.g. cocaine use, trauma and uncontrolled hypertension) are considered risk factors for AAS (Table 20.1). Atherosclerosis is the main risk factor for peptic ulcer disease (PUD).

A history of hypertension presents in around three quarters of patients presenting with acute AD.

Genetic predisposition (e.g. Marfan syndrome) to AD is an important risk factor and a family history of thoracic aortic aneurysm is also an important risk factor. It has been reported that 13–19% of patients without an identified syndrome had first-degree relatives with thoracic aortic aneurysms or AD. Data from IRAD showed that in patients younger than 40 years of age with AD, 50% had a history of Marfan syndrome. Any phenotypic features of the syndromes, such as pectus excavatum or marfanoid features among others should prompt consideration of AD as in some cases only some syndromic features present rather than the complete clinical syndrome.

CLINICAL MANIFESTATIONS

History

Chest pain is the dominant feature at presentation and occurs in >90% of patients. The pain is characterized as sharp more often than tearing or ripping in nature, and may radiate anteriorly (suggestive of type A dissection) or in the interscapular, lower back or abdominal area (suggestive of type B dissection). Limb pain or visceral discomfort may be indicative of aortic branch vessel ischemia from malperfusion. Aortic dissection can result in multiple symptoms based on its extent and presence of complications, which include syncope and focal neurological deficit, among others (Table 20.2).

Physical Examination

Patients with acute AD appear in distress. Hypertension is present in more than two-thirds of type B dissection patients and in approximately one-third of type A patients. An aortic regurgitation murmur can be heard in approximately 40% of patients with type A dissection. Pulse deficits are associated with worse outcomes, which may obscure accurate blood pressure measurements; thus, invasive intraarterial monitoring may be necessary. Jugular venous distension and pulsus paradoxus could be an indication of

Table 20.1: Risk factors for development of thoracic aortic dissection

Conditions associated with increased aortic wall stress

Hypertension, particularly if uncontrolled

Pheochromocytoma

Cocaine or other stimulant use

Weight lifting or other Valsalva maneuver

Trauma

Deceleration or torsional injury (e.g. motor vehicle crash, fall)

Coarctation of the aorta

Conditions associated with aortic media abnormalities

Genetic

Marfan syndrome

Ehlers–Danlos syndrome, vascular form

Bicuspid aortic valve (including prior aortic valve replacement)

Turner syndrome

Loeys–Dietz syndrome

Familial thoracic aortic aneurysm and dissection syndrome

Inflammatory vasculitides

Takayasu arteritis

Giant cell arteritis

Behçet arteritis

Other

Pregnancy

Polycystic kidney disease

Chronic corticosteroid or immunosuppression agent administration

Infections involving the aortic wall either from bacteremia or extension of

Adjacent infection

Source: Adapted from Hiratzka LF, Bakris GL, Beckman JA, Bersin RM, Carr VF, Casey DE Jr, et al. 2010 ACCF/AHA/AATS/ACR/ASA/SCA/SCAI/SIR/STS/SVM. Guidelines for the diagnosis and management of patients with thoracic aortic disease. A Report of the American College of Cardiology Foundation/American Heart Association Task Force on Practice Guidelines, American Association for Thoracic Surgery, American College of Radiology, American Stroke Association, Society of Cardiovascular Anesthesiologists, Society for Cardiovascular Angiography and Interventions, Society of Interventional Radiology, Society of Thoracic Surgeons, and Society for Vascular Medicine. J Am Coll Cardiol. 2010;55(14):e27-e129.

impending cardiac tamponade related to hemorrhagic pericardial effusion. Thoracic dullness to percussion and decreased breath sounds suggest pleural effusion, which is more common in the left chest. Pleural effusions may be hemorrhagic from aortic rupture or leak, or more commonly sympathetic in nature due to the intense inflammation associated with the acute tear.

Clinical Risk Markers

American College of Cardiology Foundation/American Heart Association (ACCF/AHA) guidelines proposed 12 clinical risk markers to be used as a

Table 20.2: Complications of acute aortic dissection

Cardiac
Aortic insufficiency
Pericardial tamponade
Myocardial ischemia/infarction
Congestive heart failure

Pulmonary
Pleural effusion
Aortopulmonary fistula

Neurological
Neurologic Ischemic stroke or transient ischemic attack
Spinal ischemia
Peripheral neuropathy

Renal
Renal ischemia/infarction

Gastrointestinal
Mesenteric ischemia or infarction
Aortoenteric fistula

Extremities
Limb ischemia

tool for focused bedside pretest risk assessment of acute AD. The markers are included in three risk categories:
- Condition
  - Marfan syndrome
  - Connective tissue disease
  - Family history of aortic disease
  - Known aortic valve disease
  - Recent aortic manipulation (surgical or catheter-based)
  - Known thoracic aortic aneurysm
- Pain feature (chest, back or abdominal pain)
  - Abrupt in onset, severe in intensity and quality described as ripping, tearing, stabbing or sharp
- Physical examination
  - Evidence of perfusion deficit
    - Pulse deficit
    - Systolic BP limb differential >20 mmHg
    - Focal neurologic deficit
  - Murmur of aortic regurgitation (new or not known to be old and in conjunction with pain)
  - Hypotension or shock.

The IRAD investigators have tested the sensitivity of these markers on their large registry of AD cases and concluded that it is a highly sensitive clinical tool for the detection of acute AD with a sensitivity of approximately 95%.

Guidelines suggest that the absence of any of these clinical risk markers would classify a patient as low risk for thoracic AD, making an alternative diagnosis is more likely. Nevertheless, if no alternative diagnosis can be reached and suspicion for AD is still present especially in the setting of hypotension or widening mediastinum, definitive aortic diagnostic imaging is recommended.

The presence of only one clinical risk marker places a patient in the intermediate risk category where prompt diagnostic approach is strongly recommended. In this case, expedited aortic imaging should be sought if there are no clear indications of an alternative diagnosis.

Finally, the presence of two or more clinical risk markers places a patient in the high-risk category where immediate surgical consultation and arrangement for expedited aortic imaging should be preceded without any delay.

DIAGNOSTIC EVALUATION

Biomarkers

Biomarkers may help in screening for AD cases but results should be interpreted cautiously as they are not as sensitive as definitive images and specificity is relatively low. In fact, their sensitivity is close to the suggested clinical risk marker tool model by ACC/AHA 2010 guidelines.
- **D-dimer.** Studies show that a D-dimer level of <500 ng/mL, performed within 24 hours of symptom onset, is associated with a negative likelihood ratio for acute AD of 0.07. An elevated D-dimer level has 97% sensitivity and 96% negative predictive value for identifying acute AD. On other hand, it has specificity of 56% and positive predictive value of 60%, which makes D-dimer useful screening test to rule out acute AD but not to rule in. In high-risk patients, a negative D-dimer should be interpreted with caution, as a negative test does not exclude the diagnosis of acute AD.
  - **Smooth muscle myosin heavy chain protein.** Studies show that elevated circulating smooth muscle myosin heavy chain protein can have a sensitivity of 90% and a specificity of 98% compared with healthy controls when measured within 3 hours of presentation.
  - **C-reactive protein** (CRP). An early rapid increase in CRP levels following acute AD has been observed, with levels falling rapidly 24 hours following symptom onset, which is not specific.

Chest X-ray (CXR) and Electrocardiogram (ECG)

Both are insufficient tools to rule out AD, but are helpful to exclude other etiologies. Chest X-ray is abnormal in 80–90% of patients with AD. Mediastinal widening, disparity in the caliber of the ascending and descending thoracic aortic segments, a localized bulge or angulation along the normally smooth border of the aorta, displacement of intimal calcium (especially in the region of the aortic knob) and a double density appearance may be suggestive of AD.

Associated findings may include cardiomegaly (due to pericardial effusion) and pleural effusion. Nonspecific ECG abnormalities can be seen in up to 40% of AD patients. About 15% of patients may have active ischemic changes, while findings suggestive of acute myocardial infarction are present in a minority (i.e. 3%) of cases. The presence of ST-segment elevation suggestive of myocardial infarction should be treated as a primary cardiac event without delay for definitive aortic imaging unless the patient is at high risk for AD.

Definitive Imaging

Transesophageal echocardiogram (TEE), contrast-enhanced computed tomography (CT) and magnetic resonance imaging (MRI) have very similar sensitivity and specificity for AD detection with sensitivities approaching 100%. Computed tomography is the most commonly utilized diagnostic option mainly because of its rapid access to emergency room healthcare providers. Transesophageal echocardiogram is a semiinvasive method, but it is useful for hemodynamically unstable cases and evaluating complications of AD, such as aortic regurgitation. Magnetic resonance imaging is the least used method mainly due to its limited availability in emergent situations. If a high clinical suspicion exists for acute AD but initial aortic imaging is negative, current guidelines recommend considering obtaining a second imaging study as false-negative cases may still occur.

- **CT:** Computed tomography is currently the first-line diagnostic method with sensitivity and specificity exceed >95%. It has many advantages:
  - Wide availability
  - Image the entire aorta and branch vessel involvement
  - Identifies the different types of AAS
  - The time for imaging and processing is short time.

With technology advancement, motion-free images can be generated by ECG-gated techniques similar to coronary CT angiographic imaging that minimizes radiation exposure to the patient.

Computed tomography allows evaluation of aortic valve morphology and function (although with less accuracy than echocardiogram), cardiac function, presence of pericardial effusion, as well as evaluation of the proximal coronary arteries. If appropriately acquired, an aortic CT along with complete CT coronary angiogram can be obtained in one CT acquisition.

Limitations include exposure to ionizing radiation, with associated risk especially in young patients or female sex. Iodine contrast material usage may be potentially nephrotoxic, especially in patients with diabetes mellitus or chronic kidney disease. In addition, severe allergic reactions may occur with exposure to iodine contrast.

- **Echocardiography**

Performing transthoracic echocardiography (TTE) is readily available and can be useful until more definitive diagnostic imaging becomes available. It can assess the proximal part of ascending aorta, aortic valve function, wall motion abnormalities and pericardial effusion, but performing TTE should not delay definitive imaging if indicated.

Transthoracic echocardiography is a semiinvasive diagnostic procedure that requires esophageal intubation and at least conscious sedation that can be performed at the bedside. It is useful for hemodynamically unstable patients who cannot be safely transferred to CT or MRI scanners. Images are readily available at the bedside but the procedure requires expertise. Thus, TEE is not usually the first choice for initial imaging, but it has a role if additional imaging is needed to confirm the diagnosis or for intraoperative use. Diagnostic accuracy can approach a sensitivity of 100% with a specificity of 89%, positive predictive accuracy of 89% and negative predictive accuracy of 99%.

The echocardiographic diagnosis of an AD requires the identification of a dissection flap separating true and false lumens. However, one of the major limitations of TTE and less often in TEE is the frequent appearance of artifacts that mimic a dissection flap. Many maneuvers can be performed to exclude artifacts thatinclude utilizing the color Doppler to assess the blood flow direction on both sides of the flap, obtaining multiple views with different probe angles and assessing flap motion relative to other surrounding structures. True and false lumens determination can be obtained by assessment of systolic versus diastolic expansion of each blood flow direction by color Doppler and by evaluation of the presence of echo materials that could be a sign of thrombosis of false lumen.

Identification of a pericardial effusion, overall and segmental left ventricular function and aortic valve function can be obtained by TEE or TTE. Coronary arteries ostia involvement by dissection can be evaluated by TEE. While TEE can still be useful to detect aortic wall pathology like PUD or IMH, topographic imaging by CT or MRI has better sensitivity and specificity for this purpose.

Contraindications to TEE, such as cervical spine disorders that prevent neck flexion, severe dysphagia and esophageal disorders (e.g. bleeding varices, esophageal stricture, diverticula and cancer) all must be considered when making decision regarding best definitive imaging choice.

- **Magnetic resonance imaging**

It can assess entire aorta, side branch involvement, cardiac and valvular function, and pericardial effusion without exposing the patient to either radiation or iodinated contrast. Disadvantages include prolonged duration of imaging acquisition; inability to use gadolinium contrast in patients with severe renal insufficiency; contraindication in patients with claustrophobia, metallic implants or pacemakers; and lack of widespread availability on an emergency basis. Likely as a result of these considerations, data from IRAD found that MR was the least-used imaging study, used in only 1% of patients as the initial diagnostic study although MRI has a sensitivity of 95–100% and specificity of 94–98% for detecting AD. Magnetic resonance imaging is a useful diagnostic method for long-term surveillance for patients with aortic disease.

- **Catheter-based aortic angiography**

Aortic angiography can be performed along with coronary angiography if indicated, but it is no longer the first-line diagnostic tool for many reasons, which include the following:
- Not widely available
- Invasive procedure
- Time-consuming
- Exposure to radiation and iodinated contrast
- Limited ability to diagnose IMH given a lack of visualization of luminal disruption
- Potential for false negative results when a thrombosed false lumen prevents adequate opacification to identify the dissection.

Reported sensitivities and specificities of angiography for the evaluation of acute AD are slightly lower than those for the other less invasive modalities.

The 2010 ACC/AHA thoracic aortic guidelines suggest performing preoperative coronary angiogram for patients who have confirmed acute AD but are hemodynamically stable and older than 40-year-old with either personal history of coronary artery disease or significant risk factors to assess if they benefit from coronary artery bypass grafting at the time of the indicated aortic surgery.

MANAGEMENT

Initial Acute Management

Patients with suspected or confirmed AAS should be treated promptly with intravenous medications to lower systemic blood pressure with the aim of decreasing aortic wall strain while obtaining surgical consultation and/or obtaining a definitive imaging modality. Since aortic wall strain is a function of left ventricular contraction velocity (i.e. the change in pressure over time or $\Delta P/\Delta T$), β-adrenergic receptor antagonists, with their negative inotropic and chronotropic effects, are first-line therapeutic agents. In patients with a contraindication or intolerance to β-adrenergic receptor antagonists, no-dihydropyridine calcium channel blocker, such as diltiazem or verapamil, may be effective alternatives.

Recommended targets for therapy are a systolic blood pressure ≤ 120 mm Hg and a heart rate 60 beats/minute, but medications may require titration according to clinical evidence of impaired end-organ perfusion. Administration of a direct vasodilator may be necessary as β-adrenergic receptor antagonists alone may be insufficient for achieving blood pressure control. Intravenous angiotensin converting enzyme (ACE) inhibitors or sodium nitroprusside can be used, but should not be initiated without adequate heart rate control because reflex tachycardia increases the overall aortic wall strain. Pain control by analgesic is essential as it improves blood pressure and heart rate control.

In the patient with hypotension, the differential diagnosis includes cardiogenic shock from acute myocardial infarction (resulting from extension of dissection flap to coronary arteries), hemopericardium causing cardiac tamponade or aortic rupture. In this case, volume resuscitation and/or pressor therapy may be necessary to maintain vital organ perfusion until surgery can be performed. Pericardiocentesis for relief of tamponade is not recommended, but rather to proceed with surgery emergently.

Definitive Management

Anatomical location of disease, patient comorbidities, initial complications from the dissection, and acuity of presentation are the key factors that influence surgical indications for treatment of AAS.

Surgical consultation should be considered for all AAS cases, and should be obtained emergently for any highly suspected or confirmed type A AD as in-hospital mortality with only medical therapy reaches 50-60% while immediate surgical intervention will decrease this to 20-30%. An endovascular stent-grafting only or hybrid surgical/endovascular approach is limited to only experienced centers and not recommended for type A AD since the level of evidence available is based on a limited number of published case series.

Surgical and/or endovascular treatments are indicated for type B AD only when there are complications, such as rupture, leak, extension, rapid aneurysm expansion, suboptimal blood pressure or pain control and malperfusion. In patients with a higher risk for future complications (e.g. patients with Marfan syndrome), surgical management is recommended.

Long-Term Surveillance

Having a history of AAS treated medically or surgically increases the risks of recurrent AAS and aortic aneurysms among other cardiovascular complications; thus, close clinical and imaging follow-up is important for all survivors.

Medical management includes control of blood pressure (goal ≤130/80 mm Hg) and heart rate (goal ≤60 beats/minute), statin therapy for treatment of atherosclerosis and smoking cessation. It is also important to educate patients regarding the chronic nature of this disease. Self-awareness of dissection-associated symptoms, importance of medication adherence and avoiding strenuous exercise should be emphasized.

Patients who have Marfan syndrome are very high risk of recurrent dissection or of aneurysm formation with rupture. Also patient with previous history of AD with a patent false lumen has increased risk for late complications and death.

Imaging of the entire aorta is recommended predischarge and at 1, 3, 6 and 12 months, then annually thereafter, if stable with MRI or CT.

PROGNOSIS

It has been estimated that 40% of patients with acute AD type A variant die immediately, then have risk of death of 1% per hour after presentation. It is estimated that between 5% and 20% die during or shortly after surgery.

For type B dissection, the overall in-hospital mortality rates approach 15%. For patients with uncomplicated type B dissection managed medically, 1-month survival is 90%, whereas for patients who require surgical intervention for the indications listed previously, 1-month survival is only 75%.

The 10-year actuarial survival rate of patients with AD who leave the hospital has ranged from 30% to 88%. Survival appears similar for both type A and type B dissections, presumably because adverse events, such as recurrent dissection or complications of aneurysm formation in the descending aorta, occur in both types of dissection.

AORTIC DISSECTION VARIANTS

Intramural Hematoma

The natural history of IMH is variable. The hematoma may entirely resolve in about 10%, it may convert to a classic dissection in 10–90% depending on the location or the aorta may enlarge and potentially rupture. The clinical behavior of IMH varies according to the location and mimics that of classic AD. Intra-mural hematoma of the ascending aorta has a high, early risk of complication and death with medical treatment alone and surgery is indicated as with type A AD.

Peptic Ulcer Disease

Peptic ulcer disease develop in aortic regions where atherosclerotic changes are most common; thus, it presents in descending thoracic aorta in >90% of cases. PUD may progress to aortic rupture, IMH or AD. It is recommended to treat acute PUD involving the ascending aorta as with type A AD.

SUGGESTED READING

1. Baliga RR, Nienaber CA, Bossone E, Oh JK, Isselbacher EM, Sechtem U, et al. The role of imaging in aortic dissection and related syndromes. JACC Cardiovasc Imaging. 2014;7(4):406-24.
2. Bradley A. Maron, Patrick T. O'Gara. Pathophysiology, clinical evaluation, and medical management of aortic dissection. In: Mark C, Joshua B, Joseph L (Eds). Vascular Medicine: A Companion to Braunwald's Heart Disease, 2nd edition. Philadelphia, PA: Elsevier; 2012.
3. Braverman AC. Aortic dissection: prompt diagnosis and emergency treatment are critical. Cleve Clin J Med. 2011;78(10):685-96.
4. Hagan PG, Nienaber CA, Isselbacher EM, Bruckman D, Karavite DJ, Russman PL, et al. The International Registry of Acute Aortic Dissection (IRAD): new insights into an old disease. JAMA. 2000; 283(7):897-903.
5. Hiratzka LF, Bakris GL, Beckman JA, Bersin RM, Marr VF, Carr VF, et al. 2010 ACCF/AHA/AATS/ACR/ASA/SCA/SCAI/SIR/STS/SVM. Guidelines for the diagnosis and management of patients with thoracic aortic disease. J Am Coll Cardiol. 2010;55(14):e27-129.

6. Pape LA, Tsai TT, Isselbacher EM, Oh JK, O'Gara PT, Evangelista A, et al. Aortic diameter > or = 5.5 cm is not a good predictor of type A aortic dissection: observations from the International Registry of Acute Aortic Dissection (IRAD). Circulation. 2007;116(10):1120-7.
7. Rogers AM, Hermann LK, Booher AM, Nienaber CA, Williams DM, Kazerooni EA. et al. Sensitivity of the aortic dissection detection risk score, a novel guideline-based tool for identification of acute aortic dissection at initial presentation: results from the international registry of acute aortic dissection. Circulation. 2011;123(20):2213-8.
8. Sheikh AS, Ali K, Mazhar S. Acute aortic syndrome. Circulation. 2013;128(10):1122-7.

Cardioembolic Stroke

Chapter 21

Siva Krothapalli

INTRODUCTION

Cardioembolic strokes account for about one-fifth of ischemic strokes. They are generally severe and prone to early recurrence. The risk of long-term recurrence and mortality is also high after a cardioembolic stroke. Early identification directly affects primary prevention, acute management and secondary prevention and can therefore have profound prognostic implications. The risk of early embolic recurrence in cardioembolic cerebral infarction varies between 1% and 22%. However, recurrent embolization is associated with an increased mortality of up to 70%. Alcohol abuse, hypertension, valvular heart disease, atrial fibrillation, nausea and vomiting and previous cerebral infarction are predictors of recurrent embolization.

Decreased consciousness at onset, rapid regression of symptoms (also called the spectacular shrinking syndrome), sudden onset to maximal deficit (<5 minutes), simultaneous or strokes in a sequence in multiple arterial territories (especially if bihemispheric or involving combined anterior and posterior, bilateral or multilevel posterior circulation), hemorrhagic transformation of an ischemic infarct and early recanalization of an occluded intracranial vessel all point to a cardiac origin of the stroke. Hemorrhagic transformation occurs in up to 71% of cardioembolic strokes. Decreased alertness, total circulation infarcts, proximal middle cerebral artery occlusion, hypodensity in more than one-third of the middle cerebral artery territory and delayed recanalization (i.e. >6 hours after stroke onset) together with absence of collateral flow predict hemorrhagic transformation in acute cardioembolic cerebral infarction.

Cardiac emboli (owing to their large size) flow to the intracranial vessels in most cases and cause massive, superficial, single, large striatocapsular or multiple infarcts in the middle cerebral artery. Certain clinical syndromes, such as Wernicke's aphasia or global aphasia without hemiparesis are common secondary symptoms of cardioembolism. In the posterior circulation, cardioembolism can produce Wallenberg's syndrome (i.e. a constellation of neurologic symptoms due to injury to the lateral part of the medulla), cerebellar infarctions, top-of-the-basilar syndrome (i.e. infarction of the rostral brainstem and cerebral hemispheric regions fed by the distal basilar artery), multilevel infarcts or posterior cerebral artery infarction.

In 4.7–12% of cases, cardioembolic cerebral infarction shows a rapid regression of symptoms. The dramatic improvement of an initially severe neurological deficit is thought to be due to distal migration of the embolus followed by recanalization of the occluded vessel. Headache or seizures at onset and during activity are not specific for cardioembolic strokes.

Although lacunar presentations were traditionally thought unlikely to be cardioembolic in origin, recent studies with computed tomography (CT) and magnetic resonance imaging (MRI) have shown that large artery rather than local small vessel disease may actually underlie about a quarter of these cases.

Accurate, immediate diagnosis of cardioembolism is not always possible. The clinical and radiological features suggestive of cardioembolism are highly specific but have only moderate sensitivity, and the positive predictive value does not exceed 50%. A high suspicion for cardioembolic etiology of the stroke should be maintained in patients with known emboligenic cardiac disease and in patients without classical risk factors for atheroma or small vessel disease in the right clinical setting. One of the classical descriptions of a cardioembolic stroke, albeit nonspecific in its association, involves the onset of symptoms after a Valsalva-provoking activity (e.g. enhancing right to left shunting in patients with a patent foramen ovale).

INITIAL EVALUATION AND WORKUP

A potential cardiac source of embolus can be identified by a careful history, physical examination and electrocardiogram combined with basic laboratory testing. Evidence of atrial arrhythmia, presence of murmur, signs of congestive heart failure, recent myocardial infarction (MI), signs and symptoms of diseases, such as systemic lupus erythematosus, endocarditis or neoplasia are clues to a possible emboligenic origin of stroke.

- **Standard laboratory investigations** include a complete blood count with platelet count, prothrombin time and activated partial thromboplastin time. In young patients without vascular risk factors who experience cardioembolic stroke, a prothrombotic workup including GP20210A [i.e. the prothrombin (factor II) gene] mutation, factor V Leiden mutation, protein C or S deficiency, antithrombin III deficiency, antiphospholipid antibodies, hyperhomocysteinemia and lupus anticoagulant can be considered
- **Transthoracic echocardiography** should be used as a screening test in patients in whom cardioembolism is suspected but unproven and helps in the initial assessment of the structure and function of the heart. In the absence of clinical or electrocardiographic evidence of cardiac disease, the likelihood of discovering a major cardioembolic source is <5%. However, in patients in whom the mechanism of stroke remains uncertain, transesophageal echocardiography (TEE) is appropriate in the evaluation of cardiovascular (CV) source of embolus. Transesophageal echocardiography provides improved visualization of the aortic

arch, left atrium (LA) and mitral and aortic valves. Transesophageal echocardiography performed soon after symptom onset may identify a source of embolism in 30–45% of cases. It is considered to be an inappropriate test when there is a known CV source of embolus and the results would not change management
- **Neuroimaging studies** like CT, MRI and transcranial Doppler can help confirm or establish the vascular distribution of both clinically evident and subclinical ischemic lesions. Occlusion of a large- to medium-sized artery with an otherwise normal appearance of the parent vessel may suggest cardioembolic stroke versus stroke due to intrinsic atherosclerotic disease. Magnetic resonance imaging can provide evidence for cardioembolism by showing lesions not visible on CT and can reveal cortical involvement in strokes that seem to be single lesions on CT. Diffusion-weighted imaging can also identify lacunar infarctions associated with embolic source. The neuroimaging pattern of a cardioembolic source is typically a cortical or a cortical–subcortical pattern of ischemia on diffusion weighted imaging if acute
- **Carotid ultrasonography** identifies thrombus originating from the heart and occluding the internal carotid artery as oscillating and homogeneous echoes. The suspicion for an emboligenic source of a stroke increases if angiography or transcranial Doppler shows that the artery in the territory of the infarct is patent or if they show early recanalization of a previously occluded vessel. A saline bubble study during transcranial Doppler ultrasonography can also detect right to left shunting when intravenous (IV) microbubbles are detected as they pass through the middle cerebral artery segment.

Atrial Fibrillation (AF)

Atrial fibrillation is responsible for nearly half of all cardioembolic strokes. An estimated 2.7 million Americans, including approximately 8% of the population over 80 years of age, have AF ranking as the leading cardiac arrhythmia in the elderly. The risk of developing AF increases with age, and with the increase in the aging population, the overall burden of AF and consequently stroke from AF is expected to surge in the coming decades.

The risk of stroke among people with AF can be estimated by use of validated prediction instruments, such as the $CHADS_2$ or CHA_2DS_2-VASc scores (Table 21.1). The CHA_2DS_2-VASc score helps in identifying patients at very low risk (e.g. a CHA_2DS_2-VASc score of 0 is associated with a 0% risk of stroke). The 2014 American College of Cardiology/American Heart Association/Heart Rhythm Society (ACC/AHA/HRS) guidelines for the management of AF recommend using the CHA_2DS_2-VASc score for thromboembolic risk stratification in patients with nonvalvular AF. The risk of stroke increases from 0% per year (for 0 point) to 15.2% per year (for 9 points). However, both scoring systems underestimate stroke risk for patients with a recent transient ischemic attack (TIA) or ischemic stroke and no risk factors; since in this case, the risk of stroke may be closer to 7–10% per year.

Table 21.1: Comparison of the $CHADS_2$ and CHA_2DS_2-VASc risk stratification scores for subjects with nonvalvular atrial fibrillation

$CHADS_2$	Score	CHA_2DS_2-Vasc	Score
Congestive heart failure	1	Congestive heart failure	1
Hypertension	1	Hypertension	1
Age ≥75 years	1	Age ≥75 years	2
Diabetes mellitus	1	Diabetes mellitus	1
Stroke/TIA/TE	2	Stroke/TIA/TE	2
		Vascular disease*	1
		Age 65–74 years	1
		Female sex	1
$CHADS_2$	**Adjusted stroke rate (% per year)**	**CHA_2DS_2-Vasc**	**Adjusted stroke rate (% per year)**
0	1.9	0	0
1	2.8	1	1.3
2	4.0	2	2.2
3	5.9	3	3.2
4	8.5	4	4.0
5	12.5	5	6.7
6	18.2	6	9.8
		7	9.6
		8	6.7
		9	15.2

*Vascular disease is considered prior myocardial infarction, peripheral arterial disease of aortic plaque.

TIA, transient ischemic attack; TE, thromboembolism.

Source: Adapted from January CT, Wann LS, Alpert JS, Calkins H, Cleveland Jr JC, Cigarroa JE, et al. AHA/ACC/HRS Guideline for the management of patients with atrial fibrillation: executive summary. J Am Coll Cardiol. 2014, doi: 10.1016/j.jacc.2014.03.021.

Anticoagulation therapy has been shown to be very effective in prevention of first and recurrent stroke related to AF, with antiplatelet therapy relegated to a more limited role. Similar recommendations are applied to atrial flutter and AF for purposes of secondary prevention, with patients with atrial flutter often having intervals of AF, which is associated with an increased risk for sustained AF.

If not detected on routine physical examination or electrocardiogram (ECG), in patients with acute ischemic stroke or TIA without a known diagnosis of AF, new AF is detected in approximately 10% during their hospital admission. An additional 11% are diagnosed by continuous 30-day ECG monitoring with longer monitoring protocols yielding similar rates of detection. For patients who experience an acute ischemic stroke or TIA with no other apparent cause, prolonged rhythm monitoring for up to 30 days for AF is considered reasonable within 6 months of the index event.

Pooled data from five primary prevention trials demonstrated a relative risk (RR) reduction of 68% (95% CI, 50-79%) and an absolute reduction in annual stroke rate from 4.5% for control patients to 1.4% in patients assigned to adjusted dose warfarin in prevention of thromboembolic events among patients with nonvalvular AF. This indicates the prevention of 32 ischemic strokes per year for every 1,000 patients treated. The European Atrial Fibrillation Trial (EAFT) confirmed the effectiveness of warfarin for secondary prevention. The annual risk of stroke was reduced from 12% to 4% [hazard ratio (HR), 0.34; 95% CI, 0.20-0.57]. Warfarin use has been relatively safe with an annual rate of major bleeding of 1.3% in patients on warfarin compared with 1% for patients given placebo or aspirin. The optimal intensity of oral anticoagulation for stroke prevention in patients with AF is an international normalized ratio (INR) of 2.0-3.0. For patients with ischemic stroke or TIA with paroxysmal, persistent or permanent AF, a target INR of 2.5 (range, 2.0-3.0) is recommended. The efficacy of warfarin declines significantly below an INR of 2.0. For patients with AF who experience an ischemic event despite therapeutic anticoagulation, there is no evidence that increasing the intensity of anticoagulation confers additional protection against future ischemic events, with the risk of the intracranial hemorrhage increasing dramatically as INR increases above 4.0.

An estimated RR reduction of 21% compared with placebo (95% CI, 0-38%) was seen with aspirin use in a pooled analysis of data from three trials. Although aspirin 325 mg/day was used in the Stroke Prevention in Atrial Fibrillation (SPAF 1) Trial, 75-100 mg/day is considered to offer the best balance of efficacy and safety of aspirin. The addition of clopidogrel to aspirin appears to confer additional protection, although with an increased risk of bleeding. The Atrial Fibrillation Clopidogrel Trial with Irbesartan for Prevention of Vascular Events (ACTIVE A) study compared aspirin against clopidogrel plus aspirin in 7,550 AF patients for whom vitamin K-antagonist (VKA) therapy was unsuitable. Stroke rate was reduced from 3.3% per year in the aspirin alone group compared to 2.4% per year for the combination therapy group (RR, 0.72; 95% CI, 0.62-0.83; $p < 0.001$) after a median of 3.6 years of follow-up. Major bleeding occurred in 2.0% per year with combination therapy compared to 1.3% per year with aspirin alone (RR, 1.57; 95% CI, 1.29-1.92; $p < 0.001$).

Antiplatelet therapy is less effective compared to warfarin for primary stroke prevention. ACTIVE W that evaluated the safety and efficacy of combination of clopidogrel and aspirin versus warfarin in AF patients with at least one risk factor for stroke was stopped prematurely because of clear superiority of warfarin (with goal INR 2.0-3.0) over the antiplatelet combination (RR, 1.44; 95% CI, 1.18-1.76; $p = 0.0003$).

In response to challenges with warfarin therapy with its narrow therapeutic margin and several drug or food interactions, several new oral anticoagulants have been developed. Dabigatran was the first direct thrombin inhibitor to be approved for treatment of AF in the United States. In the RE-LY(Randomized Evaluation of Long-Term Anticoagulation Therapy) trial in which >18,000 AF patients with at least one additional risk factor were randomized to dabigatran 150 mg twice daily, dabigatran 110 mg twice daily or open-label warfarin, both doses of dabigatran were noninferior to warfarin. The annual rate of stroke or systemic embolism was 1.7% in the warfarin group compared with 1.1% in the dabigatran 150 mg group (RR, 0.65; 95% CI, 0.52-0.81; $p < 0.001$). The RR for stroke or systemic embolism was nonsignificantly reduced for dabigatran 100 mg twice daily (RR, 0.84; 95% CI, 0.58-1.20) and dabigatran 150 mg twice daily (RR, 0.75; 95% CI, 0.52-1.08) compared to warfarin in a subgroup of patients with prior stroke or TIA. Dabigatran use is recommended for primary and secondary prevention of stroke in patients with nonvalvular AF.

In the ROCKET AF Trial (Rivaroxaban Once Daily Oral Direct Factor Xa Inhibition Compared With Vitamin K Antagonism for Prevention of Stroke and Embolism Trial in Atrial Fibrillation) rivaroxaban 20 mg/day was compared with adjusted dose warfarin. The primary end point of stroke or systemic embolism occurred in 269 patients assigned to the rivaroxaban group compared with 306 patients assigned to warfarin (HR with rivaroxaban, 0.88; 95% CI, 0.74-1.03; $p<0.001$ for noninferiority, $p=0.12$ for superiority) in the intention to treat analysis. Similar results were seen in patients with a prior stroke or TIA in a subgroup analysis (HR with rivaroxaban among patients with prior stroke or TIA, 0.77; 95% CI, 0.58-1.01). Rivoraxaban is recommended for use in patients with patients with nonvalvular AF for primary prevention when oral anticoagulation therapy is indicated. The 2014 stroke guidelines indicate rivaroxaban may be reasonable for use in prevention of recurrent stroke in patients with nonvalvular AF.

In the Apixaban for Reduction in Stroke and Other Thromboembolic Events in Atrial Fibrillation (ARISTOTLE) trial in which patients with nonvalvular AF and at least one other risk factor were randomized to apixaban 5 mg twice daily or adjusted dose warfarin, the primary outcome of ischemic stroke, hemorrhagic stroke or systemic embolism occurred in 212 patients assigned to apixaban (RR 0.79; 95% CI, 0.66-0.95; $p<0.001$ for noninferiority and $p = 0.01$ for superiority). Apixaban use is recommended for primary and secondary prevention of stroke in patients with nonvalvular AF.

Dose adjustments need to be made in patients with renal insufficiency with the use of the newer anticoagulants.

Guidelines indicate that it is reasonable to initiate oral anticoagulation within 14 days after the onset of neurological symptoms for most patients with a stroke or TIA in the setting of AF. However, it is reasonable to delay initiation of oral anticoagulation beyond 14 days in patients at high risk for hemorrhagic conversion (e.g. large infarct, hemorrhagic transformation on initial imaging, uncontrolled hypertension or hemorrhage tendency).

The usefulness of closure of the LA appendage with the WATCHMAN (LA appendage occlusion) device in patients with ischemic stroke or TIA and AF is uncertain at this time.

For patients with AF and a history of stroke or TIA who require temporary interruption of oral anticoagulation (especially in patients with CHADS$_2$ score of 5 or 6, stroke or TIA within 3 months or rheumatic valvular disease), bridging therapy with a low molecular weight heparin (LMWH) or unfractionated heparin is considered reasonable, depending on perceived risk for thromboembolism and bleeding.

Acute Myocardial Infarction (MI) and Left Ventricular (LV) Thrombus

With the current standard of care in patients presenting with large anterior MI, the incidence of mural thrombus has decreased and is approximately 15%, compared to 20–50% seen previously, with most thrombi occurring in patients with anterior ST segment elevation MI (STEMI) and an LV ejection Fraction <40%. The risk of embolization is considered 10–20% in patients with MI complicated by mural thrombus within 3 months in the absence of systemic anticoagulation. The risk of thrombus formation and embolization after a large MI appears to be highest during the first 1–2 weeks with a subsequent decline over a period of 3 months, with the thrombus becoming more organized, fibrotic and adherent to LV wall as time progresses.

Current guidelines indicate warfarin may be used in patients with STEMI and asymptomatic LV thrombus. The current stroke guidelines recommend the use of warfarin (target INR, 2.5; range, 2.0-3.0) in most patients with ischemic stroke or TIA in the setting of acute MI complicated by LV thrombus formation for 3 months. It is considered reasonable to start anticoagulation in patients with ischemic stroke or TIA in the setting of acute anterior STEMI without demonstrable LV mural thrombus formation but with anterior apical akinesis or dyskinesis for 3 months. In patients with ischemic stroke or TIA in the setting of acute MI complicated by LV mural thrombus formation or anterior or apical wall-motion abnormalities with an LV ejection fraction <40% who are intolerant to warfarin therapy because of nonhemorrhagic adverse events, treatment with a LMWH, dabigatran, rivaroxaban or apixaban for 3 months may be considered as an alternative to warfarin therapy for prevention of recurrent stroke or TIA.

Cardiomyopathy

The incidence of stroke is inversely proportional to LV ejection fraction. In patients with sinus rhythm and LV ejection fraction ≤35%, there is an increased rate of thromboembolic events ranging from 1.7% to 3.9% without antithrombotic therapy. Stroke rates are higher in patients with prior stroke or TIA, lower ejection fraction, LV noncompaction and peripartum cardiomyopathy. In the WARCEF (Warfarin vs. Aspirin in Reduced Cardiac Ejection Fraction) study that compared 2,305 patients with sinus rhythm, heart failure and an LV ejection fraction ≤35% randomized to aspirin 325 mg/day or warfarin with a target INR of 2.0-3.5, warfarin was associated with a reduced risk of ischemic stroke (0.72 vs. 1.36 per 100 patient-years; HR, 0.52; 95% CI, 0.33–0.82; p=0.005), albeit with an increase in the risk of major bleeding. Among patients with heart failure and sinus rhythm enrolled in four trials comparing warfarin versus aspirin, warfarin was associated with a reduced risk of ischemic stroke (RR, 0.45; 95% CI,0.24–0.86). In patients with ischemic stroke or TIA in sinus rhythm who have LA or LV thrombus, anticoagulation with warfarin is recommended for $\geq$3 months.

Patients with restrictive cardiomyopathies have an increased risk of stroke and arterial embolization attributable to LA appendage or LV mural thrombus. Systemic anticoagulation is recommended in patients with restrictive cardiomyopathy and evidence of LA or LV thrombus or history of arterial embolization.

In patients with ischemic stroke or TIA in sinus rhythm with dilated or restrictive cardiomyopathy without evidence of LA or LV thrombus, the effectiveness of anticoagulation compared with antiplatelet therapy is uncertain.

Mechanical LV assist devices (LVAD) are associated with nonhemorrhagic cerebrovascular infarction rates of 4–9% per year and the risk increases two- to threefold in patients with prior stroke or postoperative infections. Routine anticoagulation with warfarin and antiplatelet agents is recommended after LVAD implantation. In the absence of major contraindications, warfarin therapy (target INR, 2.5; range, 2.0–3.0) is considered reasonable in patients with a LVAD who have had an ischemic stroke or TIA.

Because of the paucity of data, the role of newer anticoagulation agents in the above circumstances is still considered uncertain.

Native Valvular Heart Disease

Atrial fibrillation, older age, LA enlargement, reduced cardiac output and prior embolic event are associated with increased stroke risk in patients with mitral stenosis. There is wide agreement that anticoagulation is indicated in mitral stenosis complicated by AF, prior embolism or LA thrombus. It is controversial as to whether long-term anticoagulation should be given to patients with mitral stenosis in normal sinus on the basis of LA enlargement or spontaneous contrast.

Mitral regurgitation is not associated with a significant increase in risk for first or recurrent stroke in the absence of AF.

In patients with ischemic stroke or TIA who have rheumatic mitral valve disease without atrial fibrillation or another likely cause of their symptoms, long-term warfarin therapy may be considered instead of antiplatelet therapy. In patients with rheumatic valve disease who have an ischemic stroke or TIA while being treated with adequate VKA therapy, the addition of aspirin might be considered.

In light of emerging newer data, the risk for stroke in patients with mitral valve prolapse is low (i.e. <1% annually). In patients with mitral valve prolapse who have had an ischemic stroke or TIA and who do not have AF or another indication for anticoagulation, antiplatelet therapy is recommended.

Mitral annular calcification affects women more than men and is associated with increasing age and other CV risk factors. In an analysis of patients in the Framingham Heart Study with ischemic stroke, the association with mitral annular calcification was only marginally significant (adjusted RR, 1.78; 95% CI, 1.00–3.16).

Aortic regurgitation and aortic stenosis are not known to be associated with increased risk for first or recurrent stroke in patients who are free of AF or associated mitral valve disease.

Prosthetic Valves

Patients with mechanical heart valves are at an increased risk for thromboembolic events, with the risk varying depending on the type of mechanical valve, location of the valve and other risk factors of embolism.

Current guidelines recommend anticoagulation with a VKA to achieve an INR of 2.5 (range, 2.0–3.0) in patients with a mechanical aortic valve prosthesis (such as bileaflet or Medtronic Hall single tilting disk) and no risk factors for thromboembolism. An INR goal of 3.0 (range, 2.5–3.5) is recommended when there are additional risk factors for thromboembolic events (i.e. AF, previous thromboembolism, LV dysfunction or hypercoagulable conditions) or an older-generation mechanical aortic prosthesis (e.g. ball-in-cage style or older single disc valves). The current stroke guidelines recommend warfarin therapy with an INR target of 2.5 (range, 2.0–3.0) for patients with a mechanical aortic valve prosthesis and a history of ischemic stroke or TIA before its insertion.

For patients with a mechanical *mitral* valve prosthesis and a history of ischemic stroke or TIA before its insertion, the recommended INR target is 3 (range, 2.5–3.5).

The addition of aspirin 75–100 mg/day to warfarin therapy is recommended for patients with a mechanical mitral or aortic valve prosthesis with a history of prior stroke who are at a low risk of bleeding. Increasing the dose of aspirin to 325 mg/day is considered reasonable for patients with mechanical valves who have an ischemic stroke or systemic embolism despite adequate antithrombotic therapy with a VKA and low strength aspirin. Anticoagulant therapy with oral direct thrombin inhibitors or anti-Xa agents should not be used in patients with a mechanical valve prosthesis since they have not been approved for this indication by the US Food and Drug Administration.

Bioprosthetic valves are associated with a lower rate of thromboembolism than mechanical valves. For long-term protection in patients with sinus rhythm, antiplatelet therapy is recommended. Patients who have a thromboembolic stroke after placement of a bioprosthetic valve may be at increased risk for recurrence with the annual risk for a second event being around 5%. For patients with a bioprosthetic aortic or mitral valve, a history of ischemic stroke or TIA before its insertion and no other indication for anticoagulation therapy beyond 3–6 months from the valve placement, long-term therapy with aspirin 75–100 mg/day is recommended in preference to long-term anticoagulation. For patients who have a TIA, ischemic stroke or systemic embolism despite adequate antiplatelet therapy, the addition of warfarin therapy with an INR target of 2.5 (range, 2.0–3.0) is considered reasonable.

Aortic Arch Atheroma

Atherosclerotic plaque ≥4 mm is considered an independent risk factor for recurrent stroke. In the French Study of Aortic Plaques in Stroke, aortic wall thickness including plaque ≥4 mm in the aortic arch proximal to the ostium of the left subclavian artery was an independent predictor of recurrent brain infarction (RR, 3.8; 95% CI, 1.8–7.8; $p = 0.0012$). Risk was higher if atheroma was detected in the arch. Aortic arch plaque progression is independently associated with an increased risk of stroke. Plaque morphology particularly lack of calcification may increase the risk of subsequent vascular events. Current guidelines recommend antiplatelet therapy and statin therapy in patients with an ischemic stroke or TIA and evidence of aortic arch atheroma. The role of warfarin therapy in such cases is unclear. The Aortic Arch Related Cerebral Hazard (ARCH) trial that has recently completed enrollment will study warfarin versus aspirin/clopidogrel in patients with atherothrombosis of the aortic arch and a recent cerebral or peripheral embolic event.

Patent Foramen Ovale (PFO)

Patent foramen ovale can be detected in 15–25% of the adult population. Atrial septal aneurysms are detected in 0.2–4.0% of patients examined with TEE. The association between PFO and increased risk for stroke is stronger in younger patients than in older patients. There is little and conflicting evidence regarding the role of the size of the PFO and role of atrial septal aneurysm in predicting high risk for recurrence among patients with PFO and cryptogenic stroke. There are no trials assessing whether persons found to have a PFO not associated with cerebrovascular symptoms benefit from specific medical or interventional treatments. Screening for PFO in the absence of neurological conditions is not recommended. For patients with an ischemic stroke or TIA and a PFO, who are not candidates for anticoagulation therapy, antiplatelet therapy is recommended. For patients with an ischemic stroke or TIA, and both a PFO and venous source of embolism [e.g. lower extremity deep venous thrombosis (DVT)], anticoagulation is indicated depending on stroke characteristics. If anticoagulation is contraindicated, an inferior vena cava filter is considered reasonable.

Patent foramen ovale closure is not indicated for patients with a cryptogenic ischemic stroke or TIA without evidence for DVT. In the setting of PFO and DVT, PFO closure by a transcatheter device might be considered depending on the risk of recurrent DVT.

Endocarditis

Infective and noninfective endocarditis can cause stroke. Approximately 15–35% of all patients with infective endocarditis develop clinically evident systemic emboli with the most common cause being a septic embolus resulting in ischemia often followed by hemorrhagic transformation with the risk of hemorrhagic transformation increased by anticoagulant therapy. The management of endocarditis is directed at initiating appropriate antibiotic therapy with guidance from antibiotic sensitivity data and infectious disease consultants.

The beneficial or deleterious effect of anticoagulation in patients with endocarditis is determined by clinical, bacteriologic, radiological and echocardiographic variables to strike a balance of the risk toward early recurrent stroke or intracranial hemorrhage. Current guidelines recommend that it is reasonable to temporarily discontinue anticoagulation in patients with infective endocarditis who develop central nervous system symptoms compatible with embolism or stroke irrespective of indications for anticoagulation, given the increased risk of hemorrhagic conversion. Patients on chronic oral anticoagulation could be changed to IV heparin since it is reversible with protamine if central nervous system symptoms develop.

Noninfective endocarditis can complicate systemic cancer, systemic lupus erythematosus and the antiphospholipid syndrome. Although direct evidence is lacking, antiplatelet therapy for primary prevention or anticoagulation for secondary prevention is considered reasonable.

Cardiac Masses

Atrial myxoma, a tumor of the mesenchymal cells of the heart, is a rare cause of cardioembolic stroke. It is seen more often in younger patients with stroke or TIA (1 in 250) than in older patients (1 in 750). They are usually detected on echocardiography and maybe present even without hearing a diastolic murmur or a tumor flop on auscultation. Papillary fibroelastoma is a rare cause of stroke that is also detected on echocardiography. In such cases, the ongoing risk of embolization may warrant surgical resection.

SUGGESTED READING

1. Arboix A, Alio J. Cardioembolic stroke: clinical features, specific cardiac disorders and prognosis. Curr Cardiol Rev. 2010;6(3):150-61.
2. Connolly ES Jr, Rabinstein AA, Carhuapoma JR, Derdeyn CP, Dion J, Higashida RT, et al. Guidelines for the management of aneurysmal subarachnoid hemorrhage: a guideline for healthcare professionals from the American Heart Association/American Stroke Association. Stroke. 2012;43(6):1711-37.
3. Ferro JM. Cardioembolic stroke: an update. Lancet Neurol. 2003;2(3):177-88.
4. Freeman WD, Aguilar MI. Prevention of cardioembolic stroke. Neurotherapeutics. 2011;8(3):488-502.
5. January CT, Wann LS, Alpert JS, Calkins H, Cleveland Jr JC, Cigarroa JE, et al. AHA/ACC/HRS Guideline for the management of patients with atrial fibrillation: executive summary. J Am Coll Cardiol. 2014, doi: 10.1016/j.jacc.2014.03.021.
6. Kernan WN, Ovbiagele B, Black HR, Bravata DM, Chimowitz MI, Ezekowitz MD, et al. Guidelines for the prevention of stroke in patients with stroke and transient ischemic attack: a guideline for healthcare professionals from the American Heart Association/American Stroke Association. Stroke. 2014;45:2160-236.

7. Kim AS. Evaluation and prevention of cardioembolic stroke. Continuum (Minneap Minn). 2014;20(2 Cerebrovascular Disease):309-22.
8. O'Gara PT, Kushner FG, Ascheim DD, Casey DE Jr, Chung MK, de Lemos JA, et al. ACCF/AHA guideline for the management of ST-elevation myocardial infarction: a report of the American College of Cardiology Foundation/American Heart Association task force on practice guidelines. J Am Coll Cardiol. 2013;61:e78-140.
9. Nishimura RA, Otto CM, Bonow RO, Carabello BA, Erwin JP III, Guyton RA, et al. AHA/ACC guideline for the management of patients with valvular heart disease: a report of the American College of Cardiology/American Heart Association Task Force on Practice Guidelines. J Am Coll Cardiol. 2014;63:e57-185.
10. Whitlock RP, Sun JC, Fremes SE, Rubens FD, Teoh KH. Antithrombotic and thrombolytic therapy for valvular disease: Antithrombotic therapy and prevention of thrombosis, 9th edition. American College of Chest Physicians Evidence-Based Clinical Practice Guidelines. Chest. 2012;141:e576S-600S.

Assessment of the Cardiac Patient for Noncardiac Surgery

22

Chapter

Nathan Funk

INTRODUCTION

Cardiac complications of noncardiac surgery are of great importance to surgeons and cardiovascular (CV) specialists. It is estimated that 27 million noncardiac procedures are performed annually in the United States. Major adverse cardiac events complicate approximately 1.5% of noncardiac surgeries. The same risk of complication is not shared by all patients, and it is the role of the CV specialist to identify CV risk and make all attempts to limit its effects in the perioperative period.

CARDIOVASCULAR RISK AND NONCARDIAC SURGERY

The goal of assessing CV risk preoperatively is to assist the patient in making an informed decision regarding his or her individual risk for surgery and to communicate to the surgeon the patient's risk of cardiac complications that may affect management. Given the history, physical examination and electrocardiogram (ECG), the general cardiac risk of a surgical patient can readily be estimated.

Current guidelines recommend a stepwise approach in the assessment of risk of perioperative cardiac events (Fig. 22.1). Emergent surgeries carry a high perioperative CV risk regardless of preoperative patient comorbidities. If patients have active cardiac conditions (e.g. unstable coronary syndromes, decompensated heart failure, significant arrhythmia or severe valvular disease), they are at high risk of cardiac complication and require appropriate attention to their underlying cardiac problem prior to elective operation (Table 22.1). Preoperative evaluation may require coronary angiography to assess further therapeutic options. If the surgery is low risk (Table 22.2), patients with clinical risk factors have a low rate of cardiac complications (i.e. <1%) stemming from the procedure and therefore can proceed without further workup. In patients with excess risk >1%, functional capacity is a strong predictor of perioperative events. If the patient has at least moderate functional capacity (i.e. can complete >4 METs of activity, equivalent to walking up a flight of stairs with groceries), further clinical or diagnostic risk assessment is unlikely to add more information.

While numerous clinical risk algorithms have been developed over the years, the Revised Cardiac Risk Index (RCRI) proposed by Lee et al.

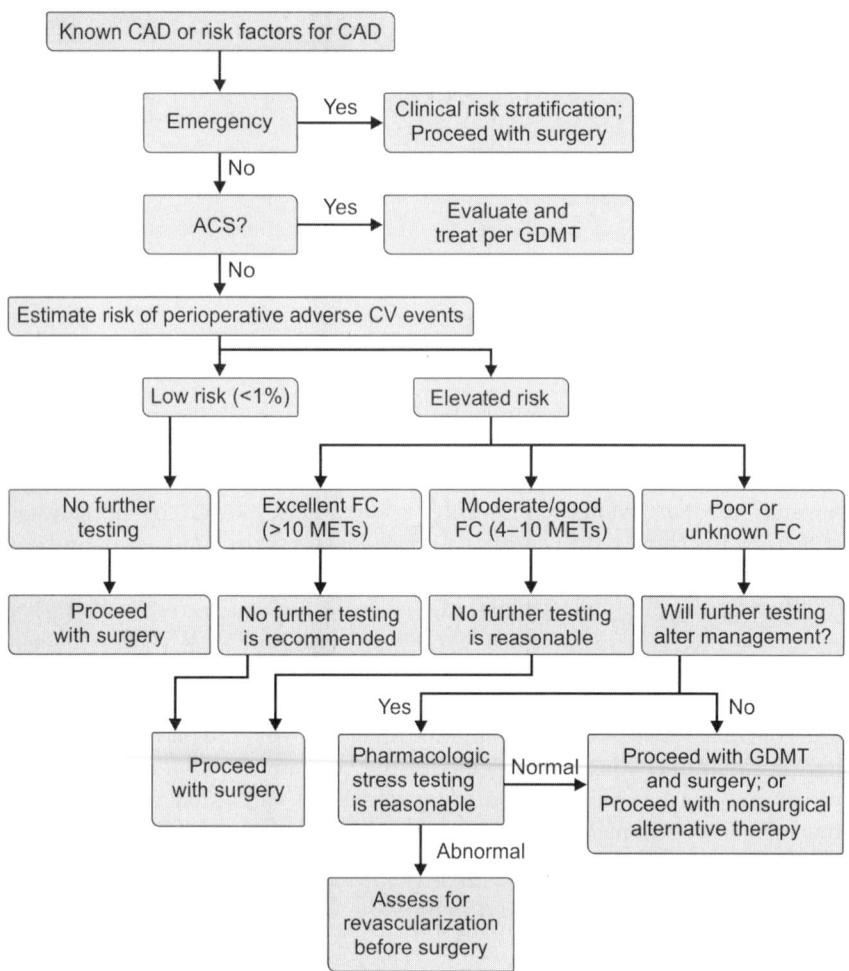

Fig. 22.1: Algorithm for determining which patients are candidates for cardiac testing.

ACS, acute coronary syndrome; CAD, coronary artery disease; CV, cardiovascular; FC, functional capacity; GDMT, guideline directed medical therapy.

Source: Adapted from Fleisher LA, Fleischmann KE, Auerbach AD, Barnason SA, Beckman JA, Bozkurt B, et al. 2014 ACC/AHA guideline on perioperative cardiovascular evaluation and management of patients undergoing noncardiac surgery: a report of the American College of Cardiology/American Heart Association Task Force on practice guideline. J Am Coll Cardiol. 2014;64(22):e77-137. doi: 10.1016/j.jacc.2014.07.944.

is the most widely used for elective noncardiac surgery (Table 22.3). This simple index assigns one point for each of six independent risk factors. As the number of risk factors increase, the risk of a major perioperative event increases. Later validation cohorts have confirmed the predictive ability of the RCRI model although showing higher levels of risk with increasing number of risk factors than originally described. In addition to the risk factors in the RCRI, comorbid conditions (e.g. tobacco abuse, advanced age, pulmonary hypertension, anemia, obstructive or restrictive lung disease or obstructive sleep apnea) may also increase the risk of cardiac and noncardiac perioperative complications.

Table 22.1: Active cardiac conditions for which the patient should undergo evaluation and treatment before noncardiac surgery

Condition	Examples
Unstable coronary syndromes	Unstable or severe angina (CCS class III or IV)*
	Recent MI†
Decompensated HF (NYHA functional class IV; worsening or new-onset HF)	
Significant arrhythmias	High-grade atrioventricular block
	Mobitz II atrioventricular block
	Third-degree atrioventricular heart block
	Symptomatic ventricular arrhythmias
	Supraventricular arrhythmias (including atrial fibrillation) with uncontrolled ventricular rate (HR >100 bpm at rest)
	Symptomatic bradycardia
	Newly recognized ventricular tachycardia
Severe valvular disease	Severe aortic stenosis (mean pressure gradient >40 mm Hg, aortic valve area <1.0 cm² or symptomatic)
	Symptomatic mitral stenosis (progressive dyspnea on exertion, exertional presyncope or HF)

*May include "stable" angina in patients who are unusually sedentary.

†The American College of Cardiology National Database Library defines recent MI as >7 days but within 30 days.

CCS, Canadian Cardiovascular Society; HF, heart failure; HR, heart rate; MI, myocardial infarction; NYHA, New York Heart Association.

Source: Adapted from Fleisher LA, Beckman JA, Brown KA, Calkins H, Chaikof EL, Fleischmann KE, et al. 2009 ACCF/AHA focused update on perioperative beta blockade incorporated into the ACC/AHA 2007 guidelines on perioperative cardiovascular evaluation and care for noncardiac surgery. Circulation. 2009;120(21): e169-276.

The clinical risk factors of patients with poor functional status undergoing intermediate to high-risk surgical procedures can be used to determine whether further risk stratification is warranted. In those with no clinical risk factors, further diagnostic testing is unnecessary and the patient can proceed to surgery. In those with clinical risk factors undergoing intermediate to high-risk surgery, one can consider further testing if the potential findings will change management. A change in management may include coronary revascularization, type of anesthesia used, extent of hemodynamic monitoring intra- and postoperative, the postoperative care setting or in the extreme circumstance, whether the procedure is performed at all.

PREOPERATIVE CARDIAC DIAGNOSTIC TESTING

The goal of preoperative diagnostic testing is to investigate symptomatic patients presenting for preoperative evaluation and/or to further risk

Table 22.2: Cardiac risk stratification for noncardiac surgical procedures

Risk stratification	Procedure examples
Vascular (reported cardiac risk* often >5%)	Aortic and other major vascular surgery
	Peripheral vascular surgery
Intermediate (reported cardiac risk generally 1–5%)	Intraperitoneal and intrathoracic surgery
	Carotid endarterectomy
	Head and neck surgery
	Orthopedic surgery
	Prostate surgery
Low† (reported cardiac risk generally <1%)	Endoscopic procedures
	Superficial procedure
	Cataract surgery
	Breast surgery
	Ambulatory surgery

*Combined incidence of cardiac death and nonfatal myocardial infarction.

†These procedures do not generally require further preoperative cardiac testing.

Source: Adapted from Fleisher LA, Beckman JA, Brown KA, Calkins H, Chaikof EL, Fleischmann KE, et al. 2009 ACCF/AHA focused update on perioperative beta blockade incorporated into the ACC/AHA 2007 guidelines on perioperative cardiovascular evaluation and care for noncardiac surgery. Circulation. 2009;120(21): e169-276.

Table 22.3: Estimated risk of a major perioperative cardiac event* based on predictors in the Lee (Revised Cardiac Risk) Index

Risk factors

- High-risk surgery (intraperitoneal, intrathoracic or suprainguinal vascular surgery)
- History of ischemic heart disease (defined as a history of myocardial infarction, positive exercise test result, current complaint of ischemic chest pain or nitrate use, or electrocardiogram showing pathologic Q waves; patients who had undergone prior coronary bypass surgery or angioplasty were included only if they had such findings after their procedure)
- History of congestive heart failure (defined as a history of heart failure, pulmonary edema or paroxysmal nocturnal dyspnea; an S3 gallop or bilateral rales on physical examination; or chest radiograph showing pulmonary vascular edema)
- History of cerebrovascular disease (stroke or transient ischemic attack)
- Use of insulin therapy for diabetes
- Preoperative serum creatinine level >2.0 mg/dL

No. of risk factors	Risk of major perioperative cardiac event, % (95% CI)
0	0.4 (0.1–0.8)
1	1.0 (0.5–1.4)
2	2.4 (1.3–3.5)
≥3	5.4 (2.8–7.9)

*Includes cardiac death, nonfatal myocardial infarction and nonfatal cardiac arrest. Not included in this table are postoperative cardiogenic pulmonary edema and complete heart block, which are included as outcomes in the Lee index. CI: confidence interval.

Source: Adapted from Devereaux PJ, Goldman L, Cook DJ, et al. Perioperative cardiac events in patients undergoing noncardiac surgery: a review of the magnitude of the problem, the pathophysiology of the events and methods to estimate and communicate risk. CMAJ. 2005;173(6):627-34.

stratify those with poor functional status and clinical risk factors planning to undergo intermediate to high-risk procedures. The routine use of echocardiography in low-risk or asymptomatic patients is not recommended. If patients present to the preoperative evaluation with cardiac symptoms, it is appropriate to investigate the underlying cause with ECG, echocardiogram or other diagnostic workup as needed prior to their procedure. An ECG is recommended in those with prior CV disease and/or those undergoing high-risk procedures.

Exercise treadmill testing has the capacity to provide useful information regarding patient function and ischemic threshold and severity. The target heart rate achieved (i.e. ≥85% maximum predicted heart rate) and the level of maximal oxygen uptake appear to be important predictors of perioperative events. While exercise treadmill testing can be useful when the patient history is in doubt, it is unlikely to add more information than self-reported exertional tolerance if the patient can perform ≥4 METs.

The addition of imaging to stress testing with either myocardial perfusion imaging (MPI) or dobutamine stress echocardiography (DSE) has the ability to further risk stratify patients with intermediate to high clinical risk undergoing intermediate to high-risk surgical procedures. Eagle et al. at the University of Michigan were able to show that in clinically intermediate risk patients, nuclear perfusion scanning resulted in successful reclassification of intermediate patients into either high- or low risk groups. The largest benefit in MPI studies is in its negative predictive value. In the above mentioned trial, patients with 1-2 clinical risk factors who had a negative MPI study had event rates similar to those with no risk factors. Most observational trials suggest that the negative predictive value of MPI is 96-100%. Dobutamine stress echocardiography shares similar benefit in reclassifying intermediate risk patients into high or low cardiac risk. The difficulty with either MPI or DSE is determining how to manage a patient with a positive test as the positive predictive value for perioperative events is low, approximately 10-20%. For patients who are at an elevated risk for noncardiac surgery, noninvasive pharmacologic stress testing is indicated if it will impact further decision making or perioperative care.

PREOPERATIVE ASSESSMENT OF PATIENTS WITH VALVULAR HEART DISEASE

If aortic stenosis is symptomatic, elective noncardiac surgery should generally be cancelled or postponed, because of increased mortality risk of about 10%. If elective surgery is not urgent, surgery can be performed after aortic valve replacement. If noncardiac surgery cannot be delayed to allow aortic valve replacement, percutaneous balloon valvuloplasty is an option to bridge the patient through noncardiac surgery until elective valve replacement can be performed. There are no data for the efficacy or safety of transcutaneous aortic valve replacement for patients with aortic stenosis undergoing noncardiac surgery. If aortic stenosis is severe, but not symptomatic, reevaluation of stenosis severity should be performed prior to surgery unless Doppler has been performed within 1 year of surgery.

Elevated risk elective noncardiac surgery with appropriate intraoperative and postoperative hemodynamic monitoring is reasonable in the following patients:
- Asymptomatic severe aortic stenosis
- Asymptomatic severe aortic regurgitation with a normal left ventricular ejection fraction
- Asymptomatic severe mitral regurgitation
- Asymptomatic severe mitral stenosis if valve morphology is not favorable for percutaneous mitral balloon commissurotomy.

REVASCULARIZATION AND NONCARDIAC SURGERY

Revascularization prior to noncardiac surgery may include coronary artery bypass grafting (CABG) or percutaneous coronary intervention (PCI). The indication for revascularization prior to noncardiac surgery has undergone revision over the past 10 years. The evidence for CABG prior to noncardiac surgery comes primarily from observational cohort studies. Considering the long-term mortality benefit from CABG for standard indications of surgical revascularization (i.e left main stenosis, three-vessel obstructive disease, two-vessel obstructive disease, including the proximal left anterior descending arter, or high risk features, such as muli-vessel disease in diabetics), surgical revascularization is generally recommended prior to non-cardiac surgery. However, the indication for PCI prior to noncardiac surgery is not as clear. The Coronary Artery Revascularization Prophylaxis (CARP) trial assessed patients who had angiographic stenosis of >70% in one or more coronary arteries prior to vascular surgery. They were randomized to medical management or revascularization (41% CABG and 59% PCI). Outcomes over 2.7 years of follow-up showed that there was no difference in mortality between the two groups. In addition, it is worth noting that perioperative elevations in myocardial enzymes were not different between the two groups. The ACC/AHA guidelines therefore do not recommend routine coronary revascularization for stable coronary artery disease (CAD) prior to noncardiac surgery. Patients with unstable coronary syndromes, non-ST elevation myocardial infarction (MI, or ST elevation MI should undergo revascularization prior to noncardiac surgery in accord with current guidelines.

PERIOPERATIVE MANAGEMENT OF CORONARY STENTS

If revascularization has been performed for any reason prior to noncardiac surgery, it is advisable to delay elective surgery at least 4-6 weeks with bare metal stenting (BMS) or 12 months with drug-eluting stent (DES) while being treated with aspirin and a thienopyridine. Not infrequently, issues arise regarding risk for in-stent thrombosis when a BMS or DES has been placed and urgent or emergent surgery is required. Only retrospective data are available for risk estimates of in-stent thrombosis. Premature discontinuation of thienopyridines is the greatest risk. Other risks include renal failure, bifurcating lesions, diabetes melliturs, and lower ejection fraction. In addition, vigilance for in-stent thrombosis should be maintained in those with high consequence for in-stent thrombosis, such as left main PCI, multivessel PC, or prior stent placement in the only remaining artery or bypass graft.

The risk associated with a short course of thienopyridine discontinuation such as for surgery is unknown; however, the risk is felt to be high and not recommended. The premature discontinuation of thienopyridine therapy is associated with a marked increase in the risk of stent thrombosis and is the leading independent predictor for stent thrombosis in multivariate analyses. Although the number of actual stent thromboses reported in individual studies is modest, the findings are noteworthy. In a large observational cohort study of patients treated with DES, stent thrombosis occurred in a striking 29% of patients in whom antiplatelet therapy was discontinued prematurely. In a single-site study of 652 patients treated with sirolimus DES, premature discontinuation of clopidogrel was associated with an approximately~30-fold greater risk of stent thrombosis, with >25% of patients who discontinued clopidogrel therapy within the first month suffering stent thrombosis. In another study of 1911 consecutive patients with DES followed up for a median of 19.4 months, 5 (7.8%) of 64 patients with premature interruption of aspirin, clopidogre, or both experienced stent thrombosis. In an analysis from the PREMIER (Prospective Registry Evaluating Myocardial Infarction: Events and Recovery) registry of 500 patients with acute MI treated with DES, the mortality rate over the next 11 months of those who stopped thienopyridine therapy was 7.5% compared with 0.7% in those who had not stopped therapy. Although the rates of stent thrombosis were not reported, it is reasonable to presume that many of the deaths were related to CAD.

As there are emerging data to suggest that the risk of stent thrombosis in the newer-generation DES stabilizes after 6 months, elective noncardiac surgery after drug-eluting stent implantation may be considered after 180 days if the risk of further delay is greater than the expected risks of ischemia and stent thrombosis. If the thienopyridine is discontinued, it is recommended to continue aspirin if possible and restart the thienopyridine as soon as possible after surgery.

The use of short-acting antithrombotic agents (e.g. glycoprotein IIb/IIIa inhibitors and heparin) is not advised in patients who require temporary interruption of anti-platelet agents.

In patients on aspirin for secondary CV prevention, its use in the perioperative period may be a source of concern for surgeons. A meta-analysis by Burger et al. showed that aspirin continuation during noncardiac surgery increased bleeding with a relative risk of 1.5. However, this did not lead to a higher level of bleeding severity with the exception of intracranial and prostate surgeries. They also demonstrated that approximately 10% of acute coronary syndrome presentations are the result of aspirin withdrawal.

Therefore, stopping aspirin in the perioperative period is not without risk and each surgical case must balance the risks and benefits of continuing versus stopping aspirin. Patients with coronary artery or other CV disease, who may be considered at moderate-to-high risk for perioperative adverse CV events, may benefit from perioperative continuation of aspirin. Such moderate-to-high-risk patients include those with ischemic heart disease, compensated or prior congestive heart failure, diabetes mellitus, renal insufficiency, or cerebrovascular disease. In addition, patients undergoing selected types of surgery associated with an increased risk for perioperative cardiovascular events, such as carotid endarterectomy and peripheral artery bypass surgery, may also benefit from perioperative continuation of aspirin. In patients considered at low risk for CV events in which there is likely to be fewer potential benefits of perioperative continuation of aspirin, interruption of aspirin may be reasonable.

PERIOPERATIVE BETABLOCKADE

Tachycardia is a predictor of postoperative myocardial ischemia, troponin T release, and long-term mortality. Beta-blockade may have other beneficial effects for arrhythmia prevention, reduction of myocardial oxygen demand, prolonged diastolic coronary filling and protection from acute plaque rupture during the increased stress of surgery. In addition, it has been shown that a β-blocker withdrawal in the perioperative period is harmful. It is, therefore, hypothesized that a β-blockade may improve surgical outcomes in noncardiac surgery. Multiple studies have attempted to reach this end with mixed results.

The POISE trial is the largest to date, which randomized 8,351 patients at risk for atherosclerotic disease to long-acting metoprolol or placebo on the day of surgery and continued this for 30 days. They showed a decrease in CV outcomes at the expense of an increase in overall mortality and an increase in the risk of cerebrovascular events. Criticisms of this study include a fixed dosing regimen without heart rate titration in advance of surgery. This one trial dominates all meta-analyses looking at the effectiveness of perioperative β-blockade.

Data in favor of β-blockade come from large retrospective cohorts that demonstrated increasing benefit with higher RCRI risk (≥3 factors) and possible harm at lower levels of risk. The DECREASE trials demonstrated benefit, but the accuracy of the data has been questioned.

In conclusion, it is not recommended to withdraw β-blockade in the perioperative period or to start β-blockade at high doses on the day of surgery. There appears to be a trend toward increased mortality and stroke for those at low to intermediate risk. However, initiation of β-blocker therapy per-operatively is reasonable in patients with intermediate- or high-risk myocardial ischemia noted in preoperative risk stratification or those with ≥3 RCRI factors. It is prudent to initiate β-blocker therapy in β-blocker naïve patients 2–7 days before surgery to allow optimal dosing and titration to avoid hemodynamic instability from hypotension and/or bradycardia. Beta-blocker therapy should be continued in patients undergoing surgery who have been on β-blockade chronically.

PERIOPERATIVE STATIN USE

Statins have become a cornerstone of management for patients with established CAD in preventing cardiac events. Not only are there benefits to lowering cholesterol levels, but there are additional pleiotropic benefits, such as effects on vascular inflammation, endothelial function and atherosclerotic plaque stabilization. For these reasons, their benefit in the perioperative period has been hypothesized. Most of the data in support of their use have been in observational cohorts in patients who already had an indication for their use. The utility of starting patients who do not otherwise have an indication to be on a statin surrounding the time of surgery is still in question.

PERIOPERATIVE ANTICOAGULATION MANAGEMENT

The need for anticoagulation management surrounding surgical procedures is a commonly encountered scenario in patients with atrial arrhythmias, mechanical valves, or prior venous thromboembolism (VTE). There are a limited number of procedures that can be done while on anticoagulation (e.g. dental extraction, cataract surgery, joint aspiration, arteriograph, and minor skin procedures). The risk of procedural bleeding must be balanced with the risk of a thrombotic event. Patients may be stratified into risk categories of low, moderate and high risk of embolization: patients classified as high risk have a >10% annual risk for thromboembolism, patients classified as moderate risk have a 5 10% annual risk for thromboembolism, and patients classified as low risk have a 5% annual risk for thromboembolism (Table 22.4). In low-risk patients, warfarin should be stopped 5 days prior to surgery.

Several procedures do not require cessation of warfarin. In patients requiring a minor dental procedure, warfarin may be stopped 2-3 days before the procedure. An alternative is to continue warfarin and coadminister a prohemostatic mouthwash, such as the antifibrinolytic and tranexamic acid. In patients who require minor dermatologic procedures, warfarin can be continued around the time of the procedure with optimization of local hemostasis. In patients who require cataract surgery, warfarin can be continued around the time of the surgery.

Most anticoagulant therapy is still performed using warfarin, although the use of newer oral anticoagulants (OACs), such as direct thrombin inhibitors (e.g. dabigatran) and factor Xa inhibitors (e.g, apixaban, rivaroxaban, edoxaban) is increasing rapidly. The newer OACs should be discontinued 1-2 days prior to the planned surgical procedure and restarted when the risk of postprocedural bleeding is deemed appropriately low.

Those at high risk for thrombotic events include mechanical prosthetic valves (mitral position or aortic valve ball-in-cage and single tilting disks),

Risk stratum	Indication for VKA therapy		
	Mechanical heart valve	Atrial fibrillation	VTE
High*	Any mitral valve prosthesis Any caged-ball or tilting disc aortic valve prosthesis Recent (within 6 months) stroke or transient ischemic attack	$CHADS_2$ score of 5 or 6 Recent (within 3 months) stroke or transient ischemic attack Rheumatic valvular heart disease	Recent (within 3 months) VTE Severe thrombophilia (e.g. deficiency of protein C, protein S or antithrombin; antiphospholipid antibodies; multiple abnormalities)
Moderate	Bileaflet aortic valve prosthesis and one or more of the of following risk factors: atrial fibrillation, prior stroke or transient ischemic attack, hypertension, diabetes, congestive heart failure, age >75 years	$CHADS_2$ score of 3 or 4	VTE within the past 3–12 months Nonsevere thrombophilia (e.g. heterozygous factor V Leiden or prothrombin gene mutation) Recurrent VTE Active cancer (treated within 6 months or palliative)
Low	Bileaflet aortic valve prosthesis without atrial fibrillation and no other risk factors for stroke	$CHADS_2$ score of 0–2 (assuming no prior stroke or transient ischemic attack)	VTE >12 months before and no other risk factors

*High-risk patients may also include those with a prior stroke or transient ischemic attack occurring 3 months before the planned surgery and a $CHADS_2$ score 5, those with prior thromboembolism during temporary interruption of VKAs, or those undergoing certain types of surgery associated with an increased risk for stroke or other thromboembolism (e.g. cardiac valve replacement, carotid endarterectomy, major vascular surgery).

$CHADS_2$, congestive heart failure, hypertension, age ≥75 years, diabetes mellitus and stroke or transient ischemic attack; VKA, vitamin K antagonist; VTE, venous thromboembolism.

Source: Adapted from Douketis JD, Spyropoulos AC, Spencer FA, Mayr M, Jaffer AK, Eckman MH, et al. Perioperative management of antithrombotic therapy: antithrombotic therapy and prevention of thrombosis, 9th ed: American College of Chest Physicians evidence-based clinical practice guidelines. Chest. 2012;141(Suppl 2) e326S-50S.

atrial fibrillation with elevated $CHADS_2$ score of 5-6, recent VTE within the last 3 months, thrombophilia or recent stroke. If a bridging strategy for a surgical procedure is pursued, warfarin should be stopped 5 days prior to the planned procedure with either low molecular weight heparin or unfractionated heparin beginning when the international normalized ratio (INR) falls <2. In patients receiving subcutaneous low molecular weight heparin, the last preoperative dose should be given approximately 24 hours before surgery (instead of 12 hours). In patients at high bleeding risk after surgery, LMWH can be resumed at 48-72 hours after surgery (rather than 24 hours).

In patients at moderate risk, the decision for bridging should be individualized. For example, a patient with atrial fibrillation and prior stroke and one additional stroke risk factor (i.e. congestive heart failure, hypertension, age ≥75 years, diabetes mellitus) would have a $CHADS_2$ score of 3 and would be classified as being in the moderate-risk group in the classification, but could be perceived as high risk because of the prior stroke. In addition, patients with remote (i.e. >1 year ago), but severe VTE associated with pulmonary hypertension may be perceived as high risk, even though they would be classified as low risk. An example of moderate-risk category patients who do not need bridging are those undergoing surgery with high-bleeding risk, such as carotid endarterectomy.

In patients who require temporary interruption of oral anticoagulants before surgery, the medication can be resumed approximately 12–24 hours after surgery (i.e. the evening of surgery or the next morning) and when there is adequate hemostasis.

PERIOPERATIVE MANAGEMENT OF PACEMAKERS

The use of electrocautery during surgical procedures in most cases delivers unipolar current between the cautery tip and an indifferent pad usually placed on the patient's skin. The current has the potential to interfere with the pacing, sensing or defibrillation capabilities of the device. Interference has decreased considerably with the use of bipolar device leads, but is still a consideration when cautery is going to be used in the vicinity of the leads of the device. If the patient is not pacemaker-dependent or electrocautery will be performed in a remote location from the device, no interrogation or reprogramming is needed. If the patient is pacemaker-dependent, then either reprogramming the device to asynchronous DOO or VOO pacing or placing a magnet over the device is appropriate. If the patient has an implantable cardioverter defibrillator (ICD), then either a magnet can be placed over the device or the tachy-therapies can be turned off for the procedure and restarted following completion of the case. In most ICDs, placing a magnet over the device will disable the tachy-therapies, but will not affect the pacing function of the leads. If a patient is pacemaker-dependent and has an ICD, device reprogramming is required rather than simply placing a magnet over the device.

PREOPERATIVE ASSESSMENT OF CANDIDATES FOR KIDNEY OR LIVER TRANSPLANTATION

The transplantation population is on average younger than the general population. Therefore, achieving a functional status of 4 METs may not be as predictive for perioperative events. Noninvasive testing may be considered in kidney transplantation candidates with no active cardiac conditions given their multiple CAD risk factors, regardless of functional status. In addition, an assessment of left ventricular (LV) function is recommended in the pretransplant evaluation since there is a strong relationship between LV ejection fraction and outcomes. If Doppler echocardiography demonstrates that the RV systolic pressure is ≥45 mm Hg, there should be consideration of further evaluation because of the increased risk of posttransplant complications. If right heart catheterization confirms pulmonary artery (PA) hypertension (i.e. mean PA pressure $\geq$25 mm Hg, pulmonary capillary wedge pressure $\leq$15 mm Hg and pulmonary vascular resistance of >3 Wood units) in the absence of an identified secondary cause (e.g. obstructive sleep apnea, left heart disease), it is reasonable to refer to a pulmonary hypertension specialist for consideration of advanced vasodilator therapies. In patients needing percutaneous coronary intervention before transplant surgery (e.g. if symptoms of myocardial ischemia are present), a drug eluting stent may be considered. Some centers consider the bleeding risk of kidney transplantation to be low and will operate while patients continue to take dual antiplatelet therapy.

The overall risk of CAD is lower in candidates for liver transplantation compared to renal transplantation candidates. However, mortality has been reported as high as 50% in patients with CAD undergoing liver transplantation. Therefore, noninvasive stress testing may be considered in these transplant candidates, having no active symptoms but risk factors for CAD, regardless of functional class. Several cardiopulmonary problems are unique to liver transplantation candidates [e.g. portopulmonary hypertension and hepatopulmonary syndrome (HPS)]. Transthoracic echocardiography for all liver transplant candidates is recommended to assess chamber sizes, LV hypertrophy, systolic and diastolic function, LV outflow tract obstruction, valve function, PA systolic pressure, intracardiac shunting and pericardial effusion. The presence of severe pulmonary hypertension is associated with a marked decrease in survival among liver transplantation candidates and recipients. Two-dimensional Doppler echocardiography is an effective screening tool for pulmonary hypertension in this patient group. Because of the margin of error for Doppler, a PA systolic pressure estimate of 45 mm Hg may be reasonable to pursue further evaluation with right heart catheterization. If significant pulmonary hypertension is documented (refer to criteria above in the section on renal transplantation), referral to pulmonary hypertension specialist may be considered. A mean PA pressure of $\geq$35 mm Hg has traditionally been considered a contraindication to liver transplantation. Hepatopulmonary syndrome is defined as evidence of intrapulmonary vascular shunting, hypoxemia at rest and chronic liver disease. There are no effective medical treatments for HPS, but with liver transplant, pulmonary shunting decreases substantially. Hepatopulmonary syndrome patients who undergo transplant have no worse outcomes compared to other liver transplant patients.

SUMMARY

Improving the perioperative care of the cardiac patient undergoing noncardiac surgery is the goal of the preoperative evaluation. The challenge is to determine how to use preoperative risk assessments, diagnostic tests and additional therapy to care for the surgical patient. Several trials have called into question the utility of preoperative revascularization and perioperative β-blockade. Balancing the risk of perioperative bleeding with thrombotic events is an important issue for patients with the coronary stents and for those with other indications for anticoagulation. Ideally, the care of the patient having noncardiac surgery involves a multidisciplinary effort between surgeons and consultants grounded in effective communication and teamwork.

SUGGESTED READING

1. Anderson JL, Adams CD, Antman CD, Bridges CR, Califf RM, Casey DE Jr, et al. 2012 ACCF/AHA focused update incorporated into the ACCF/AHA 2007 guidelines for the management of patients with unstable angina/non-ST-elevation myocardial infarction: a report of the American College of Cardiology Foundation/American Heart Association Task Force on Practice Guidelines. J Am Coll Cardiol. 2013;61(23):e179-347.
2. Burger W, Chemnitius JM, Kneissl GD, et al. Low-dose aspirin for secondary cardiovascular prevention-cardiovascular risks after its perioperative withdrawal versus bleeding risks with its continuatio- review and meta-analysis. J Intern Med. 2005;257(5):399-414.
3. Deberaldini M, Arcanjo AB, Melo E, da Silva RF, Felicio HC, Arroyo PC Jr, et al. Hepatopulmonary syndrome: morbidity and survival after liver transplantation. Transplant Proc. 2008; 40(10):352-16.
4. Devereax P J, Goldman L, Cook DJ, et al. Perioperative cardiac events in patients undergoing noncardiac surgery: a review of the magnitude of the problem, the pathophysiology of the events and methods to estimate and communicate risk. CMAJ. 2005;173(6):627-34.
5. Douketis JD, Spyropoulos AC, Spencer FA, Mayr M, Jaffer AK, Eckmann MH, et al. Perioperative management of antithrombotic theray: aAntithrombotic therapy and prevention of thrombosis, 9th ed: American College of Chest Physicians evidence-based clinical practice guidelines. Chest. 201241(2 Supl 2): e326S-50S.
6. Eagle KA, Coley CM, Newell JB, Brewster DC, Darling RC, Stranss HW, et al. Combining clinical and thallium data optimizes preoperative assessment of cardiac risk before major vascular surgery. Ann Intern Med. 1989;110(11):859-66.
7. Fleisher LA, Beckman JA, Beckman JA, Brown KA, Calkins H, Chailkof EL, Fleischmann KE, et al. 2009 ACCF/AHA focused update on perioperative beta blockade incorporated into the ACC/AHA 2007 guidelines on perioperative cardiovascular evaluation and care for noncardiac surgery. Circulation. 2009;120(21):e169-276.
8. Fleisher LA, Fleischmann KE, Auerbach AD, Barnason SA, Beckman JA, Bozkurt B, et al. 2014 ACC/AHA guideline on perioperative cardiovascular evaluation and management of patients undergoing noncardiac surgery. J Am Coll Cardiol. 2014;doi: 10.1016/j.jacc.2014.07.944.
9. Grines CL, Bonow RO, Casey DE, Gardner TJ, Lockhart PB, Moliterno DJ, et al. Prevention of premature discontinuation of dual antiplatelet therapy in patients with coronary artery stents. Circulation. 2007;15:813-8.
10. POISE study group, Devereaux PJ, Yang H, Yusuf S, Guyatt G, Leslie K, et al. Effects of extended-release metoprolol succinate in patients undergoing non-cardiac surgery (POISE trial): a randomised controlled trial. Lancet. 2008;371(9627):1839-47.
11. Iakovou I, Schmidt T, Bonizzoni E, Ge L, Sangiorgi GM, Stankovic G, et al. Incidence, predictors, and outcome of thrombosis after successful implantation of drug-eluting stents. JAMA. 2005;293(17):2126-30.

12. Kushner FG, Hand M, Smith SC, King SB, Anderson JL, Antman EM, et al. 2009 focused updates: ACC/AHA guidelines for the management of patients with ST-elevation myocardial infarction (updating the 2004 guideline and 2007 focused update) and ACC/AHA/SCAI guidelines on percutaneous coronary intervention (updating the 2005 guideline and 2007 focused update). J Am Coll Cardiol. 2009;54(23):2205-41.
13. Lee TH, Marcantonio ER, Mangione CM, Thomas EJ, Polanczyk CA, Cook EF, et al. Derivation and prospective validation of a simple index for prediction of cardiac risk of major noncardiac surgery. Circulation. 1999;10(10):1043-9.
14. Lentine KL, Costa SP, Weir MR, Robb JF, Fleisher LA, Kasiske BL, et al. Cardiac disease evaluation and management among kidney and liver transplantation candidates: a scientific statement from the American Heart Association and the American College of Cardiology Foundation: endorsed by the American Society of Transplant Surgeons, American Society of Transplantation, and National Kidney Foundation. Circulation. 2012;126(5):617-63.
15. Lindenauer PK, Pekow P, Wang K, Mamidi DK, Gutierrez B, Benjamin EM, et al. Perioperative beta-blocker therapy and mortality after major noncardiac surgery. N Engl J Med. 2005;353(4):349-61.
16. London MJ, Hur K, Schwgrtz GG, et al. Association of perioperative beta-blockade with mortality and cardiovascular morbidity following major noncardiac surgery. JAMA. 2013;309(16):1704-13.
17. Mangano DT, Goldman L. Preoperative assessment of patients with known or suspected coronary disease. N Engl J Med. 1995;333(26):1750-6.
18. McFalls EO, Ward HB, Moritz TE, Goldman S, Krupski WC, Littooy F, et al. Coronary-artery revascularization before elective major vascular surgery. N Engl J Med. 204;351(27):2795-804.
19. O'Neil-Callahan KG, Katsimaglis G, Tepper MR, Ryan J, Mosby C, Ioannidis JP, et al. Statins decrease perioperative cardiac complications in patients undergoing noncardiac vascular surgery: the Statins for Risk Reduction in Surgery (StaRRS) study. J Am Coll Cardiol. 2005;45(3):336-42.
20. Raval Z, Harinstein ME, Skaro AI, Erdogan A, DeWolf AM, Shah SJ, et al. Cardiovascular risk assessment of the liver transplant candidate. J Am Coll Cardiol. 2011;58(3):223-31.
21. Snowden, CP, Prentis JM, Anderson JM, Roberts DR, Randles D, Rentom M, et al. Submaximal cardiopulmonary exercise testing predicts complications and hospital length of stay in patients undergoing major elective surgery. Ann Surg. 2010;251(3):535-41.

Dyslipidemias

23
Chapter

Byron F Vandenberg

INTRODUCTION

Lipoproteins are macromolecular complexes that carry lipids and proteins in plasma. The hydrophobic core of lipoproteins contains triglyceride and cholesterol esters. The outer surface contains mainly phospholipids and small amounts of free cholesterol and protein. Classes of lipoproteins are defined by their physical and chemical characteristics, particularly by their flotation characteristics during ultracentrifugation. The three major classes of lipoproteins are low-density lipoprotein (LDL), very low-density lipoprotein (VLDL) and high-density lipoprotein (HDL). Very low-density lipoprotein carries both triglycerides and cholesterol and is derived from the liver. In hypertriglyceridemia, VLDL is elevated. Low-density lipoprotein is derived from the catabolism of VLDL and is the predominant cholesterol-carrying lipoprotein; LDL is removed from the circulation primarily by the LDL receptors on the surface of liver cells. The risk of atherosclerotic cardiovascular (CV) disease increases as the level of LDL-cholesterol (LDL-C) increases. When LDL-C infiltrates into the arterial wall, it initiates and promotes atherosclerosis. Another triglyceride-rich lipoprotein is the chylomicron that carries triglycerides derived from dietary fat. While chylomicrons are apparently not atherogenic, chylomicron remnants may be.

Intermediate-density lipoprotein (IDL), LDL and VLDL carry apolipoprotein B, which serves as a ligand to attach to hepatic receptors. Non-HDL-C provides an estimate of these three atherogenic lipoproteins and is calculated as the difference between total cholesterol and HDL-C. However, a target goal for non-HDL has not been established in recent guidelines.

A number of guidelines have been published for the management of dyslipidemias. These include guidelines from the American College of Cardiology/American Heart Association (ACC/AHA), the International Atherosclerosis Society and the European Society of Cardiology/European Atherosclerosis Society. In addition, organizations in other countries have developed guidelines. For this chapter, the ACC/AHA guidelines were the major resource for management recommendations. Since these guidelines did not address the management of patients with hypertriglyceridemia, recommendations from the Endocrine Society are provided.

Statin therapy is recommended for individuals at increased ASCVD risk who are most likely to experience a net benefit in terms of the potential for

ASCVD risk reduction and the potential for adverse effects. Other approaches to treatment of blood cholesterol have been advocated, including "treat to target" (such as LDL-C <70 mg/dL or LDL-C <100 mg/dL). While this strategy has been widely used over the past 15 years, current clinical trial data and guidelines do not indicate specific targets.

SECONDARY PREVENTION/PATIENTS WITH ATHEROSCLEROTIC CV DISEASE

High-intensity statin therapy (Table 23.1) should be initiated or continued as first-line therapy in women and men aged 75 years or younger with clinical ASCVD, unless contraindicated. Clinical ASCVD includes acute coronary syndromes, history of myocardial infarction (MI), stable or unstable angina, coronary or other arterial revascularization, stroke, transient ischemic attack or peripheral arterial disease presumed to be of atherosclerotic origin. When high-intensity statin therapy is contraindicated or when characteristics predisposing to statin-associated adverse effects are present, moderate-intensity statin should be used as the second option if tolerated. Moderate-intensity statin therapy should be considered for individuals older than 75 years of age with clinical ASCVD, since it is not clear that there is additional reduction in ASCVD events from high-intensity statin therapy.

In patients not currently on a statin, initial evaluation includes a fasting lipid panel, hepatic transaminase (ALT), creatinine kinase (CK) (if indicated, such as those with a personal or family history of statin intolerance or muscle disease, clinical presentation or concomitant drug therapy that might increase the likelihood of myopathy) and evaluation for other secondary causes of LDL-C elevation. Secondary causes include dietary issues (e.g. intake of saturated or trans fats, weight gain or anorexia), use of certain drugs (Table 23.2), some diseases (e.g. hypothyroidism, biliary obstruction or nephrotic syndrome), obesity and pregnancy. In addition, patients should be screened

Table 23.1: High-moderate- and low-intensity statins

High-intensity statins (≥50% reduction in LDL-C)	Moderate-intensity statins (30 to <50% reduction in LDL-C)	Low-intensity statins (<30% reduction in LDL-C)
Atorvastatin 40–80 mg Rosuvastatin 20–40 mg	Atorvastatin 10–20 mg Rosuvastatin 5–10 mg Simvastatin 20–40 mg Pravastatin 40–80 mg Lovastatin 40 mg Fluvastatin XL 80 mg Fluvastatin 40 mg bid Pitavastatin 2–4 mg	Simvastatin 10 mg Pravastatin 10–20 mg Lovastatin 20 mg Fluvastatin 20–40 mg Pitavastatin 1 mg

LDL-C, low-density lipoprotein cholesterol.

Source: Adapted from Stone NJ, Robinson J, Lichtenstein AH, Bairey Merz CN, Blum CB, Eckel RH, et al. 2013 ACC/AHA guideline on the treatment of blood cholesterol to reduce atherosclerotic cardiovascular risk in adults: a report of the American College of Cardiology/American Heart Association task force on practice guidelines. Circulation. 2014;129(Suppl 2):S1-45.

Table 23.2: Effect of selected drugs on LDL-cholesterol and triglyceride levels

Drug	LDL cholesterol	Triglycerides
Alcohol	No effect	Increased
Estrogens	Decreased	Increased
Androgens, testosterone	Increased	Increased
Progestins	Increased	Decreased
Glucocorticoids	No effect	Increased
Cyclosporines	Increased	Increased
Tacrolimus	Increased	Increased
Thiazide diuretics	Increased	Increased
Beta-blockers	No effect	Increased
Sertraline	Increased	Possible increase
Protease inhibitors	No effect	Increased
Valproate and related drugs	No effect	Increased
Isotretinoin	No effect	Increased

LDL, low-density lipoprotein.

Source: Adapted from Brunzell JD. Clinical practice. Hypertriglyceridemia. N Engl J Med. 2007;357:1009-17.

Table 23.3: Clinical characteristics associated with increased risk for statin adverse effects

Characteristics predisposing individuals to statin adverse effects:
- Multiple or serious comorbidities, including impaired renal or hepatic function
- History of previous statin intolerance or muscle disorders
- Unexplained ALT elevations three or more times ULN
- Patient characteristics or concomitant use of drugs affecting statin metabolism
- Age >75 years

Additional characteristics that could modify the decision to use higher statin intensities:
- History of hemorrhagic stroke
- Asian ancestry

Source: Adapted from Stone NJ, Robinson J, Lichtenstein AH, Bairey Merz CN, Blum CB, Eckel RH, et al. 2013 ACC/AHA guideline on the treatment of blood cholesterol to reduce atherosclerotic cardiovascular risk in adults: a report of the American College of Cardiology/American Heart Association task force on practice guidelines. Circulation. 2014;129(Suppl 2):S1-45.

for characteristics that are associated with increased risk of an adverse effect (Table 23.3).

During statin therapy, it is reasonable to measure CK in individuals with muscle symptoms and liver functions tests if symptoms suggesting hepatotoxicity arise (e.g. unusual fatigue or weakness, loss of appetite, abdominal pain, dark-colored urine or jaundice).

After initiation of statin therapy, a follow-up lipid panel is recommended 4–12 weeks later to determine the patient's adherence. Then, surveillance testing should be performed every 3–12 months as clinically indicated.

Decreasing the statin dose may be considered when two consecutive values of LDL-C are <40 mg/dL, although there is no evidence that an excess of adverse events occurs when LDL-C is below this level.

Statins are listed as pregnancy category X and should not be used in women of childbearing potential unless these women are using effective contraception and are not nursing.

In addition to statin therapy, lifestyle modifications for LDL-C lowering are recommended. Dietary modifications include a low-fat diet (Table 23.4), avoiding trans fats and limiting the intake of saturated fats to 5–6% of total calories, since these fats are associated with increased LDL-C levels. Examples of trans-fatty acids are bakery shortening and stick margarine, and examples of saturated fatty acids are fatty beef, lamb, pork, poultry with skin, cream, butter, cheese and other dairy products, and palm and coconut oil. Unsaturated (mono- and polyunsaturated) fatty acids do not increase LDL-C levels and are an alternative to saturated fatty acids.

Table 23.4: Diet advice for adults who would benefit from LDL-C lowering

- Aim for a dietary pattern that achieves 5–6% of calories from saturated fat
- Reduce percent of calories from trans fat
- Consume a dietary pattern that emphasizes the following:
    - intake of vegetables, fruits and whole grains;
    - includes low-fat dairy products, poultry, fish, legumes, nontropical vegetable oils and nuts; and
    - limits intake of sweets, sugar-sweetened beverages and red meats
- Adapt this dietary pattern to appropriate calorie requirements, personal and cultural food preferences and nutrition therapy for other medical conditions (including diabetes mellitus)
- Achieve this pattern by following plans, such as the DASH dietary pattern, the USDA Food Pattern or the AHA Diet:

	DASH (for 2,100 calorie plan)	AHA	USDA
Total fat	27%		20–35%
Saturated fat	6%	<7%	<10%
Trans fat		<1%	As low as possible
Protein	18%		
Carbohydrate	55%		
Cholesterol	150 mg	<300 mg	<300 mg
Fiber	30 g		
Sodium	<2,300 mg	<2,400 mg	<2300 mg

DASH, Dietary Approaches to Stop Hypertension; AHA, American Heart Association; USDA, United States Department of Agriculture.

Source: Adapted from Eckel RH, Jakicic JM, Ard JD, de Jesus JM, Miller NH, Hubbard VS, et al. 2013 AHA/ACC guideline on lifestyle management to reduce cardiovascular risk: a report of the American College of Cardiology/American Heart Association task force on practice guidelines. Circulation. 2014;129(Suppl 2): S76-99.

Patients should engage in aerobic physical activity to reduce LDL-C and non-HDL-C: 3–4 sessions a week, lasting on average 40 minutes per session, and involving moderate-to-vigorous intensity physical activity.

PRIMARY PREVENTION

Since statin therapy reduces ASCVD events regardless of risk factor characteristics in both primary and secondary prevention. A global ASCVD risk assessment is recommended to guide initiation of statin therapy. The Pooled Cohort Risk Assessment Equations predict stroke as well as coronary heart disease events in non-Hispanic Caucasian and African American women and men aged 40–79 years with or without diabetes who have LDL-C levels 70–189 mg/dL. This risk calculator is derived from the ARIC (The Atherosclerosis Risk In Communities study), CHS (the Cardiovascular Health Study) and CARDIA (Coronary Artery Risk Development In young Adults) and the Framingham original and offspring cohorts. In patients from populations other than African Americans and non-Hispanic Whites, the risk equations for non-Hispanic Whites may be considered when estimating risk.

In patients with high estimated 10-year ASCVD risk, primary prevention with statins reduces total mortality as well as nonfatal ASCVD events. The ACC/AHA guidelines selected 7.5% as a threshold for statin treatment.

A downloadable spreadsheet enabling estimation of 10-year and lifetime risk for ASCVD and a Web-based calculator are available at: http://my.americanheart.org/cvriskcalculator.

If, after quantitative risk assessment, a decision to initiate statin therapy is otherwise unclear, additional factors may be considered to inform treatment decision making. These factors include primary LDL-C ≥160 mg/dL or other evidence of genetic hyperlipidemias; family history of premature ASCVD with onset <55 years of age in a first-degree male relative or <65 years of age in a first-degree female relative; high-sensitivity C-reactive protein >2 mg/L; CAC score ≥300 Agatston units or ≥75 percentile for age, sex, and ethnicity; ankle-brachial index <0.9; or elevated lifetime risk of ASCVD.

It is reasonable to assess traditional ASCVD risk factors every 4–6 years in adults aged 20–79 years who are free from ASCVD and estimate the 10-year ASCVD risk every 4–6 years in adults aged 40–79 years who are free from ASCVD. There is a paucity of data available for individuals aged 21–39 years and few data were available for individuals older than 75 years of age.

Assessing 30-year or lifetime ASCVD risk based on traditional risk factors may be considered in adults aged 20–59 years without ASCVD and who are not at high short-term risk. Treatment strategies based on lifetime ASCVD risk are problematic because of the lack of data on long-term follow-up of trials >15 years, the safety and ASCVD event reduction when statins are used for periods >10 years and treatment of individuals younger than 40 years.

Prior to initiating statin therapy, patients should be screened for characteristics that may be associated with an increased risk of adverse side effects with statin therapy, as discussed in the secondary prevention section.

Significant statin adverse effects are rare but should be considered especially in the evaluation of their use for primary prevention in low-risk groups. The rate of excess diabetes varies by statin intensity. For moderate-intensity statins, approximately 0.1 excess case of diabetes per 100 statin-treated individuals per year has been observed, and approximately 0.3 excess cases of diabetes 100 statin-treated individuals per year have been observed for high-intensity statins. The long-term adverse effects of statin-associated cases of diabetes over a 10-year period are unclear and are unlikely to be equivalent to an MI, stroke or ASCVD death. Myopathy (~0.01 excess case per 100) and hemorrhagic stroke (~0.01 excess case per 100) make minimal contributions to excess risk from statin therapy.

Although ASCVD events are reduced by moderate- and high-intensity statin therapy for those with a 5% to <7.5% estimated 10-year ASCVD risk, the potential for adverse effects may outweigh the potential for ASCVD risk reduction benefit when high-intensity statin therapy is used in this risk group. However, for moderate-intensity statin therapy, the ASCVD risk reduction exceeds the potential for adverse effects.

STATIN INTOLERANCE

Myalgias are a common adverse effect of statins. If the symptoms are mild to moderate, the statin can be discontinued until the symptoms can be evaluated. Initial evaluation should include assessment for other conditions that might increase the risk for muscle symptoms (e.g. hypothyroidism, reduced renal or liver function, rheumatologic disorders, such as polymyalgia rheumatica, steroid myopathy, vitamin D deficiency or a primary muscle disease).

If muscle symptoms resolve, and if no contraindication exists, the patient may be given the original or a lower dose of the same statin to establish a causal relationship between the muscle symptoms and statin therapy. If a causal relationship exists, the statin should be discontinued, and when muscle symptoms resolve, start a low dose of a different statin or an intermittent dose of a long-acting statin (such as atorvastatin or rosuvastatin). Then, if a low or intermittent dose is tolerated, the dose can be gradually increased as tolerated. However, if muscle symptoms or elevated CK level does not resolve completely after 2 months, consider another etiology of the muscle symptoms.

If the muscle symptoms are severe, the statin should be discontinued and the patient evaluated for the possibility of rhabdomyolysis by checking CK, creatinine and urinalysis for myoglobinuria.

Nonstatin cholesterol-lowering drugs [such as ezetimibe, bile acid sequestrants (BAS) and niacin] are alternative pharmacologic agents to lower LDL-C in statin-intolerant patients. However, there is a paucity of evidence supporting their use to reduce events related to ASCVD.

Ezetimibe blocks the absorption of cholesterol in the intestine and lowers LDL-C by 15–25%. However, ezetimibe has not been tested in randomized controlled trials against placebo as monotherapy or when combined with a statin. It is reasonable to obtain baseline hepatic transaminases before initiating ezetimibe. When ezetimibe is coadministered with a statin, monitoring of transaminase levels is recommended as clinically indicated. Ezetimibe should be discontinued if ALT elevations are persistently more than three times the upper limit of normal.

Bile acid sequestrants are large polymers that bind the negatively charged bile acids and bile salts in the small intestine. As bile acids decrease, hepatic cholesterol is converted to bile acid and there is a compensatory increase in LDL receptors. Monotherapy with BAS lowers LDL-C by 5–30% in a dose-dependent manner. It is reasonable to use BAS with caution if baseline triglyceride levels are <300 mg/dL, but a fasting lipid panel should be evaluated 4–6 weeks after initiation of therapy. Bile acid sequestrants should not be used in individuals with baseline fasting triglyceride levels ≥300 mg/dL or type III hyperlipoproteinemia, because severe triglyceride elevations might occur. A fasting lipid panel should be obtained before BAS is initiated, 3 months after initiation and every 6–12 months thereafter. Bile acid sequestrants should be discontinued if triglycerides exceed 400 mg/dL.

Nicotinic acid produces an average 5–20% reduction in LDL-C and its use is discussed in the hypertriglyceridemia section.

FAMILIAL HYPERCHOLESTEROLEMIA

Adults aged 21 years or older with primary, severe elevations of LDL-C (≥190 mg/dL) have a high lifetime risk for ASCVD events. This is due to their lifetime exposure to markedly elevated LDL-C levels arising from genetic causes. Thus, at age 21, these individuals should receive statin therapy if they have not already been diagnosed and treated before this age. Although in most clinical trials, individuals with LDL-C ≥190 mg/dL were not included due to their need for treatment, extensive evidence shows that each 39 mg/dL reduction in LDL-C by statin therapy reduces ASCVD risk by about 20%. Patients with primary elevations of LDL-C ≥190 mg/dL require even more substantial reductions in their LDL-C levels and intensive management of other risk factors to reduce their ASCVD event. Therefore, it is reasonable to use high-intensity statin therapy to achieve at least a 50% reduction. It is recognized that maximal statin therapy might not be adequate to lower LDL-C sufficiently to reduce ASCVD event risk in individuals with primary severe elevations of LDL-C. Therefore, in addition to a maximally tolerated dose of statin, nonstatin cholesterol-lowering medications are often needed to lower LDL-C to acceptable levels in these individuals.

Because the hypercholesterolemia in these high-risk individuals is often genetically determined, family screening is especially important in this group to identify additional family members who would benefit from assessment and early treatment.

DIABETES MELLITUS

Moderate-intensity statin therapy is recommended for persons with diabetes mellitus, 40–75 years of age. A high-intensity is recommended for individuals with diabetes mellitus and a ≥7.5% estimated 10-year ASCVD risk since they are at a substantially increased lifetime risk for ASCVD events and death. Moreover, individuals with diabetes mellitus experience greater morbidity and worse survival following the onset of clinical ASCVD and high-intensity statins reduce ASCVD events more than moderate-intensity statins.

In diabetes patients younger than 40 years or older than 75 years of age, statin therapy should be individualized based on considerations of ASCVD risk reduction benefits, the potential for adverse effects and drug–drug interactions, and patient preferences.

VERY HIGH TRIGLYCERIDES, SEVERE HYPERTRIGLYCERIDEMIA AND THE CHYLOMICRONEMIA SYNDROME

A very high triglyceride level is defined as a triglyceride level >500 mg/dL (after a 12-hour fast) and severe hypertriglyceridemia is usually defined as a level ≥1,000 mg/dL, which is also the suggested threshold associated with an increased risk for pancreatitis. In patients with severe hypertriglyceridemia, the lipoprotein lipase (LPL) removal system is saturated. If a fat-rich meal is consumed, triglycerides can rapidly increase, placing the patient at risk of pancreatitis due to chylomicronemia. Secondary causes of hypertriglyceridemia that may increase the risk of pancreatitis include acquired disorders of metabolism [e.g. hypothyroidism, pregnancy (especially in the third trimester) and poorly controlled diabetes mellitus], diet (e.g. excess alcohol or high saturated fat intake), drugs, and renal and liver disease.

There are a number of familial disorders associated with elevated triglycerides. While the levels of triglycerides vary in these disorders, there is a central role of LPL, which is needed for the hydrolysis of plasma triglyceride to free fatty acid.

Patients who are heterozygous for LPL deficiency (also known as type V Fredrickson class) present with triglyceride levels >1,000 mg/dL. However, in association with excess alcohol, steroids, estrogens, poorly controlled diabetes mellitus, hypothyroidism, renal disease or the third trimester of pregnancy, triglyceride levels can exceed 2,000 mg/dL and produce elevated chylomicrons, placing the patient at increased risk for pancreatitis.

Familial combined hyperlipidemia (also known as type IIB Fredrickson class) present with multiple lipoprotein abnormalities (including elevated triglycerides and LDL-C) due to increased free fatty acids returning to the liver, resulting in hepatic overproduction of VLDL, which is exacerbated with weight gain. Non-HDL-C levels, in addition to LDL-C, may serve as a basis for identifying which of these patients are at increased risk for CV disease.

Familial dysbetalipoproteinemia (also known as type III Fredrickson class) is due to a gene mutation in an apolipoprotein gene (i.e. APOE) leading to the accumulation of cholesterol-rich VLDL because of decreased hepatic uptake of VLDL and reduced conversion of VLDL to IDL and LDL particles.

The diagnosis is suggested when total cholesterol and triglyceride levels are nearly equivalent and in the range of 300–1,000 mg/dL. Additional factors such as obesity, type 2 diabetes mellitus or hypothyroidism are generally required for clinical expression of this dyslipidemia, which includes palmar xanthomas, orange lipid deposits in the palmar creases and increased ASCVD risk. The elevated triglycerides may be very responsive to adhering to a low-carbohydrate diet.

Familial hypertriglyceridemia (also known as type IV Fredrickson class) is due to isolated high VLDL levels with triglyceride levels most commonly in the 200–500 mg/dL range and related to increased triglyceride synthesis. The LDL-C and HDL-C levels are typically low. The expression of the disorder is accentuated by the presence of a secondary factor such as obesity or insulin resistance. The presence of a secondary factor places them at increased risk of further elevations in triglycerides, the chylomicronemia syndrome and pancreatitis. There may be an elevated risk of CV disease, but it is at least partially related to the increased prevalence of obesity and metabolic syndrome in these patients.

Familial chylomicronemia (also known as type 1 Fredrickson class) is a very rare disorder, manifesting in young patients who have very low or undetectable levels of LPL (when presenting with the homozygous mutation).

Patients with triglyceride levels >500 mg/dL should receive triglyceride-lowering medications, with a fibrate as first-line therapy. This is in addition to intensive therapeutic lifestyle changes to prevent pancreatitis. However, no randomized, placebo-controlled trial has been completed to verify this presumed benefit. Statins may be a reasonable second-line drug treatment. Fibrates and omega-3 PUFA have similar and partially overlapping mechanisms so that the incremental triglyceride lowering of adding omega-3 PUFA may not be additive to background fibrate therapy.

The chylomicronemia syndrome is associated with pancreatitis. The risk increases with triglyceride levels >2,000 mg/dL, and can be prevented by maintaining triglyceride levels <1,000 mg/dL. Proposed mechanisms include a release of excess fatty acids from the chylomicrons, exceeding the binding capacity of albumin in pancreatic capillaries. Treatment includes moderate to severe dietary fat restriction and fibrates. The Endocrine Society does not recommend heparin infusion or plasmapheresis as treatment for very severe hypertriglyceridemia (i.e. triglyceride level >2,000 mg/dL).

Dietary management of hypertriglyceridemia is directed at a reduction of dietary fat and simple carbohydrates. Replacement of saturated fats with mono- and polyunsaturated fats, weight loss (since a weight loss of 5–10% is associated with a 20% reduction in triglycerides), avoiding high-carbohydrate diets (e.g. maintaining carbohydrate intake at ≤50% of total calories) and limiting the intake of added sugars and fructose are recommended. Most of these goals can be accomplished by regular exercise, reducing the intake of total calories and following a low calorie Mediterranean-style diet pattern [which includes fruits, vegetables, nuts, whole grains (as a source of dietary fiber and reduced intake of simple carbohydrates), olive oil (as a source of

Table 23.5: Effect of lipid-lowering therapies on triglyceride reduction

Drug	Triglyceride reduction (%)
Fibrates	30–50
Immediate-release niacin	20–50
Omega-3 PUFA	20–50
Extended-release niacin	10–30
Statins	10–30
Ezetimibe	5–10

PUFA, polyunsaturated fatty acids.

Source: *Adapted from* Miller M, Stone NJ, Ballantyne C, Bittner V, Criqui MH, Ginsberg HN, et al. Triglycerides and cardiovascular disease. Circulation. 2011;123:2292-333.

fat calories) and lean meats and fish (which limit the intake of saturated fatty acids)]. Patients with severe hypertriglyceridemia should abstain from alcohol intake.

Potential therapies for lowering triglyceride levels include fibrates, niacin, omega-3 polyunsaturated free fatty acids (PUFA), statins and ezetimibe (Table 23.5).

Statins may be beneficial especially in the setting of an LDL-C that merits treatment. At least two statin trials (the 4S and CARE trials) demonstrate that patients with higher triglyceride levels at baseline had greater risk reduction with statin therapy (although this has not been a consistent finding in other statin trials).

Among the available drug therapies for hypertriglyceridemia, fibrates offer the most triglyceride reduction. Fibrates increase fatty acid oxidation, increase LPL synthesis and reduce expression of apolipoprotein C3 (APOC3). This apolipoprotein blocks the uptake of lipoproteins by receptors in the liver and may impair LPL activity. These actions result in decreased production and increased catabolism of VLDL. Since there may be an increased incidence of cholesterol gallstones, fibrates are contraindicated in patients with liver and gallbladder disease. Dosing should be adjusted in patients with renal insufficiency. Renal status should be evaluated before fenofibrate initiation, within 3 months after initiation and every 6 months. Fenofibrate should not be used if moderate or severe renal impairment, defined as glomerular filtration rate (GFR) <30 mL/min/1.73 m². If GFR is between 30 and 59 mL/min/1.73 m², the dose of fenofibrate should not exceed 54 mg/day. If, during follow-up, the GFR decreases persistently to ≤30 mL/min/1.73 m², fenofibrate should be discontinued.

When fibrates are added to statin therapy, the fibrate of choice is fenofibrate since there is an increased risk of rhabdomyolysis with the statin-gemfibrozil combination. While monotherapy with a fibrate has been shown to reduce CV risk in patients with high triglycerides and low HDL (in post-hoc subgroup analysis), the benefit of adding a fibrate to background therapy of a statin is less clear. For example, in the Action to Control Cardiovascular

Risk in Diabetes (ACCORD) trial, the addition of fenofibrate to a statin in patients with type 2 diabetes mellitus showed only a nonsignificant ($p = 0.06$) trend in reducing CV events in the subgroup analysis of patients with triglycerides >204 mg/dL and HDL <34 mg/dL. However, statin trials have demonstrated that high-risk statin-treated patients who continue to have elevated triglyceride levels have an increased risk for CV disease.

Niacin at doses of 500–2,000 mg per day is effective in lowering triglycerides. If an extended release preparation is used, the starting dose is 500 mg per day, which can be titrated to the maximum of 2,000 mg per day over 4–8 weeks, with the dose increasing not more than weekly. Niacin decreases triglyceride formation by inhibiting an enzyme that transfers the third fatty acid to glycerol. In addition, there is decreased secretion of VLDL and LDL. Peripheral effects on decreasing free fatty acid mobilization from adipose tissue appear to be minor. However, niacin contributes to the release of prostaglandin from cells in the skin leading to vasodilation that can result in cutaneous flushing, but can be minimized by ingesting niacin after a meal and after ½ hour from taking aspirin. Patients should be monitored for liver function tests, worsening of glucose tolerance and hyperuricemia. Niacin should not be used if the patient has an ALT more than two to three times the upper limit of normal, new onset atrial fibrillation, persistent hyperglycemia, acute gout or unexplained abdominal pain or gastrointestinal symptom. Niacin is contraindicated in patients with active peptic ulcer disease.

Niacin has been shown to reduce progression of carotid disease. In the AIM-HIGH outcome trial, the addition of niacin to patients on background statin therapy, LDL <80 mg/dL and median triglyceride level of 160 mg/dL (range of 125–400 mg/dL) did not demonstrate a benefit in reducing CV events in the study. However, caution is warranted in the generalization of the results since the study was limited to patients with treated LDL-C to <80 mg/dL and the potential for benefit in patients with high triglycerides and LDL-C >80 mg/dL cannot be excluded based on this trial.

The marine-derived omega-3 PUFAs [i.e. eicosapentaenoic acid (EPA) and docosahexaenoic acid (DHA)] lower triglycerides in a dose-dependent manner, with a 5–10% reduction in triglycerides for every 1 g of EPA/DHA consumed, and there is greater efficacy in individuals with higher triglyceride levels before treatment. The omega-3 PUFAs reduce hepatic secretion of triglyceride-rich VLDL particle, reduce the triglyceride content of secreted VLDL particles and increase triglyceride clearance from the blood by lowering the concentration APOC3 (an inhibitor of LPL activity). However, the extent to which triglyceride lowering through this supplementation reduces CV risk remains to be determined. In the Japan EPA Lipid Intervention Study (JELIS), subgroup analysis of primary prevention patients with triglycerides >150 mg/dL and HDL-C <40 mg/dL treated with EPA up to 1.8 g per day on a background of a very low-dose statin had a 53% reduction in CV events compared to statin monotherapy. However, triglyceride levels were only reduced by 5% suggesting that the benefit was not related to triglyceride-lowering effects. Finally, omega-3 PUFA may increase LDL-C, but this may be related to a specific omega-3 fatty acid. Recent studies (i.e. the MARINE and ANCHOR studies) have demonstrated that products containing EPA alone lack the LDL-C elevating effect of products containing DHA.

Orlistat is an inhibitor of intestinal lipase and reduces fat absorption, which may be helpful in patients with fasting hyperchylomicronemia. It has been used in combination with fibrates with additive effects on triglyceride lowering. Side effects include bloating, diarrhea, incontinence, and oily leakage related to the amount of fat ingested in the diet.

METABOLIC SYNDROME AND/OR HIGH TRIGLYCERIDES

The plasma triglyceride level reflects the concentration of the triglyceride-carrying lipoproteins, VLDL and chylomicrons. Hypertriglyceridemia results from increased triglyceride production, reduced triglyceride catabolism or both. However, the independence of triglyceride level as a causal factor in promoting CV disease is debatable. Meta-analyses have demonstrated that after adjustment for standard risk factors and for HDL-C and non-HDL-C, the associations for both CV disease and stroke are no longer significant. However, there is increased risk when elevated triglycerides are associated with low HDL-C or type 2 diabetes mellitus. The mechanism for increased CV event risk may be due to the remnants of delipidated VLDL and chylomicrons or the presence of small, dense LDL particles that are associated with increased atherogenicity.

A therapeutic target for triglyceride level has not been established since there is insufficient evidence to support a lowering of CV risk by lowering triglyceride levels when baseline levels are high, 200–499 mg/dL. However, there is evidence of benefit of fibrate therapy based on post-hoc subgroup analyses from clinical trials, not specifically designed to evaluate treatment in a hypertriglyceridemic populations (discussed previously in the section on severe hypertriglyceridemia).

The potential atherogenicity of high triglycerides can be assessed by the level of non-HDL-C (i.e. total cholesterol—HDL-C), a measure of the apolipoprotein B containing particles, including LDL, VLDL and IDL. Elevations in non-HDL-C are associated with increased CV risk. While target goals for non-HDL-C have not been established, the International Atherosclerosis Society suggests that an optimal non-HDL-C is <130 mg/dL.

The hypertriglyceridemia associated with type 2 diabetes mellitus is due to increased hepatic VLDL production and defective removal of chylomicrons and chylomicron remnants, which often reflect poor glycemic control. With insulin resistance, there is increased free fatty acid flux to the liver and de novo hepatic lipogenesis. Therapy with metformin or a thiazolidinedione improves peripheral insulin sensitivity, leading to inhibition of lipolysis in adipose tissue and a decrease in plasma free fatty acid levels. Side effects of thiazolidinediones include weight gain and risk of heart failure and macular edema.

The hypertriglyceridemia associated with chronic kidney disease is primarily related to the reduced catabolism of the triglyceride remnant lipoproteins (i.e. chylomicrons and VLDL) due to reduction in activity of lipoprotein lipase and hepatic triglyceride lipase (which catabolizes IDL to LDL). Other factors that accompany chronic kidney disease such as diabetes mellitus, metabolic syndrome, obesity and marked proteinuria may exacerbate the hypertriglyceridemia.

Metabolic syndrome is diagnosed when three or more of the following risk factors are present: increased waist circumference [>40 inches in men (>35 inches in Asian men), >35 inches in women (>31 inches in Asian women)], elevated triglycerides ($\geq$150 mg/dL), low HDL-C (<40 mg/dL in men and <50 mg/dL in women), elevated blood pressure ($\geq$130 mm Hg, $\geq$85 mm Hg or taking antihypertensive medication because of history of hypertension) or elevated fasting glucose (>100 mg/dL or taking medication to control blood sugar). Metabolic syndrome is associated with central obesity and insulin resistance. Increased visceral fat is associated with insulin resistance, hyperinsulinemia and elevated free fatty acids, which leads to secretion of triglyceride-containing lipoproteins, VLDL and LDL.

Patients should be screened for hypertriglyceridemia as part of a fasting lipid panel at least every 5 years.

SUMMARY

Statin therapy is recommended for secondary prevention, familial hypercholesterolemia, diabetes mellitus and primary prevention if 10-year risk of ASCVD is >7.5% (Table 23.6). Management of hypertriglyceridemia involves initial assessment for secondary causes and combined diet and drug therapy to achieve a triglyceride level <500 mg/dL.

Table 23.6: Recommendations for statin use

	Moderate-intensity statin	High-intensity statin
Clinical ASCVD	Age > 75 years, or not candidate for high-intensity statin	Age <75 years
LDL-C > 190 mg/dL	Not candidate for high-intensity statin	Yes
Diabetes mellitus, type 1 or 2 (age 40–75 years), and no ASCVD	10-year risk score <7.5%	10-year risk score >7.5%
10-year risk >7.5%, no ASCVD and LDL-C 70–189 mg/dL	Moderate to high intensity	Statin

Definitions of statin intensity: Moderate intensity lowers LDL-C (low-density lipoprotein cholesterol) by approximately 30–< 50% and high intensity lowers LDL-C by approximately $\geq$50%.

Definition of Clinical ASCVD (atherosclerotic cardiovascular disease): acute coronary syndrome, history of myocardial infarction, stable or unstable angina, coronary or other arterial revascularization, stroke, transient ischemic attack or peripheral arterial disease presumed to be of atherosclerotic origin.

SUGGESTED READING

1. Berglund L, Brunzell JD, Goldber AC, Goldberg IJ, Sacks F, Murad MH, et al. Evaluation and treatment of hypertriglyceridemia: an endocrine Society clinical practice guideline. J Clin Endocrinol Metab. 2012;97:2969-89.
2. Brunzell JD. Clinical practice. Hypertriglyceridemia. N Engl J Med. 2007;357:1009-17.
3. Eckel RH, Jakicic JM, Ard JD, de Jesus JM, Miller NH, Hubbard VS, et al. 2013 AHA/ACC guideline on lifestyle management to reduce cardiovascular risk: a report of the American College of Cardiology/American Heart Association task force on practice guidelines. Circulation. 2014;129(Suppl 2):S76-99.
4. Goff DC, Lloyd-Jones DM, Bennett G, Coady S, D'Agostino RB, Gibbons R, et al. 2013 ACC/AHA guideline on the assessment of cardiovascular risk: a report of the American College of Cardiology/American Heart Association task force on practice guidelines. Circulation. 2014;129(Suppl 2):S49-73.
5. Goldberg AC, Hopkins PN, Toth PP, Ballantyne CM, Rader DJ, Robinson JG, et al. Familial hypercholesterolemia: screening, diagnosis and management of pediatric and adult patients. J Clin Lipidol. 2011;5:133-40.
6. Grundy SM, Arai H, Barter P, Bersot TP, Betteridge DJ, Carmena R, et al. An International Atherosclerosis Society position paper: global recommendations for the management of dyslipidemia—full report. J Clin Lipidol. 2014;8(1):29-60.
7. Maki KC, Bays HE, Dicklin MR. Treatment options for the management of hypertriglyceridemia: strategies based on the best-available evidence. J Clin Lipidol. 2012;6:413-26.
8. Miller M, Stone NJ, Ballantyne C, Bittner V, Criqui MH, Ginsberg HN, et al. Triglycerides and cardiovascular disease. Circulation. 2011;123:2292-333.
9. Stone NJ, Robinson J, Lichtenstein AH, Bairey Merz CN, Blum CB, Eckel RH, et al. 2013 ACC/AHA guideline on the treatment of blood cholesterol to reduce atherosclerotic cardiovascular risk in adults: a report of the American College of Cardiology/American Heart Association task force on practice guidelines. Circulation. 2014;129(Suppl 2):S1-45.
10. Vandenberg BF. Drugs for dyslipidemias. In: Chatterjee K and Topol E (Eds). Cardiovascular Drugs. New Delhi, India: Jaypee Brothers Medical Publishers; 2013. pp. 184-231.

Index

Page numbers followed by *f* refer to figure, *t* refer to table

A

Airway 36
  mass 36
Alcoholism 142
Aldosterone antagonists 55, 56
Aldosterone receptor blocker therapy 69
Aldosterone, low 99
Alveolar hypoventilation disorders 103
Alveolitis 36
American College of Cardiology 32, 214, 297
American College of Chest Physicians Practice Guidelines 155
American Heart Association 51, 65, 210, 297, 300
American Thoracic Society 35, 39
Amitriptyline 209
Amlodipine 17, 95
Amphetamines 48
Amyloidosis 67, 182
Anemia 3, 9, 36, 37, 194
Aneroid devices 86
Angina pectoris 8
  typical 13
  unstable 20
Angiotensin-converting enzyme (ACE) 56, 95
  inhibitors 18, 53-56, 68, 95, 231
Angiotensin-receptor blockers 53, 54, 56, 58, 93, 94, 231, 251
Ankle-brachial index 251
Anthracyclines 48
Anti-inflammation 116
Anti-ischemic therapy 28
Anti-platelets therapy 252
Antithrombotic regimens 232
Antithrombotic therapy 76, 153
Anxiety 9
Aortic angiography, catheter based 267
Aortic arch atheroma 280
Aortic coarctation 98
Aortic disease 263
Aortic dissection 1, 4, 182, 194, 259
  classification 260
  variants 269
Aortic jet velocity 120
Aortic manipulation 263
Aortic regurgitation 118, 122, 123t, 124t, 288
Aortic stenosis 9, 118, 121, 121t, 288
  severity, classification of 120t
Aortic syndrome 259
Aortic ulcer 259
Aortic valve 120, 157
  disease 118, 263
  replacement 121t, 124t
Aortoiliac lesions 254t
Arrhythmia 31, 36, 49, 52, 82, 182, 285
Arrhythmic syncope 184t, 194
Arrhythmogenic right ventricular cardiomyopathy 184, 185
Arrhythmogenic right ventricular dysplasia 48
Arterial blood gases 108
Arterial blood pressure 85
Arterial hypertension 112
Arteriovenous fistulae 9
Artery disease 250
Arthralgia 135
Arthritis 135
Ascites 49
Aspergillus fumigatus 143
Aspirin 25, 169
Asthma 36-38
Atrial fibrillation 48, 52, 75, 131, 154f, 220, 223, 224, 227, 230, 231, 243f, 273
Atrial flutter 240

Atrial natriuretic peptide 45
Atrial pressure 67
Atrial rate 241
Atrial tachycardia 240
Atrioventricular block 211, 217
Atrioventricular dissociation 244f
Atrioventricular nodal re-entrant tachycardia 239, 239f
Atrioventricular node 211f
Auscultation 172
Autonomic failure 182

B

Bacteremia 133
Balloon atrial septostomy 112, 115
Becker muscular dystrophy 48
Behçet arteritis 262
Bendroflumethiazide 95
Bezold-Jarisch reflex 209
Bicuspid aortic valve 118, 122, 125, 262
Bioprosthetic valves 149
Bjork-Shiley tilting disk valve 150
Blood cultures 137
Blood gas analysis 107
Blood pressure 73, 84, 121
Blood tests 167
Blood volume 85
Bradyarrhythmia 197, 205
  causes of 184
Bradycardia 16, 17, 75
Brain abscess 135
Brain natriuretic peptide 39, 45, 195
Bronchiolitis obliterans 36
Bronchitis 36
Brugada criteria 245
Brugada pattern 184
Brugada syndrome 185, 200
Bruit, abdominal 98
Bundle branch block 8, 47, 184, 192, 195, 220, 244

C

Calcium channel blocker 15, 52, 94-96, 112, 113
Canadian Cardiovascular Society 285
Candesartan 53, 56, 95
Cardiac arrhythmia 183
Cardiac computed tomographic angiography 11
Cardiac emboli 271
Cardiac enlargement 49

Cardiac implanted electronic device infections 145, 146
Cardiac index 51
Cardiac magnetic resonance imaging 110, 174
Cardiac masses 197, 281
Cardiac resynchronization therapy 58-60
Cardiac risk index, revised 283
Cardiac sarcoid 185
Cardiac syncope 183, 197
Cardiac tamponade 182
Cardiac troponins 23
Cardioembolic stroke 271
Cardiogenic shock 16, 31, 75, 75t
Cardiomyopathy, dilated 9, 75, 126, 185
Cardioverter defibrillator, internal 59
Carotid sinus 182
  syncope 182
Carotid ultrasonography 273
Cataplexy 186
Central nervous system 135
  disorders 36
Central venous pressure 81
Cerebral emboli 135
Chagas disease 209
Chemotherapy 48
Chest pain 1, 13, 166
  causes of 1t
  musculoskeletal 6
  nonanginal 13
Chest radiography 108, 167
Chest wall injury 36
Chest X-ray 264
Chlorthalidone 95
Cholecystitis 1
Chordae tendineae 126
Chylomicronemia syndrome 304
Cirrhosis 142
Cocaine 48, 262
Colchicine 169
Combination therapy 114
Complete blood count 50
Complete heart block 217, 218, 218f
Congenital abnormalities 200
Congenital cardiomyopathies 103
Congenital heart disease 103, 107, 126, 144
Congestive heart failure 38, 52, 274, 294
Connective tissue disease 103, 107, 263

Consciousness, transient loss of 181, 188
Constipation 16
Constrictive pericarditis 174, 175f, 176
    management of 179f
    transient 178
Contrast-enhanced computed tomography 265
Coronary angiography 11
Coronary artery
    revascularization prophylaxis 288
    disease 1, 8, 13t, 14t, 36, 47, 48, 194, 250, 284, 288
    bypass grafting 11, 21, 288
Coronary obstruction 9
Coronary stents, perioperative management of 288
Coronary syndrome 1, 2, 20, 21f, 38, 43, 284, 285
Corrigan's pulse 123
Corticosteroids 170, 262
Costochondritis 1, 6
Coxiella burnetii 136, 143
C-reactive protein 264
Critical aortic stenosis 75
Critical limb ischemia 250, 256
Cushing's reflex 209
Cushing's syndrome 98
Cyclic guanosine monophosphate 69

D

Daytime somnolence 98
Debakey and Stanford classification systems 260, 260f
Deep venous thrombosis 280
Degenerative disease 126
Dehydration 182
Density lipoprotein, intermediate 297
Device therapy 58
Diabetes mellitus 48, 143, 182, 252, 274, 292, 303, 309
Diaphragmatic disorders 36
Diastolic blood pressure 84
    low 123
Diastolic dysfunction, assessment of 65
Dietary therapy 18
Digoxin 57, 68, 113
Diphtheria 209
Dissection syndrome 262
Distention, abdominal 36
Diuretics 55, 96, 111
Dizziness 17

Dobutamine 77
Docosahexaenoic acid 307
Dopamine 77
Drop attacks 186
Duke criteria, modified 136t
Duke treadmill score 10
Dyslipidemias 297
Dyspepsia 17
Dyspnea 5, 35, 36, 38t, 49

E

Echocardiography 23, 76, 109, 167, 172, 177, 193, 265
Ectopic atrial tachycardia 48
Edema 38, 49
Ehlers-Danlos syndrome 262
Eicosapentaenoic acid 307
Ejection fraction 14, 50
Electrocardiogram 2, 8, 92, 107, 119
Electrocardiographic ambulatory monitoring 190
Emphysema 36
Enalapril 56, 95
Endocarditis 75, 280
    noninfective 126
Endomyocardial fibrosis 126
Endothelin receptor antagonist 112, 114
Enoxaparin 26
Enterococcal endocarditis 140
Epilepsy 187t
Epileptic seizures 186
Eprosartan 95
Erythrocyte sedimentation rate 135
Esophageal diseases 6
Esophageal spasm 1
European Respiratory Society Task 39
Excessive dietary salt intake 92
Exercise stress testing 193
Exercise therapy 253
Exploratory thoracotomy 178
Extensive ischemia 13
Extracorporeal circulatory support 80
Extracorporeal membrane oxygenation 80, 115

F

Familial hypercholesterolemia 303
Familial thoracic aortic aneurysm 262
Femoral popliteal lesions 255t
Fibrillation, ventricular 75
Fibrosing mediastinitis 103

Fibrothorax 36
Focal neurologic deficit 263
Fondaparinux 26
Foramen ovale 280
Fosinopril 56
Fulminant myocarditis 75

G

Gastroesophageal reflux 1, 36, 37
Gastrointestinal lesions 143
Gastrointestinal malignancy 133
Gastrointestinal procedures 162
Gaucher's disease 103
Gene therapy 116
Genitourinary disorders 142
Genitourinary procedures 162
Giant cell arteritis 262
Gingival hyperplasia 16
Global aphasia 271
Glomerular filtration rate 306
Glomerulonephritis 135
Glycogen storage disease 103
Goiter 98
Graves' disease 201
Guideline directed medical therapy 59-61, 284

H

HACEK group of organisms 141
Haemophilus aphrophilus 134, 136, 141, 143
Haemophilus parainfluenzae 134, 136, 141, 143
Headache 16, 17, 98
Heart block 75
Heart catheterization 110, 173
Heart disease 103
Heart failure 38, 43, 50*f*, 54, 66, 63, 92, 285
 acute 57, 75
 chronic 75
 decompensated 16, 52*t*, 64
 exacerbation 3
 stages of 65
 treatment of 56
Heart rate 285
Heart Rhythm Society 210
Heart transplantation 61
Heart conduction system 206*f*
Hematologic disorders 103
Hemoglobin 81

Hemolysis 163
Hemolytic anemia, chronic 103
Hemorrhage 182
Hepatic transaminase 298
Hepatojugular reflux 49
Hepatopulmonary syndrome 294
High density lipoprotein 297
His bundle 218
His-Purkinje system 211
Hodgkin's lymphoma 166
Holter monitoring 190, 191
Hong Kong Diastolic Heart Failure Study 69
Human immunodeficiency virus (HIV) 104
 infection 103
Hydrochlorothiazide 95, 96
Hyperaldosteronism 99
Hyperkalemia 209
Hyperparathyroidism 161
Hypertension 9, 48, 52, 84, 88, 89, 99, 161, 251, 262, 274
 causes of 98
 classification of 87, 88*t*
 management 94*f*
 pulmonary 102
 treatment of 95
Hypertensive crisis 3
Hypertensive heart disease 209
Hyperthermia 9
Hyperthyroidism 9, 36
Hypertriglyceridemia 304, 309
Hypertrophic cardiomyopathy 1, 9, 184, 185
 obstructive 75
Hypervagotonia 209
Hyperviscosity 9
Hypoglycemia 209
Hypokalemia 99
Hypotension 16, 17, 73, 263
Hypothermia 209
Hypothyroidism 36, 209
Hypoxemia 9, 111, 209

I

Ibuprofen 169
Idiopathic pulmonary arterial hypertension 112
Immune complex phenomena 135
Implantable cardioverter defibrillator 58, 145, 293

Implantable intracardiac defibrillator 193
Indapamide 95
Infection 48, 52, 209
Infective endocarditis 133, 136, 141, 144
Inflammation
 biomarkers of 46
 markers of 168
Influenza vaccine 18
Inotropes 77
Inotropic therapy 58
International Registry of Aortic Dissection 260
International Study of Infarct Survival 27
Interstitial lung disease 103
Intra-aortic balloon pump 78
Intracardiac pressures, diastolic equalization of 173
Intracardiac shunt 36
Intracellular dysfunction 74
Intracranial hypertension 209
Intramural hematoma 259, 269
Intravenous angiotensin converting enzyme inhibitors 267
Intravenous vasodilator therapy 57
Irregular narrow complex tachycardia 241
Ischemia 52, 182, 194
Ischemic attack, transient 186, 273, 292
Ischemic heart disease 9f, 10f, 15f, 126
Ivabradine 17, 70

J

Janeway lesions 135
Joint National Committee 88, 93
Jugular venous distension 38
Jugular venous pressure 175f
 elevated 49, 172
Junctional ectopic tachycardia 240

K

Kidney
 disease 84
 dysfunction 92
Korotkoff sound 89
Kussmaul's sign 172
Kyphoscoliosis 36

L

Large ischemic burden 31
Laryngeal disease 36

Limb ischemia 256
Lipids 252
Lipoprotein lipase 304
Lipoprotein, low density 297
Lisinopril 56, 95
Listeria monocytogenes 142
Lithium 209
Liver function tests 50
Liver transplantation 293
Loeys-Dietz syndrome 262
Loop diuretics 96
Losartan 56, 95
Luminous phenomena 177
Lung diseases, developmental 103
Lung transplantation 115
Lyme's disease 209, 219f
Lymphangioleiomyomatosis 103
Lymphangitic carcinomatosis 36

M

Macrocirculation 73
Marfan's syndrome 122, 126, 262, 263
Matrix remodelling, biomarkers of 46
Maximal impulse, point of 90
Mean arterial pressure 81
Medtronic-hall tilting disk valve 150
Meningitis 143
Mercury sphygmomanometers 85
Metabolic acidosis 36
Metabolic disorders 103
Metabolic syndrome 308
Metastatic disease 36
Methotrexate 170
Metoprolol 95
Microorganisms, demonstration of 136
Microvascular disease 9
Milrinone 78
Mitral annular calcification 126
Mitral regurgitation 75, 82, 118, 125, 126t, 128t, 129, 288
Mitral repair 128
Mitral stenosis 118, 129, 131, 288
 severity, classification of 130t
 surgical repair of 131t
Mitral valve 126, 157
 disease 118
 inflow 67
 prolapse 1, 126, 200
 replacement 128t
 stenosis 157t
 surgery 128, 131

Multiarray ablation catheter 230
Multidrug-resistant *Streptococcus viridans* 134
Multiple system atrophy 182
Murmurs 49, 91
Muscular dystrophies 185
Myeloproliferative disorders 103
Myocardial dysfunction 126
Myocardial infarction 1, 12, 22, 24, 24*f*, 25*t*, 32, 47, 59, 60, 75, 200, 272, 277, 285, 298
   mechanical complications of 75
   universal classification of 22*t*
Myocardial ischemia 31, 200
Myocardial stretch, biomarkers of 45
Myocarditis 3, 48, 185, 209
Myocardium, ventricular 218
Myocyte injury, biomarkers of 46
Myxedema 209

N

Narrow complex tachycardias 238
Native valve oxacillin-resistant staphylococci endocarditis 139
Nausea 17
Neisseria gonorrhoeae 142
Neuromuscular disorders 37
New York Heart Association 44, 51, 54, 60, 131, 285
Nicotine replacement therapy 252
Nitrendipine 95
Nitroglycerin 28, 77
Noncardiac surgery 156, 283
Non-Hodgkin's lymphoma 166
Noninvasive stress testing risk stratification 12*t*
Nonparoxysmal junctional tachycardia 240
Nonsteroidal anti-inflammatory drugs 97
Nonvalvular atrial fibrillation 274*t*
Norepinephrine 77

O

Obesity 37, 92
Obstructive pulmonary disease 37, 38, 103
Oral anticoagulants 111, 232
Orthopnea 119
Orthostatic hypotension 183, 197
Orthostatic vital signs 189
Oscillometric method 86
Osler's nodes 135
Oxygen 111

P

Pacemakers, perioperative management of 293
Pain, abdominal 263
Palpitation, management of 202*f*
Pancreatitis 1
Papillary muscle 126
Parachute mitral valve 126
Paravalvular regurgitation 162
Parkinson's disease 182
Paroxysmal atrioventricular block 218*f*
Paroxysmal nocturnal dyspnea 119
Paroxysmal supraventricular tachycardia 239
Partial thromboplastin time 26
Patch monitors 191
Pedal edema 16, 17
Peptic ulcer disease 1, 261, 269
Percutaneous coronary intervention 288
Percutaneous mitral balloon commissurotomy 288
   valvuloplasty 131
Pericardial disease 36, 165
Pericardial friction rub 167
Pericardiectomy 170
Pericarditis 1, 5, 165, 209
Perindopril 56
Peripheral arterial disease 16
   lower extremity 250
Peripheral circulation 91
Peripheral edema 16
Perivalvular infection 134
Permanent junctional reciprocating tachycardia 48, 242
Persistent atrial fibrillation 229
Persistent bacteremia 134
Persistent pulmonary hypertension 103
Petechiae 135
Pheochromocytoma 98, 262
Phosphodiesterase-5 inhibition 69, 114
Phrenic nerve 36
Pneumonia 38, 143
Pneumonitis 36
Pneumothorax 36, 38
Polycystic kidney disease 262
Polyunsaturated fatty acids 306
Portal hypertension 103

Portopulmonary hypertension 294
Postcardiac injury 166
Postmyocardial infarction pericarditis 166
Postpartum cardiomyopathy 75
Postpericardiotomy 166
Postural orthostatic tachycardia syndrome 183, 200
Potassium sparing diuretics 96
Prehypertension 88
Progressive atrioventricular block 219*f*
Prophylactic implantable cardioverter defibrillator 53
Prosthetic cardiac valves 144
Prosthetic valve 139-141, 239
    staphylococci endocarditis
        oxacillin-resistant 140
        oxacillin-sensitive 139
    thrombosis 159
    types of 149
Proton pump inhibitors 169
Proximal nail bed splinter hemorrhages 135
Pseudomonas aeruginosa 142
Psychogenic pseudosyncope 186
Pulmonary arterial hypertension 1, 102, 103, 109*f*
    treatment of 112*f*
Pulmonary artery 106*f*
    catheterization 52, 76
    pressures 109*f*
    systolic pressure 130, 176
    wedge pressure 104
Pulmonary capillary
    hemangiomatosis 103
    wedge pressure 51, 57, 81
Pulmonary edema 36
Pulmonary embolism 1, 3, 4, 38, 182, 194
Pulmonary endothelial cells 106
Pulmonary fibrosis 36
Pulmonary function tests 108
Pulmonary histiocytosis 103
Pulmonary hypertension 36, 102-104, 107*f*, 116*t*, 182
    classification of 103*t*
Pulmonary vascular disease 37
Pulmonary vein ablation catheter 229*f*
Pulmonary veno-occlusive disease 103
Pulmonic valve autotransplantation 151
Pulse 89
    deficit 263
    pressure 90
Pulsus paradoxus 167, 172
Pulsus parvus 119
Pulsus tardus 119
Purkinje fibers 218

Q

Quinapril 56
Quincke's pulse 123

R

Radiation heart disease 126
Ramipril 56
Ranolazine 17, 18, 70
Recurrent paroxysmal atrial fibrillation 225
Recurrent pericarditis 170
Red blood cells 81
Reflex syncope 181, 194
Regular narrow complex tachycardias 239
Renal dysfunction, biomarkers of 46
Renal insufficiency 161
Renin angiotensin-aldosterone system 55, 116, 231
Renovascular hypertension 99
Resistant hypertension 96
    evaluation and treatment of 97
Restrictive lung diseases 37
Retinal damage 98
Retinal hemorrhage 98
Retinopathy 92
Revascularization therapy 253
Rheumatic heart disease 75, 118, 126
Rheumatoid arthritis 166
Rose rule 195
Ross procedure 151

S

San Francisco syncope rule 195
Sarcoidosis 103
Schistosomiasis 103
Scrotal edema 49
Sepsis 3
Septal defect, ventricular 75, 81
Serologic tests 137
Shallow breathing 166
Shock 73, 263
    management of 81*f*
Sick sinus syndrome 16
Sinoatrial exit block 207*f*

Sinoatrial nodal re-entrant tachycardia 241
Sinus arrest 205, 206f
Sinus bradycardia 16, 184, 207, 208f
    causes of 209t
Sinus node dysfunction 75, 205, 207, 220
Sinus pause 205, 206f
Sinus tachycardia 240
Situational syncope 182
Skin disorders 142
Sleep apnea 98, 209
Sleep disordered breathing 103
Snoring 98
Sodium diet, low 92
Solid organ transplant 143
Soluble guanylate cyclase stimulators 112, 114
Spinal cord disorders 36
Spine, osteoarthritis of 1
Spironolactone eplerenone 56
Spodick's sign 167
Spontaneous myocardial infarction 22
Staphylococcal bacteremia 146
Staphylococci endocarditis 139
Staphylococcus
    S. aureus 134, 136, 142, 161
    S. epidermidis 134
Starr-Edwards caged-ball valve 150
Stem cells 116
Streptococci endocarditis 139
Streptococcus
    S. bovis 133, 136, 139
    S. pneumoniae 142
    S. viridans 134, 161
Streptokinase 30
Stress cardiomyopathy 75
Stroke 186, 292
Structural valve deterioration 151, 160
Subclavian steal syndrome 182
Substance abuse 52
Supportive therapy 111
Supraventricular arrhythmia 185
Swedish Doppler echocardiographic study 69
Sympathetic nervous system 116
Syncope 181, 187t, 189t, 198
    classification of 181, 182t
    evaluation of 188f
    study 195
    types of 181
Systemic disorders 103
Systemic embolization 134
Systemic hypertension 84
Systemic lupus erythematosus 166
Systemic neuromuscular disorders 36
Systemic vascular resistance 81
Systolic blood pressure 84
Systolic dysfunction 49t
    causes of 48t
Systolic heart failure, stages of 51f

T

Tachyarrhythmia 197, 238, 238f
Tachy-Brady syndrome 206
Tachycardia 9, 38, 48, 75
    ventricular 75, 184, 185, 243
Takayasu arteritis 262
Therapeutic hypothermia 80
Thiazide diuretics 96
Thoracic aortic aneurysm 263
Thoracic aortic dissection, development of 262t
Thrombocytopenia, heparin induced 26
Thromboembolic disease 36
Thromboembolic pulmonary hypertension, chronic 103, 107
Thyroid
    Disorders/ disease 37, 98, 103
    stimulating hormone 50
Tissue Doppler imaging 66, 67
Tissue plasminogen activator 30
Tracheal stenosis 36
Tracheomalacia 36
Trandolapril 56
Trans-Atlantic Inter-Society Consensus Classification 254
Transesophageal echocardiography 127, 137, 138, 157, 272
Transthoracic echocardiography 59, 60, 119, 137, 265, 272
Trimetazidine 17
Tropheryma whipplei 141
Truncal obesity 98
Turner syndrome 262

U

Unfractionated heparin 26, 155

V

Valsalva maneuver 65-67
Valsartan 56, 95
Valvular heart disease 36, 52, 75, 103, 133, 182, 278, 285, 287

Valvular obstruction 197
Valvular regurgitation 135
Vasculitis 36
Vasodilation 116
Vasopressors 77
Vasovagal reflex 200
Vasovagal syncope 182, 188, 195
  treatment of 196t
Veno-occlusive disease 36
Venous pressure, elevation of 167
Venous thromboembolism 292
Ventricular diastolic dysfunction 103
Ventricular ejection fraction 43, 59, 60, 121, 122
Ventricular failure 36
Ventricular hypertrophy 3, 98, 184, 195
Ventricular infarction 31
Ventricular interaction, enhancement of 176
Ventricular systolic dysfunction 103
Veteran's Administration Cooperative Study 27
Viral cultures 168
Virchow's triad 4
Vitamin K antagonist 138, 292

W

Wallenberg's syndrome 271
Wernicke's aphasia 271
White coat hypertension 88
Wide complex tachycardia 240, 243